Innovative Ultrasound Imaging Techniques

SCIENCES

Image, Field Director – Laure Blanc-Féraud

Imagery in Life Sciences, Subject Head – Françoise Peyrin

Innovative Ultrasound Imaging Techniques

Biomedical Applications

Coordinated by
S. Lori Bridal

iSTE

WILEY

First published 2024 in Great Britain and the United States by ISTE Ltd and John Wiley & Sons, Inc.

ISTE Ltd
27-37 St George's Road
London SW19 4EU
UK

www.iste.co.uk

John Wiley & Sons, Inc.
111 River Street
Hoboken, NJ 07030
USA

www.wiley.com

Library of Congress Control Number: 2023943621

British Library Cataloguing-in-Publication Data
A CIP record for this book is available from the British Library
ISBN 978-1-78945-163-4

ERC code:
LS7 Applied Medical Technologies, Diagnostics, Therapies and Public Health
LS7_1 Imaging for medical diagnosis

Contents

1

Principles of Ultrasound Imaging and Signal Analysis

S. Lori BRIDAL
CNRS, INSERM, Laboratoire d'Imagerie Biomédicale (LIB), Sorbonne Université, Paris, France

1.1. Introduction: probing living systems with ultrasound

A primary objective of medical imaging is to reveal something about a patient that cannot be evaluated by other means, while imposing as few constraints as possible on the operator and the patient during the imaging process. Ultrasound has many qualities relative to other imaging modalities that help it to contribute towards this goal. In addition to practical advantages such as portability and relative affordability, the nature of interactions between biological media and mechanical waves, and the speed of these interactions give ultrasound a unique place in the biomedical imaging armamentarium.

Within the power and amplitude ranges authorized for diagnostic ultrasound imaging, its innocuous nature has made it the method of choice for prenatal screening. Diagnostic ultrasound is also widely applied for cardiovascular imaging and to examine the liver, kidney, muscles, prostate, thyroid and superficial vessels. Spatial resolution can be adjusted within a range from about a millimeter to hundreds of micrometers, depending on the selected transducer and the explored depth. Images are constantly refreshed on the monitor in real time to provide a continuous sequence of images from the scanned regions. Conventional systems

---

For a color version of all the figures in this chapter, see www.iste.co.uk/bridal/innovative.zip.

Innovative Ultrasound Imaging Techniques,
coordinated by S. Lori BRIDAL. © ISTE Ltd 2024.

offer imaging frame rates on the order of 50 images per second, and ultrafast systems can acquire data at frame rates reaching 20,000 images per second. Images are created from the sensitive detection of echoes returned from scattering structures of a tissue or organ and are presented on a grayscale where strongly reflecting interfaces or scattering structures are brighter. The resulting B-mode (brightness mode) images can be used to visualize the morphology of structures within the body – even those that are rapidly moving, like the beating heart. Doppler mode tracks the movement of red blood cells, and estimated values can be presented on a color scale overlaid on the morphological image to map out information about the blood flow speed, direction or concentration. Specially adapted ultrasound systems can deliver much higher acoustic intensity or power than that used for diagnostic imaging to a position that is selected by focusing. This can be applied, for example, to destroy a cancerous lesion or a kidney stone in zones that are difficult to reach with more conventional interventions.

This very versatile modality has a few notable limitations. Due to the relatively limited differences between the acoustic properties of soft biological tissues and the speckle pattern caused by the interference of echoes returned simultaneously to the transducer from sub-resolution-sized scattering structures, contrast between different types of tissues can be limited. This can hamper the detection of lesions or other anomalies. Compound imaging coherently adds echoes backscattered from the same imaged plane acquired from slightly different angles to reduce the effect of speckle. Image sequences are typically obtained in a single plane so that screening for anomalies relies on a sweep (most-often performed by hand) of the image plane through the volume of interest. Image placement and interpretation are very operator-dependent, so diagnosis can be influenced by the operator's choices and expertise. Growing capacities for three-dimensional ultrasound alleviate these limitations to some degree but, for full-body screening, ultrasound is still outranked by techniques like positron emission or X-ray tomography. Key ultrasound imaging advantages and limitations are summarized in Figure 1.1. Research is underway to curtail limitations and further empower ultrasound's ability to probe living systems.

Consider a typical ultrasound image (see Figure 1.2). The source of ultrasound, the ultrasonic probe, is positioned against the body (at the top of the image in Figure 1.2), and the cross-section of the body in the line of sight of the probe is mapped out in grayscale beyond this surface. Echoes from zones farther from the probe return to the probe later than echoes from more superficial regions so that, along the propagation axis, the echo time delay describing the lapse of time between the emission of the ultrasound pulse and echo reception, Δt_{echo}, is related to the average speed of sound propagation in the medium, c, and the depth, D, of the echogenic structure simply by relating the round-trip travel time to the depth:

$$2D = c \cdot \Delta t_{echo} \quad [1.1]$$

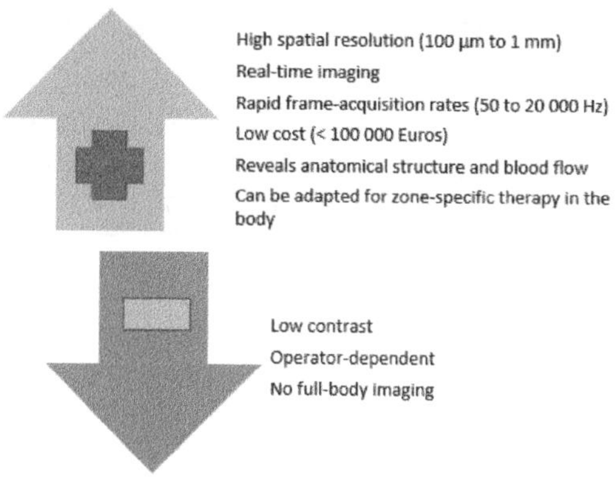

Figure 1.1. *Key advantages and limitations of ultrasound*

The on-screen display identifies the type of ultrasound probe used to make the image (ultrasonic frequency and other salient characteristics). The mechanical index and thermal index can also be displayed to show that imaging safety limits have been respected and that the system is operating under conditions that will not create either cavitation or significant heating in the body. The number of images recorded per unit time, which is referred to as the frame rate, is typically presented in units of Hz or frames per second (fps). If we look more closely at the image, we may note that there are some bright and well-defined boundaries where the ultrasound wave has been reflected from surfaces between different types of tissues or organs. Zones in between such clear boundaries present a speckled brightness pattern instead of a uniform level of gray. Also, deeper regions can present a lower, average brightness than the more superficial regions of the same organ because the ultrasonic wave reaching these deeper zones and the echoes returned from them are more strongly attenuated.

This first chapter will present the basic concepts behind the formation of ultrasound images and, for each key aspect of ultrasound imaging, the subsequent chapters will provide deeper insight into specific ultrasonic techniques and a look at the most promising current innovations that are moving these techniques forward towards the next generation of ultrasound imaging.

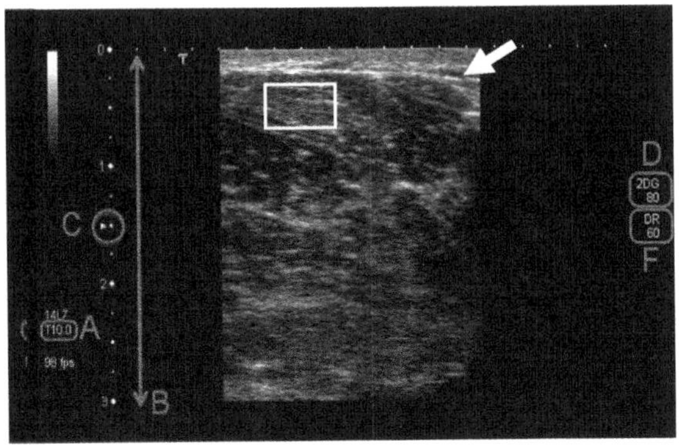

Figure 1.2. *Ultrasound B-mode image with an on-screen display of probe and imaging settings. In this case, the probe is a linear array transducer with a frequency range from 7 to 14 MHz (probe label, 14L7). The selected central transmit frequency in MHz (A), imaging depth in cm (B), focal position marked by arrowheads (C), gain in dB (D) and display dynamic range in dB (F) are shown on-screen. The white arrow designates a bright echo from a boundary, and the white box outlines a zone of speckle pattern. No decrease in the average brightness of the speckle pattern with depth is apparent in this image because time gain compensation (gain that increases as a function of depth) has been applied*

1.2. Ultrasound probes

1.2.1. *Piezoelectric materials: electro-acoustic conversion*

Creating and detecting ultrasonic signals relies on the use of piezoelectric (PZT) materials. In 1880, Pierre and Jacques Curie discovered that applying a mechanical constraint along a selected axis of certain types of crystals led to the creation of an electrical potential across the crystal ("Piezo" comes from a Greek word for pressure). PZT materials are dielectric, which means that they are poor conductors of electric current. Thus, if the specifically arranged, electrical charges associated with the atoms within them are displaced minutely, a global charge distribution is created such that the crystal presents a net charge or electrical potential across its opposite faces. This is known as the direct piezoelectric effect (see Figure 1.3(a)). It works the other way too. The negative charges within the PZT material shift by a tiny amount to counter-act an electric field applied across the material, and this induces a tiny global deformation of the material's thickness in response to an applied electric potential. This is known as the inverse piezoelectric effect (see Figure 1.3(b)). By alternating positive and negative electric potentials across the crystal, the PZT can be made to mechanically vibrate. PZT materials provide the means for the electro-acoustic conversion used to generate and receive ultrasound signals.

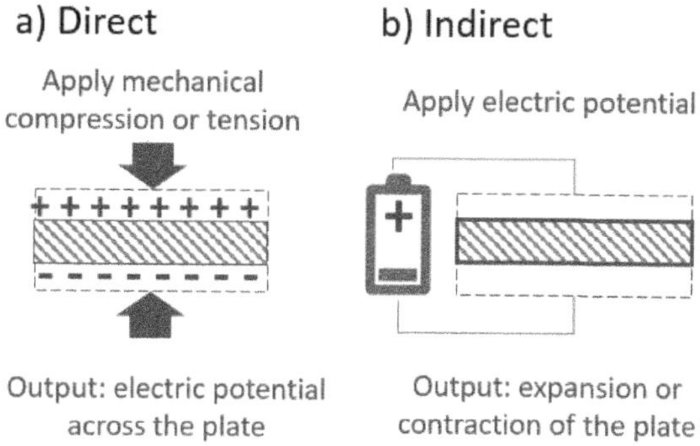

Figure 1.3. *Direct and indirect (or inverse) piezoelectric effects are used for electro-acoustic conversion*

1.2.2. *Transducers*

The handheld ultrasonic probe generally contains an assemblage of PZT elements within its tip that are arranged geometrically to best adapt to the desired scanning conditions needed for the organ or zone to be examined. This ultrasonic transducer array of PZT elements converts electrical energy into acoustic energy and vice versa. For linear transducer arrays, the PZT elements are aligned in a row and the transducer will produce a rectangular set of scan lines. In a convex array, the PZT elements are arranged in a curvilinear fashion (along the arch of a curve) so that the scan lines can fan out from the ultrasound source to evaluate a zone that widens with depth. This can be very useful for the evaluation of large organs at greater depths within the body or for situations where there is only a limited space on the body's surface through which to transmit sound. A position on the body where the transducer can be placed to provide a pathway for wave propagation within the body without the obstruction of the transmitted signals is known as an acoustic window. For example, for cardiac imaging, the transducer has to be placed in the limited space between the ribs to achieve effective ultrasonic transmission. Matrix arrays have PZT elements arranged across a rectangular, 2D grid so that 3D imaging of full volumes can be performed. Other arrangements may be designed to image from within cavities or for specialized applications. Diagrams of some of the possible element arrangements are shown in the next chapter in Figure 2.3.

Each PZT element is electrically connected by depositing a thin layer of conductive material on its surfaces so that there is a positive electrode on the back of the element and a ground electrode on the front. Electrical impedance matching is necessary to optimize the electromechanical coupling between the system electronics and the PZT element. The rear side of each PZT element is adhered to a backing. For imaging, the backing properties are designed to absorb ultrasound propagating within the housing of the transducer. This backing is also important for damping the resonance of the transducer so that the length of transmitted pulses can be limited in time (shorter pulse duration, higher bandwidth). The face plate of the ultrasound probe is designed to optimize the transmission of ultrasound from the PZT elements of the transducer into the body. To do this, quarter wavelength matching layers with an acoustic impedance, Z_{match}, between that of the transducer material, Z_{PZT}, and that of the body's superficial tissue, Z_{body}, are embedded in this interface ($Z_{match} = \sqrt{Z_{PZT} \times Z_{body}}$). Finally, an acoustic coupling gel is used to prevent air-spaces between the ultrasonic probe and the patient, because even a thin layer of air will interfere strongly with the effective transmission of ultrasound.

The characteristic acoustic impedance of a material, denoted as Z, has a definition analogous to Ohm's law (voltage = impedance times current) that relates the acoustic impedance to the local particle displacement, $\dot{u} = \frac{du}{dt}$, and pressure, p, produced by a propagating acoustic wave:

$$Z = \frac{p}{\dot{u}} \quad [1.2]$$

Since the pressure at a specific point caused by an acoustic wave is related to the material's density, ρ, the wave's speed, c, and the particle displacement as described by:

$$p = \rho \cdot c \cdot \dot{u} \quad [1.3]$$

the characteristic acoustic impedance can also be expressed in terms of the density and the speed of sound in the medium of propagation, which is the PZT material in this case:

$$Z = \rho \times c. \quad [1.4]$$

1.2.3. *Modeling the transducer response*

The transducer crystal can vibrate resonantly after excitation with a brief impulsion, or it can be forced to vibrate at a selected driving frequency. The level of damping will determine the system's tendency to resist oscillation and the rate of decay of mechanical oscillations after the application of an electrical impulsion across the crystal's electrodes. This behavior is reminiscent of the familiar response of a damped harmonic oscillator (see Figure 1.4(a)), for which Hooke's law relates the force, F_S, on a mass attached to a spring with a positive spring constant, k [N m^{-1}], to the displacement of the mass, x, relative to its initial equilibrium position at $x = 0$:

$$F_S = -k \cdot |x| \qquad [1.5]$$

Such a system will oscillate at some natural resonance frequency after excitation with an impulsion. It can also be driven to oscillate with a time-varying force $F(t) = a\, sin\, \omega t + b\, cos\, \omega t$, where a and b are constants and ω is the angular frequency of the applied oscillations. As illustrated in Figure 1.4, the oscillations produced by the applied force are subject to mechanical damping.

Damped harmonic oscillator systems can be simulated with an equivalent circuit model. To build intuition about this kind of model, consider the very simple RLC circuit where a time-varying voltage produces a current, $i(t)$, in a circuit composed of a capacitor, a resistor and an inductor in series (see Figure 1.4(b)). In the circuit, energy is stored in an electric field across the capacitor. The inverse of electrical capacitance, $1/C$, is analogous to the spring constant, k, of the mass–spring system. Energy can also be charged in the magnetic field as current flows through the inductor. The electric inductance, L, is analogous to the mass on the spring (or the equivalent mass of a transducer system). The energy is dissipated by the electrical resistance, R, which is analogous to mechanical damping. Finally, the applied electrical potential, $V(t)$, in the circuit is analogous to the applied mechanical force, $F(t)$, used to drive the mass–spring system. The oscillating mass–spring, the transducer and the circuit all exhibit resonant behavior. For the circuit, this resonance can be varied by changing the values or the arrangement of R, L, C components.

Equivalent circuit models can be used to simulate the properties (frequency bandwidth, sensitivity, driven and natural resonant frequencies, etc.) that will be obtained for a specific transducer design (choice of piezoelectric material, thickness, acoustic and electrical matching). The model is based on parallel and series RLC components (resistors, capacitors and inductors) that represent transducer properties, such as the mechanical damping, the mass, elastic compliance and electrostatic capacitance between the faces of the PZT element. Two classic equivalent circuit models for transducers, and the characteristics that they can be used to evaluate, are explained in more detail in Chapter 2.

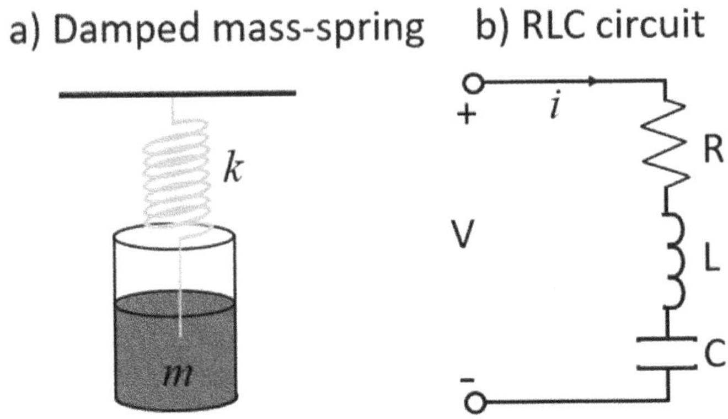

Figure 1.4. *Damped harmonic oscillators: a) spring and mass in oil, b) RLC circuit*

1.2.4. *Frequency and period of oscillation*

In the mass–spring and RLC circuit analogies, the driving force can be a sinusoidally oscillating force at an angular frequency of ω. The frequency, f, measured in Hz (hertz) designates the number of oscillatory cycles per second (e.g. if the spring is vibrating at 1 Hz, the movement will complete a full cycle from the lowest position of the mass to the highest position of the mass and back again to the lowest position in one second). The angular frequency, ω, describes an angular displacement per unit time in units of radians per second. The two quantities are related by a simple equation:

$$\omega = 2\pi f = \frac{2\pi}{\tau} \qquad [1.6]$$

As the mass moves through the different stages of its oscillation, the angular frequency describes the rate of change of the phase as a function of time of the sinusoidal waveform that would map out the amplitude of the displacement of the mass relative to its equilibrium position, as illustrated in Figure 1.5. The period of oscillation, τ, describes how long it takes for a complete cycle of oscillation and is the inverse of the frequency of the oscillation:

$$\tau = \frac{1}{f} \qquad [1.7]$$

By describing the fractional number of oscillatory periods that have occurred at time, t, as $\frac{t}{\tau}$, the displacement of the mass as a function of time can be written using a sinusoidal function, where the position of the oscillating mass relative to the equilibrium position at $x = 0$ at any time, t, is:

$$x(t) = x_{max} \sin\left(2\pi\frac{t}{\tau}\right) = x_{max} \sin(\omega \cdot t). \quad [1.8]$$

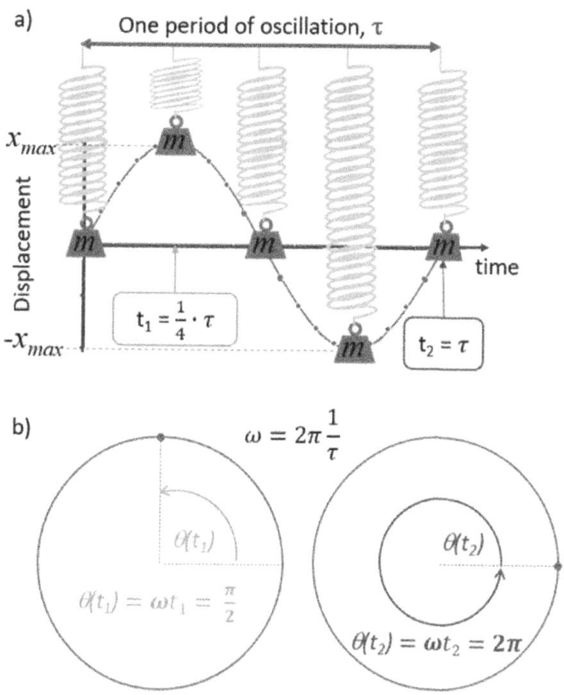

Figure 1.5. *Relating linear and angular frequency. a) As the mass oscillates about its equilibrium position, the linear frequency of oscillation, f, is the number of cycles per second, which is the inverse of the period of oscillation, τ. b) Angular frequency, ω, in units of radians per second can be used to express the cyclical nature of the motion. A period of oscillation is completed after each full rotation of 2π*

1.2.5. *Transducer resonant frequency and bandwidth*

For ultrasonic transducers, the thickness of the PZT elements is tailored to respond optimally at a selected resonant frequency, $f_{PZT\ Res}$. If we excite a piezoelectric plate of thickness, **t**, with an electrical impulse, the plate will have a natural, thickness-mode resonance frequency when the round-trip distance of vibration $2t$ is equal to the speed of sound in the material, c_{PZT}, times the time required for one cycle of vibration (one period) τ:

$$2t = c_{PZT}\tau \text{ so that } f_{PZT\ Res} = \frac{c_{PZT}}{2t} \qquad [1.9]$$

A thicker crystal has a lower thickness-mode resonance frequency, and a thinner crystal resonates at a higher frequency. For the PZT elements used for biomedical ultrasound, this frequency is typically in the MHz range for excitation with an electrical impulse or gated excitation voltage, and the longitudinal mechanical wave created by the oscillation is in the ultrasonic range – at frequencies much too high to be heard with the human ear.

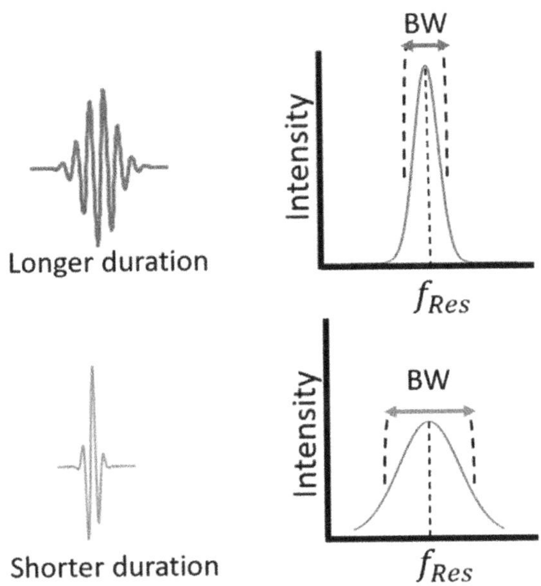

Figure 1.6. *At a fixed frequency, the less highly damped pulse has a longer duration in time and a narrower bandwidth, BW, in the frequency domain than a more highly damped one*

An ultrasound pulse created with a piezoelectric plate of thickness **t** will, in general, contain a range of frequencies with peak energy at the thickness-mode resonance frequency, $f_{PZT\ Res}$, of the PZT plate. By taking the Fourier transform of the pulse, the amplitude of the energy in the pulse can be represented in the frequency domain based on its weighted frequency content, as shown in Figure 1.6. The range of the significant frequency response included in the transmitted pulse is referred to as the bandwidth. It is inversely related to the pulse duration, which is influenced by the frequency of the transducer and its damping. The bandwidth can be defined as the range of frequencies within which the intensity is greater than or equal to -3 dB of the peak spectral amplitude. If the pulse has not been detected directly, but rather evaluated based on the reflection from a perfect reflector, the same bandwidth can be identified by searching for the range of frequencies within -6 dB of the peak of the Fourier transform of the reflected pulse (50% of the spectrum's peak amplitude). The more strongly damped the PZT plate, the shorter the pulse and the wider the bandwidth, but the pulse also contains less energy when it is strongly damped.

1.3. Longitudinal ultrasound waves

1.3.1. *Vibrations along the axis of wave propagation*

A pulse generator emits an electric pulse that is used to excite the PZT elements in the ultrasound transducer so that the energy in the electrical pulse is converted to a mechanical vibration that is coupled into the body as a mechanical wave. Ultrasound propagates into the body in the form of a longitudinal, compressional wave. Thus, as the energy of the wave is transmitted from the transducer into the medium and moves through the medium where ρ_0 and p_0 are, respectively, the ambient density and pressure in the medium, the molecules are displaced slightly from their equilibrium positions along the axis parallel to the propagation of the wave to temporarily form zones of compression (molecules are closer together than usual so the material is effectively denser $\rho = \rho_0 + \Delta\rho$, $\Delta\rho > 0$ and the local pressure is increased, $p = p_0 + \Delta p$, $\Delta p > 0$) alternating with zones of rarefaction (molecules are farther apart than usual so the material is effectively less dense $\rho = \rho_0 + \Delta\rho$, $\Delta\rho < 0$ and the local pressure is decreased, $p = p_0 + \Delta p$, $\Delta p < 0$). The local particle displacement leads to a modification of the local pressure and the local density as the medium is compressed or rarefied. This is diagrammed in Figure 1.7 for a continuous wave. The distance labeled with the symbol λ in the figure corresponds to the acoustic wavelength, the distance between positions where the particle displacement is at the same point in the cyclic motion or, stated differently, the distance between two points of matched phase and amplitude. In this illustrated case, the wavelength is shown between two zones of maximum compression. It should be kept in mind that zones of maximum rarefaction, maximum compression and all the relative levels of compression and rarefaction in between can be considered to have an approximately homogeneous local pressure and density on a scale $<< \lambda$.

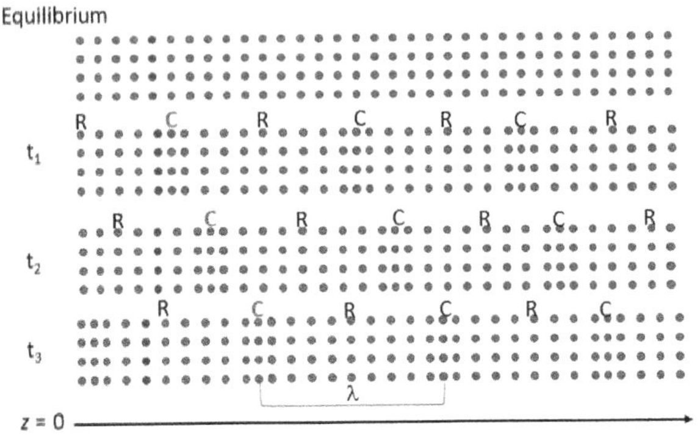

Figure 1.7. *The molecules or particles of a material, represented by the blue disks, at equilibrium (top row). Imagine that a transducer placed flush against the particles at z = 0 is creating a continuous vibration that propagates along the z axis. Zones of compression, C, and rarefaction, R, are formed in the propagation medium. Each compressive and rarefactive disturbance propagates steadily to deeper positions in the material as a function of time, t. A set of particles is labeled with red disks to illustrate that the particles vibrate about their fixed equilibrium position as the wave's energy propagates in z*

1.3.2. *The 1D, elastic wave equation*

Ultrasonic waves are mechanical waves that result from the transfer of energy in the form of a traveling disturbance in the density and pressure of the propagation medium. The wave propagates as this disturbance moves away from the source. Hooke's law, Newton's second law of motion and the continuous medium theorem are used to express this disturbance in the form of the wave equation. If we consider infinite plane waves in a lossless elastic medium, the propagation of this local disturbance in the density and pressure within the propagation medium can be considered in one dimension for simplicity. Consider the 1D propagation medium as a row of atoms or particles where each has mass, m, and they are elastically coupled to one another by springs where each spring has the same elastic constant, k. Unperturbed by a sound wave, the particles are equally separated by a distance a. The elastic force on particle n exerted by its two neighbors is:

$$F^{eq.}_{(n-1)\rightarrow n} = k\{(n-1)\cdot a - n\cdot a\} = -ka \qquad [1.10]$$

$$F^{eq.}_{(n+1)\rightarrow n} = k\{(n+1)\cdot a - n\cdot a\} = ka \qquad [1.11]$$

The net force on particle *n* at equilibrium is therefore the sum of equations [1.10] and [1.11] such that:

$$F^{eq.}_{(n-1)\to n} + F^{eq.}_{(n+1)\to n} = -ka + ka = 0. \quad [1.12]$$

If the first particle in this chain is moved slightly away from its equilibrium position by some force (our vibrating ultrasound transducer), its displacement will exert a force on its neighbor via the connecting spring, and a series of displacements will be transferred from one particle to the next to propagate farther and farther along the chain of particles (see Figure 1.8). Once the disturbance has passed by a region, the restoring force of the springs between the particles will return them to their equilibrium positions.

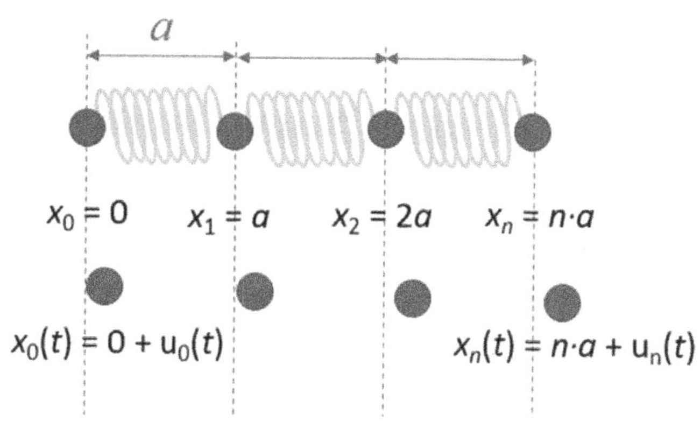

Figure 1.8. *Each particle is initially at a position $x_n = n{\cdot}a$. When displaced from equilibrium, the perturbed position for each can be written as $x_n = n{\cdot}a + u_n(t)$, where $u_n(t)$ is the displacement at time t relative to the particle's equilibrium position*

Since the forces between particles at equilibrium cancel each other out, the net force will only depend on the relative extension or compression of the "springs" between a particle and each of its neighbors. The additional force imposed by particle *n*-1 on particle *n* is thus:

$$F_{(n-1)\to n}(t) = k\big(u_{n-1}(t) - u_n(t)\big) \quad [1.13]$$

The additional force due to the displacement of particle *n*+1 on particle *n* is:

$$F_{(n+1)\to n}(t) = k\big(u_{n+1}(t) - u_n\,(t)\big) \quad [1.14]$$

So, the overall force on particle n as a function of time is:

$$F_{(n-1)\to n}(t) + F_{(n+1)\to n}(t) = k\big(u_{n-1}(t) - u_n(t)\big) + k\big(u_{n+1}(t) - u_n(t)\big)$$

$$= -k\big(2 \cdot u_n(t) - u_{n-1}(t) - u_{n+1}(t)\big) \qquad [1.15]$$

Since the relative displacements that occur at the particles n-1, n and n+1 in the medium occur on the scale of the spacing between atoms in matter (a scale of Angstroms or 10^{-10} meters), and since transducers create vibrations in biological media with characteristic lengths on the order of hundreds of millimeters or micrometers (> 10^{-4} meters), there should only be a very small difference in the relative displacements between atoms n-1, n and n+1. The medium can therefore be considered as a continuum where the displacement can be characterized for every position x as $u(x, t)$ and a second-order Taylor expansion can be applied to estimate the displacements at the positions $x_{n-1} = x_n - a$ and $x_{n+1} = x_n + a$:

$$u_{n-1}(t) \to u(x_{n-1}, t) \cong u(x_n, t) - \frac{\delta u}{\delta x} a + \frac{1}{2}\frac{\delta^2 u}{\delta x^2} a^2 \qquad [1.16]$$

$$u_{n+1}(t) \to u(x_{n+1}, t) \cong u(x_n, t) + \frac{\delta u}{\delta x} a + \frac{1}{2}\frac{\delta^2 u}{\delta x^2} a^2 \qquad [1.17]$$

Partial derivatives are used since the displacement depends on both time, t, and position, x. Using equations [1.16] and [1.17], equation [1.15] becomes:

$$F_{(n-1)\to n}(t) + F_{(n+1)\to n}(t) = -k\big(2 \cdot u(x_n, t) - u(x_{n-1}, t) - u(x_{n+1}, t)\big)$$

$$= -k\left(2 \cdot u(x_n, t) - \left[u(x_n, t) - \frac{\delta u}{\delta x} a + \frac{1}{2}\frac{\delta^2 u}{\delta x^2} a^2\right] - \left[u(x_n, t) + \frac{\delta u}{\delta x} a + \frac{1}{2}\frac{\delta^2 u}{\delta x^2} a^2\right]\right)$$

$$= k \cdot \frac{\delta^2 u}{\delta x^2} a^2 \qquad [1.18]$$

From Newton's second law of motion, the force on a moving object equals its mass times its acceleration. The elastic force described above can thus be related to the acceleration of the particle motion to obtain the one-dimensional wave equation for a wave in an elastic medium

$$m \frac{\delta^2 u}{\delta t^2} = k \cdot \frac{\delta^2 u}{\delta x^2} a^2$$

$$\frac{\delta^2 u}{\delta x^2} - \frac{m}{a^2 k}\frac{\delta^2 u}{\delta t^2} = 0 \qquad [1.19]$$

Consider now a block of material. Hooke's law for a bar of material states that the force, $F_\perp$, per unit area, *S*, applied perpendicularly to the surface of the material is equal to Young's modulus, *E*, times the relative deformation of the material along its length, *l*:

$$\frac{F_\perp}{S} = E \cdot \frac{\Delta l}{l} \qquad [1.20]$$

For the chain of particles, Hooke's relation is expressed as:

$$F_\perp = k \cdot (u_{n+1} - u_n) \qquad [1.21]$$

Consider that the surface area, *S*, of the face of a material can be divided into tiny squares of surface area, a^2, where each of these squares contains one of the particle chains. The force due to a tiny displacement of this surface will be multiplied by the number of chains of particles that are being disturbed $n = S/a^2$. For the application of a force to a surface area of material, therefore, the equation above, expressed in terms of the elastic constant between individual particles, *k*, is:

$$F_\perp = \frac{S}{a^2} k \cdot (u_{n+1} - u_n) \qquad [1.22]$$

$$\frac{F_\perp}{S} \cong \frac{k}{a^2} \cdot \left(\frac{\delta u}{\delta x} a\right) \cong \frac{k}{a} \cdot \left(\frac{\delta u}{\delta x}\right) \qquad [1.23]$$

It is practical to rewrite the wave equation in equation [1.19] using the relations $E \cong k/a$ and $\rho = m/a^3$ to refer to quantities that characterize material properties for the continuous medium:

$$\frac{\delta^2 u}{\delta x^2} - \frac{ma}{a^3 k}\frac{\delta^2 u}{\delta t^2} = 0 \qquad [1.24]$$

$$\frac{\delta^2 u}{\delta x^2} - \frac{\rho}{E}\frac{\delta^2 u}{\delta t^2} = 0 \qquad [1.25]$$

1.3.3. *The propagating wave*

The development in the previous section was made considering that the displacement could be described by a plane wave. Its general solution is:

$$u(x, t) = f_1(t+x/c) + f_2(t-x/c) \qquad [1.26]$$

where f_1 describes a propagation towards negative x and f_2 describes a propagation towards positive x (at a speed of c). Taking the partial derivatives of this solution that are found in the wave equation (equation [1.25]):

$$\frac{\delta^2 u}{\delta t^2} = u(x,t) \qquad [1.27]$$

$$\frac{\delta^2 u}{\delta x^2} = \frac{1}{c^2} u(x,t) \qquad [1.28]$$

and putting equations [1.27] and [1.28] into the wave equation [1.25], the following is obtained:

$$\frac{1}{c^2} u(x,t) - \frac{\rho}{E} u(x,t) = 0 \qquad [1.29]$$

$c = \sqrt{\frac{E}{\rho}} = \sqrt{\frac{1}{\rho k}}$, where κ is the compressibility of the medium that relates the change in pressure to the change in density, $\kappa = \frac{dp}{d\rho}$. Thus, the speed of sound, c, in the medium is related to the density and compressibility of the medium. A more rigid material with low compressibility will typically exhibit a higher longitudinal speed of sound than a less rigid (more compressible) material.

The particle displacement shown in Figure 1.7 can be presented in terms of density, pressure or particle displacement at a given position as a function of time, as shown in Figure 1.9. At any selected position in the medium, the time it takes for the vibration to complete a full cycle is the period of the wave, τ. The frequency is the number of cycles per unit time so that the frequency is related to the period according to $\tau = \frac{1}{f}$. Since the period is the time for one full cycle of vibration to occur and since the wave is traveling at a speed of c, the wavelength (distance between two points of matched phase and amplitude) can be expressed in terms of the speed of the wave propagation times the wave period $\lambda = c \cdot \tau$, or as the speed of wave propagation divided by the wave frequency: $\lambda = \frac{c}{f}$. As a function of time, the perturbation repeats itself every period. As a function of position, the perturbation pattern is repeated every wavelength.

A sine wave is a simple solution to the wave equation. For a continuous waveform advancing towards positive x, the pressure can thus be described by a sinusoidal function so that $p(x,t) = p_{max} \sin\left(2\pi\left[\frac{t}{\tau} - \frac{x}{\lambda}\right]\right) = p_{max} \sin\left(\omega\left[t - \frac{x}{c}\right]\right)$.

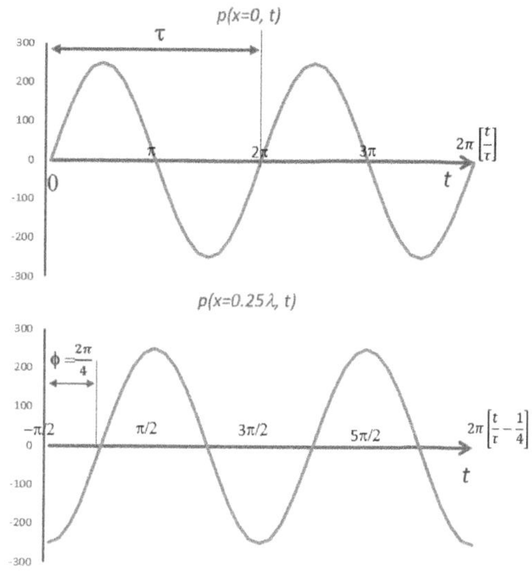

Figure 1.9. *At a fixed position x in the medium, the pressure, p, as a function of time for a continuous wave is described by* $p(x,t) = p_{max}\sin\left(2\pi\left[\frac{t}{\tau}-\frac{x}{\lambda}\right]\right)$. *At other positions in the medium (e.g. x = 0.25λ in the bottom graph), the pressure presents the same periodicity, but is offset in time by a phase φ = 2π(x/λ)*

1.4. Pulse-echo ultrasound

1.4.1. *Ultrasonic pulses*

For imaging, pulses of ultrasonic waves are transmitted into the medium instead of continuous waves. The pulse generator emits a brief electrical pulse to excite the transducer. That brief change in electrical potential is converted to an ultrasound pulse through the inverse piezoelectric effect. Pulses can be represented as Gaussian-modulated sinusoidal waves (a gated portion of an oscillating wave):

$$p(x,t) = p_{max}e^{\frac{-\sigma^2\left[t-\frac{x}{c}\right]^2}{2}}\sin\left(\omega\left[t-\frac{x}{c}\right]\right) \quad [1.30]$$

Such pulses will be sent repeatedly at a rate that is consistent with the time needed to explore the full depth of the region:

$$2\times[Maximum\ depth\ to\ explore] \leq c\times[time\ between\ two\ pulses] \quad [1.31]$$

The pulse duration, *PD*, is the time between the "beginning" and the "end" of the ultrasound pulse. A specific level can be chosen in dB (e.g. -20 dB) to precisely establish what amplitude levels relative to the peak amplitude correspond to the effective beginning and end of the envelope of the pulse. The *PD* is illustrated relative to the pulse repetition interval, T_{PRI}, in Figure 1.10. The pulse duration is typically on the order of a few periods of acoustic oscillation ($PD = [\# \, cycles] \times \tau$ is on the order of a few microseconds for MHz range ultrasound) so that the pulse contains only a small number of wavelengths. The pulse repetition interval is much longer (hundreds of microseconds to milliseconds) so that each pulse can complete the round-trip time to and back from the deepest region to explore before the next pulse is initiated.

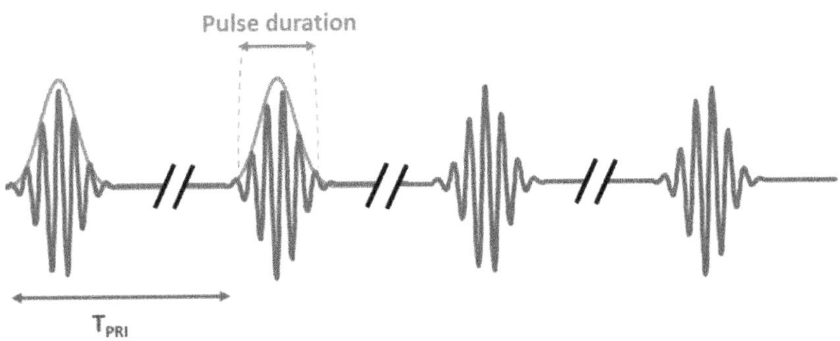

Figure 1.10. *Gaussian-modulated pulse repeated at a pulse repetition interval of T_{PRI}. The black break points show that the time scale is not continuous between pulses because the pulse repetition interval is much longer than the pulse duration. The pulse repetition frequency is the inverse of the pulse repetition interval*

1.4.2. *Pressure and intensity*

The pressures used for ultrasonic imaging are limited, as described with respect to the mechanical index (equation [1.41]). Thus, depending on the frequency, pulse pressures are in the 100 kPa to a few MPa pressure range. This can be compared to the equilibrium or atmospheric pressure, which is 100 kPa. Therapeutic ultrasound can use much higher pressures in the megaPascal range.

Intensity is defined as power per unit area. For a continuous acoustic wave creating cyclical changes in the pressure and the particle displacement of a medium, the average power transported per unit area is:

$$\hat{I} = \frac{1}{\tau}\int_0^{\tau} p\,(t) \times \dot{u}\,(t)dt = \frac{1}{2}p_{max} \cdot \dot{u}_{max} \qquad [1.32]$$

When considering the intensity for pulsed ultrasound, the temporal-averaged intensity is found based on the average intensity during an individual pulse multiplied by the active fraction of the duty cycle, where the duty cycle is the pulse duration divided by the pulse repetition interval:

$$Temporal - average\ intensity = Avg.pulse\ intensity \times \frac{PD}{T_{PRI}} \qquad [1.33]$$

The geometrical distribution of the energy in the ultrasound beam can also be considered. There are regulatory limits on the spatial average temporal average (SATA) and other associated parameters used to characterize the acoustic intensity delivered during imaging.

1.4.3. *Central frequency choice*

The central frequency of the ultrasonic pulse can be adapted to the application. For a fixed level of damping, the pulse length can be essentially limited to a fixed number of wavelengths. Since high-frequency transducers create shorter wavelengths, they can provide shorter pulses and improved axial resolution. Higher frequencies can provide a better spatial resolution, but they are also more strongly attenuated in biological media. To image the abdominal organs or the heart, frequencies near 2 MHz are generally used. Imaging of more superficial regions, such as the breast, can call upon higher frequency transducers (approximately 10 MHz). To examine structures in the eye or to image small animals, the frequencies can be further increased to more than 20 MHz. For therapy, frequencies near 1 MHz are often chosen.

1.4.4. *Attenuation*

The attenuation, generally expressed in dB per cm, describes the exponential loss of signal as a function of the total propagation distance through an attenuating medium that is due to both scattering and absorption processes. This limits the depth that can be effectively imaged. To estimate the signal loss due to attenuation, it is important to apply the coefficient appropriately for the relative loss of amplitude or intensity:

$$Pressure\ amplitude\ (z) = p_{max}(z=0)e^{-\left(\frac{Attenuation\ in\ dB/cm}{8.686}\cdot z\right)} \quad [1.34]$$

$$Intensity\ (z) = I_{max}(z=0)e^{-\left(\frac{Attenuation\ in\ dB/cm}{4.343}\cdot z\right)} \quad [1.35]$$

The attenuation of ultrasonic signals in biological media is stronger for higher frequencies (shorter wavelengths) so the signal-to-noise ratio decreases more rapidly with depth for higher frequencies. In most biological materials within the range of frequencies used for diagnostic imaging, the attenuation can be expressed as a factor of proportionality in dB/cm-MHz. Thus, for a given medium, the number of decibels lost per cm of propagation distance is twice as high at 10 MHz as compared to 5 MHz. Attenuation also depends on the type of media encountered along the propagation path. Ultrasound loses relatively little of its energy as it progresses through water: about 0.01 dB/cm at 5 MHz. Tissues like breast or liver attenuate about 3 dB/cm for an ultrasonic wave at 5 MHz. Lungs and bones attenuate very strongly (tens of dB/cm at 5 MHz) so that it becomes very difficult to transmit ultrasound through these materials.

1.4.5. *Propagation speed*

Within most soft tissues in the body, sound propagates at a speed of approximately 1,540 m/s. There are subtle differences, however, between the speed of propagation in different types of biological tissues. Transmission through layered soft tissues can degrade images due to an effect called phase aberration. For example, the speed of sound in a layer of fat is slightly lower than that in more muscular tissue so that waves propagating through different thicknesses of fat will present slight phase offsets with respect to each other. Phase aberration and methods to correct it are described in Chapter 8. The speed of sound can also be modified by anisotropic properties within the medium. For example, within muscles, the fibers can be arranged in a regular arrangement about a specific axis. This is particularly true within the Achilles tendon. Ultrasound will propagate significantly faster along the direction aligned with muscle or tendon fibers than along the direction perpendicular to the fiber orientation.

1.4.6. *Nonlinear propagation effects*

As shown in Figure 1.7, the wave itself modifies the local pressure (and density) in the medium it is propagating through. The zones that are denser have faster sound speed than zones at lower density. In general, this effect is negligible, but if the relative change in pressure/density produced by the wave is strong or if the wave is propagating across a large distance, the wave can become distorted due to this nonlinear effect. The higher the pressure amplitudes in the wave, the more quickly nonlinear components will accumulate. More highly compressible propagation media (like fatty tissue) are also prone to enhancing nonlinear propagation.

During nonlinear wave propagation, the frequency content of the wave will be modified so that high-frequency components accumulate. This will change (increase) the attenuation of the wave and also lead to harmonic content. The shift in the spectral content due to higher frequency, nonlinear tissue harmonics can be used to improve the resolution (tissue-harmonic imaging) of finer details and improve imaging from deeper regions.

1.4.7. *Reflection, transmission and refraction*

As for transducer materials, biological materials also have an acoustic impedance that is related to the density of the material multiplied by its speed of sound. At a smooth interface with dimensions >> λ that is between two media with different characteristic impedances, Z_1 and Z_2, a fraction of the intensity in an ultrasonic plane wave will be reflected back towards the transducer, while the rest will be transmitted across the interface and continue propagating away from the transducer, as diagrammed in Figure 1.11. If the interface is perpendicular to the direction of wave propagation, the fraction of the reflected intensity is:

$$R_I = \frac{(Z_2 - Z_1)^2}{(Z_2 + Z_1)^2} \qquad [1.36]$$

And the remaining fraction is transmitted:

$$T_I = 1 - R_I \qquad [1.37]$$

Very strong reflections occur at interfaces between tissues and gas-filled regions of the body (gas-filled bowel, for example). A much smaller part of the intensity, typically less than 0.1%, is reflected from boundaries between soft tissues.

If the interface is not perpendicular to the direction of wave propagation so that the incident wave arrives at an angle of θ_i with respect to the interface, the reflected wave will be reflected and the transmitted signal will be refracted at an angle determined by the relative speeds of sound in the two materials:

$$\theta_t = \left[\frac{c_2}{c_1} \sin \theta_i\right] \quad [1.38]$$

where c_1 and c_2 represent the speed of sound in the first and second tissues encountered. Thus, the greater the difference in the speed of sound between the two media, the more strongly the transmitted sound will be refracted or deviated from its original path. In this case, the fraction of reflected intensity can be expressed as:

$$R_I = \frac{(Z_2 \cos \theta_i - Z_1 \cos \theta_t)^2}{(Z_2 \cos \theta_i + Z_1 \cos \theta_t)^2} \quad [1.39]$$

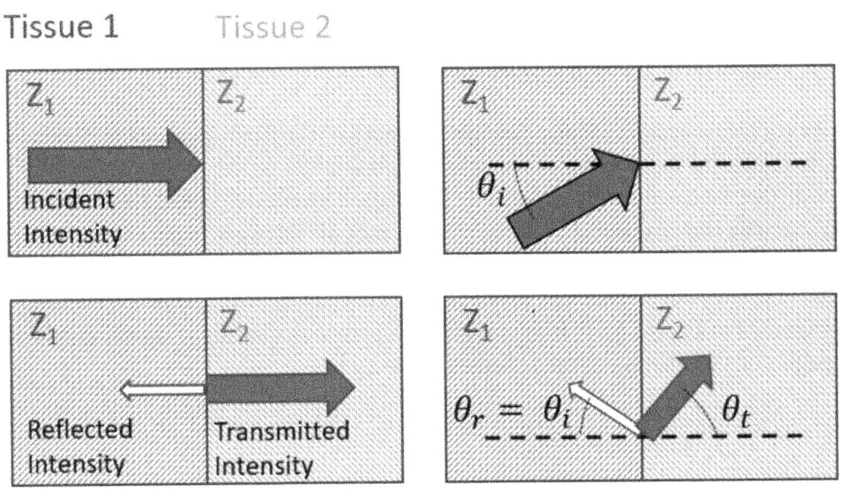

Figure 1.11. *Intensity of the energy in an ultrasonic plane wave incident upon a smooth interface with dimensions much greater than that of the ultrasound wavelength will be partially reflected and partially transmitted according to equations [1.36] and [1.37] for perpendicular incidence, and according to equations [1.39] and [1.37] if the wave intersects the interface at an angle θ_i, with refraction of the transmitted wave according to equation [1.38]*

1.4.8. *Scattering and acoustic speckle*

When the variation of the acoustic impedance occurs for a structure that is on the order of the same size or smaller than the wavelength of the interrogating ultrasound pulse, the sound is not reflected but scattered. As the name implies, scattering redirects part of the incident intensity in many directions. Since intensity is expressed in terms of the power per unit area, a scattering cross-section can be defined for any scattering object to conveniently express how much power will be scattered by the object for any given incident intensity. In other words, by calculating the product of the object's scattering cross-section and the incident intensity, the total power scattered by the object is found:

$$\text{scattered power} = \text{incident intensity x scattering cross-section} \quad [1.40]$$

For a rigid spherical scatterer with a radius a that is much smaller than the ultrasound wavelength, the scattering cross-section increases as a function of frequency, f, (f^4) and also as a function of the scatterer's radius, a, (a^6). The scattering cross-section is also greater when there is a more marked difference between the compressibility and density of the scatterer and the surrounding medium. The scattered signals from blood are about 20 dB lower than those from tissue parenchyma.

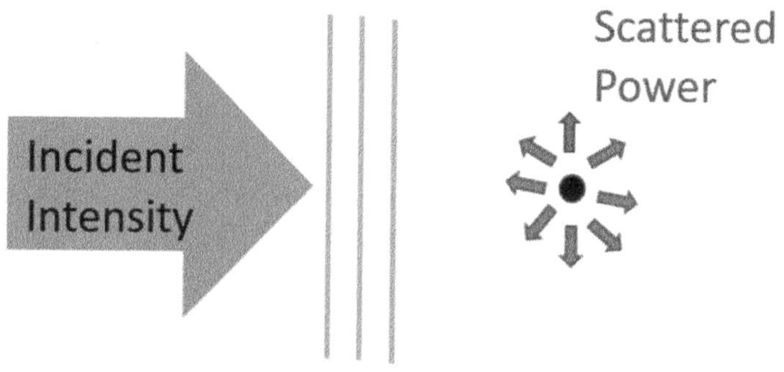

$$\sigma_{Total} = \frac{P_{Total\ scattered}}{I_{Incident}} \qquad \sigma_{B.S.} = \frac{P_{Backscattered}}{I_{Incident}}$$

Figure 1.12. *A structure much smaller than the acoustic wavelength scatters part of the incident intensity in many directions. The part of the power backscattered towards the transducer can be related to the incident intensity by the backscatter cross-section, $\sigma_{B.S}$*

Since the ultrasound probe is used in pulse-echo mode to detect scattering, the backscattered power that is returned for detection by the transducers in the probe is the only part of the scattered intensity that is of interest. This can be calculated based on the part of the power returned within a limited solid angle oriented back towards the transducer probe. Thus, in general, it is the backscatter cross section describing this portion of the total scattered power that is of interest.

For a cellular-sized structure in the body, the backscatter cross section is very small (on the order of 10^{-18} cm^2), but since the ultrasound probe will receive power scattered from many such tiny scattering structures simultaneously, a detectable signal can be obtained. Because these scattering structures are arranged in a random fashion on a scale that is very small compared to the ultrasonic wavelength, the signals returned to the probe will interfere with each other. Whether the interference is positive or negative will depend on the random spatial organization of the scattering structures. This interference between echoes from the fluctuations of the acoustic impedance due to tiny structures in the tissue that are much smaller than the ultrasonic wavelength results in a grainy pattern on ultrasound images that is referred to as ultrasonic speckle. Experienced radiologists can perceive different speckle patterns and integrate this information into their diagnostic process. However, the speckle pattern also reduces the level of contrast between different types of media.

1.4.9. *Cavitation and the mechanical index*

The peak negative pressure used for ultrasonic imaging in tissue must be limited to avoid the risk of creating cavitation. In effect, if the negative pressure (rarefaction) created by the ultrasonic wave is too strong, pockets of gas can be created.

The mechanical index, MI, is defined as:

$$MI = \frac{derated\, peak\, rarefactional\, pressure\; (MPa)}{\sqrt{center\; frequency\; of\; the\; pulse\; (MHz)}} \quad [1.41]$$

To obtain the derated peak rarefactional pressure, in general, the pulse pressure is initially measured with a calibrated hydrophone placed at the desired distance from the transducer in a water path. The attenuation coefficient for the biological tissue to be imaged with the transducer is then applied to estimate the derated pressure. The FDA imposed limitation on the MI for diagnostic ultrasound is 1.9.

1.4.10. *Heating and the thermal index*

The heat absorbed by the medium must be limited during imaging. As the wave is attenuated, part of its energy is absorbed by the medium and this leads to heating.

Heating can become significant if the ultrasound waves have a high intensity or if the media interacting with the ultrasound are highly attenuating.

The thermal index, TI, is defined as:

$$TI = \frac{Power\ output\ (Watts)}{Power\ required\ to\ raise\ temperature\ by\ 1°C\ (Watts)} \qquad [1.42]$$

The power required to raise the temperature by 1°C depends on the type of medium that is being insonified. For example, tissues that are well perfused with blood will require more power to induce heating than poorly vascularized tissues. Strongly absorbing materials such as bone will heat more readily.

A TI < 1 is considered to be safe for early fetal screening. The FDA limit for the spatial peak temporal average intensity is 720 mW/cm^2 during fetal imaging. Using a heating model, more precise estimates of the temperature rise can be obtained for different depths, types of tissues or exposure times.

1.4.11. *Radiation pressure*

Acoustic radiation pressure is produced when momentum from the acoustic wave is transferred to an absorbing or reflecting medium to create a displacement. This uniaxial force can be produced by focusing bursts of compressional ultrasound within a medium. Radiation pressure can be used, for example, to create push and release forces that act as sources for shear wave elastography techniques, as described in section 3.4.2.

1.5. Forming an image

1.5.1. *An array of signals that can be viewed in many ways*

Each ultrasonic pulse sent into the medium propagates deeper and deeper into the tissue. When it is reflected or scattered by inhomogeneities in the medium, echoes are created with a tiny fraction of the intensity of the interrogating ultrasound wave. These low-intensity echoes propagate back to the transducer, which sensitively detects the tiny vibrations and re-converts them into electrical signals which are then processed by the system.

A single scan line is referred to as an A-mode signal. The echoes returned to the probe are converted into relative amplitudes associated with a specific line of sight. The relative amplitude of this signal, related to the relative echogenicity of structures encountered by the ultrasonic pulse, is recorded as a function of time. This fast time scale describes the propagation of the ultrasonic pulse to successive depths. Thus, the depth of each echogenic structure can be estimated by echo-ranging according to equation [1.1].

A single scan line can be presented as a function of time in M-mode to look along a single line of sight. The position of echoes on the M-mode will be displaced as objects move over time. Adjacent M-mode lines are separated in time on the scale of the pulse repetition interval, T_{PRI}.

For a B-mode image, scan lines from adjacent lines of sight are assembled to form an image within a plane where stronger echoes are displayed as brighter levels of gray. The time required to form such an image is known as the frame-rate.

When a sequence of images is acquired, signals acquired along a specific line of sight can be compared between consecutive image frames. The time between matched lines-of-sight from consecutive images is determined by the time required to acquire each image (the inverse of the number of frames per second, FPS).

1.5.2. *Diffraction and natural focusing*

Diffraction describes how the waves from a finite source spread out and interfere with each other. For a simple, continuous wave (CW) single-element transducer with finite dimensions, every point on the transducer's surface can be considered as a source of spherical wavelets according to the Huygens principle. These wavelets propagate outward, away from the source and interfere constructively and destructively when individual wavelets are strongly out of phase with each other. This interference is very strong when the wavelets are close to the source (in the near field or in the Fresnel zone) so that the pressure wave is very irregular in the near field. The diffraction of the source also leads to side lobes. A larger transducer element diameter or longer wavelengths will lead to reduced side lobes.

The near-field boundary is at the axial position of the last maximum in field pressure. This occurs at a position that is approximately equal to the square of the radius of the transducer element divided by the wavelength of the transmitted wave. At this "natural focus", there is constructive interference of the wavelets from the source. The transducer surface can be shaped to place the constructive interference at a desired point referred to as the focal point. Beyond the near-field boundary lies the far field or the Fraunhofer zone in which the approximately planar wavefront diverges and decreases steadily in intensity.

1.5.3. *Electronic focusing versus ultrafast plane waves*

Ultrasound arrays are made up of hundreds of transducer elements. Each individual PZT element has a width on the order of the ultrasound wavelength and is mechanically and electrically isolated so that each element can be activated with different time delays to steer or focus the array's beam. Since the intensity of the field is increased in the focal zone, the backscattered power (echoes) from structures in these zones is increased and objects near the focal zone can be detected with greater sensitivity. This method of conventional focused imaging applies selected delays for a sub-set of the array elements to focus the acoustic pulse along one line of sight within the imaged medium. Echoes returned from that line of sight are reconverted into electrical signals by the elements of the transducer and processed to form one collected scan line. If 256 adjacent scan lines are focused and collected to reconstruct an image of the medium, it is necessary to wait the time needed for 256 acoustic round trips from the transducer to the deepest point in the image and back to the transducer to obtain all the information needed to form the image. For focused ultrasound imaging, frame rates are typically on the order of 30–50 frames/s.

Plane-wave imaging does not apply time delays to focus the emitted beam on a specific zone of the image. All structures within the scan plane are more uniformly insonified, and echoes returned from all regions of the scan plane will be on the same basic footing in terms of echo intensity. Plane-wave imaging can provide much higher scanning rates because the entire plane is insonified with ultrasound in a single shot and then all the echoes from all regions of the imaged plane are collected. Echoes from multiple scattering structures can have the same pulse-echo propagation times. For example, echoes from a deep region along the direct line of sight for one of the elements of the transducer will be returned to that element at the same time as echoes from a more shallow zone at some angle off of the central axis. Thus, computer analysis must be applied to interpret the signals and form an image. This single-shot and off-line numerical reconstruction process is much faster than conventional focused ultrasound, but the contrast of the reconstructed image is much lower. Contrast can be recuperated, however, if several plane waves with slightly different angles of incidence are used to insonify the medium and then the final image reconstruction is based on this multi-angle plane-wave dataset. Use of multiple angles reduces the frame rate but, in general, only a few tens of angled plane waves are needed to recuperate image contrast upon reconstruction. Thus, the final frame rate is still much more rapid than for conventional focused ultrasound, which must form hundreds of focused scan lines to form an image. For plane-wave imaging, the fundamental limitation on the frame rate comes from the time required for one round trip from the transducer to the deepest zone in the image and then back again. This can be further divided by the number of plane-wave angles acquired to improve contrast in the reconstructed image. For example, if the frame rate for a single-angle plane-wave acquisition is 18,000 frames/s, the frame rate for plane-wave image reconstruction using such plane-wave acquisitions along 40 slightly different angles would be 450 frames/s.

1.5.4. *Key technical innovations*

Data analysis is now faster and largely software-based thanks to GPU (Graphical Processing Unit) technology. Coupled with the recent development of open platform ultrasound systems, more flexible programming of new and ultrafast sequences is now possible with access to emission and receive data. Programmable and ultrafast ultrasound systems are the key behind shear wave elastography, functional ultrasound imaging of the rat brain and ultrafast ultrasensitive Doppler, discussed briefly in section 4.4.3.

Ultrasound is also becoming more portable. For example, CMUT probes consist of tiny membranes printed on an integrated circuit that provide an electro-mechanical connection with the membrane's movement. CMUTs can do lots of processing within the probe itself and be connected to an iPad or iPhone for mobile ultrasound. Three-dimensional imaging systems with a 2D transducer matrix are also becoming more prevalent. This is a key to reducing operator dependence due to image-plane choice from ultrasound evaluations.

1.5.5. *Time gain compensation*

Since attenuation leads to a relationship between the probe frequency and the accessible depth, and since this effect has an impact on the frequency content of the propagating wave, time gain compensation can be applied to amplify signals returning from deeper regions more strongly than signals returning from less deep regions. The gain at each depth can be adjusted by the operator.

1.5.6. *Contrast-to-noise ratio*

Objects with uniform composition will appear speckled on ultrasound images, and this makes the detection of irregularities more difficult. Clutter due to reverberations, sidelobes and other artifactual signal sources can lead to echoes that are out-of-place and therefore can mask the detection of structures of interest. These effects limit the contrast-to-noise ratio and can limit the sensitivity to detect small diameter or low contrast irregularities.

1.5.7. *Beam volume and spatial resolution*

The spatial resolution is defined based on the minimum separation between two different objects that allows them to be discriminated from each other. For an ultrasound array, this resolution is different for each of the three dimensions concerned by the image: the lateral dimension running parallel to the axis of the array, the axial dimension along the axis of ultrasound propagation and the elevational or out-of-plane dimension.

The lateral resolution is limited by the wavelength, λ, and the geometry of the transmitting elements in the array because the extent of the zone into which we can focus energy will determine how far apart objects must be along the lateral axis in order to be resolved:

$$Lateral\ Res. \approx \frac{1.22 \cdot \lambda \cdot Focal\ length}{Transmitting\ aperature\ diameter} \qquad [1.43]$$

In depth, echoes received from two objects that are aligned along the axial direction must return to the transducer at times that are sufficiently separated to distinguish the signals scattered from each object. This is determined by the spatial pulse length, which is usually on the order of 1.5–2 wavelengths. The spatial pulse length, *SPL*, and the pulse duration, *PD*, are very simply related:

$$SPL = [\#\ cycles\ in\ pulse] \times \lambda = [\#\ cycles\ in\ pulse] \times \tau \times c = PD \times c \qquad [1.44]$$

The axial resolution is given by:

$$Axial\ Res. = \frac{c \times PD}{2} = \frac{SPL}{2} \qquad [1.45]$$

The elevational resolution is perpendicular to the image plane. For a linear array, this out-of-plane resolution is a function of the PZT element height and the characteristics of the fixed focal lens on the face of the transducer array.

1.5.8. *Pulse repetition frequency and frame rate*

The pulse repetition frequency, PRF (the fastest rate at which ultrasound pulses can be sent and received to interrogate a region), is the inverse of the time-to-echo from the deepest region of the image:

$$PRF = \frac{1}{T_{PRI}} = \frac{1}{TE_{Max\ depth}} = \frac{c}{[greatest\ distance\ of\ interest] \times 2} \qquad [1.46]$$

For example, for 6 cm (or 60 mm), the $TE_{Max\ depth}$ is 80 microseconds and the PRF is 1/(80 µs) or 0.0125 pulses per µs (12.5 kHz or 12,500 pulses per second).

The time required to scan an entire image is only limited by the $TE_{Max\ depth}$ and the number of times such a round trip is necessary to form an image:

$$Time\ per\ image = [\#\ scan\ lines] \times TE_{Max\ depth} = \frac{\#\ scan\ lines}{PRF} \quad [1.47]$$

If focusing along 256 scan lines is required to construct a single image, the time to acquire one image will be equal to the number of scan lines (the number of pulses we need to create and detect in pulse-echo mode) divided by the PRF. So, 256 divided by 12.5 pulses per millisecond, which is 20.48 milliseconds per image (0.02048 seconds per image). The number of image frames per second, FPS, that can be acquired is simply the inverse of the number of seconds needed to acquire each image

$$FPS = \frac{1}{Time\ per\ image\ [seconds]} \quad [1.48]$$

In the example considered above where 20.48 milliseconds are required per image (0.02048 seconds per image), the FPS is approximately 48.8 frames per second. The FPS is directly proportional to the PRF and inversely proportional to the number of sequential transmit events required to scan the imaged region.

If a full image is scanned with a single pulse-echo event initiated by transmitting simultaneously with all the array elements at once using plane-wave imaging, the time per image is simply 1/PRF, or 80 µs per image (0.00008 seconds per image) for the example considered above, so that the FPS for such a plane-wave system would be 12,500 images per second. This series of examples show that focusing along 256 scan lines to image a 6 cm depth can provide about 49 frames per second, while plane-wave ultrasound can acquire data from the same zone at a rate of up to 12,500 frames per second. Plane-wave ultrasound provides an enormous time resolution advantage.

1.6. Imaging modes to further probe living systems

1.6.1. *Doppler*

If a source creates a sound wave while moving towards an observer, the observer will encounter the successive peaks and troughs of the waves more frequently due to the source's motion (see Figure 4.1), and the observer will perceive a higher frequency than the frequency emitted by the source. The opposite is also true. If the source is moving away from the observer, the observer will detect a sound with a lower frequency than that emitted by the source. The Doppler shift is perceived when a rapidly moving vehicle emitting a sound (for example, a car honking) passes an observer.

For continuous wave Doppler, a transducer transmits an ultrasonic wave with a frequency of f_0 that propagates at a speed of c_0 towards moving red blood cells that then scatter echoes as they move. This scattered wave is detected by a confocally aligned receiver, as diagrammed in Figure 4.2. The moving red blood cells intersect the incident ultrasonic wave while they are moving, so that the frequency of the incident wave on the red blood cells is shifted due to the component of their velocity along the propagation axis of the incident wave, $v(cos\ \theta)$. Then, the red blood cells scatter echoes in all directions as they continue to move, so that the frequency detected by the receiver has been shifted a second time due to the component of the velocity of the source scattering waves that lies along the beam axis of the receiving transducer, $v(cos\ \emptyset)$. The overall Doppler frequency shift of the received signal, Δf_D, is linearly proportional to the blood flow velocity, v, as described in the CW Doppler equation:

$$\Delta f_D \approx \frac{v(cos\ \theta + cos\ \emptyset\ )}{c_0} f_0 \qquad [1.49]$$

To estimate the blood flow velocity from the Doppler frequency shift, the angles, θ and $\emptyset$, between the transmit and receive beams relative to the direction of the blood flow must be known (see Figure 4.2). The Doppler frequency shift detected from physiological blood flow using an ultrasound system operating at frequencies in the MHz range will fall within the audible range, at frequencies of a few kHz so that the information can be conveyed audibly. If the depth of the vessel allows the use of a higher transmit frequency, f_0, the intensity of backscatter from the rather weakly scattering red blood cells can be increased and, since the Doppler shift is proportional to f_0, a greater Doppler frequency shift can be obtained for a given blood flow velocity. The Doppler shift is also greater and subject to less error when the transducer beams and the direction of blood flow are well aligned (θ and ϕ are very small angles). CW Doppler is sensitive to all movements within the confocally aligned region of the two transducer beams, and a range of Doppler shifts corresponding to a range of velocities within the region of overlap between the two transducers will be obtained. It may be necessary to apply a high pass filter to exclude the detection of movement from strongly scattering but slowly moving tissue.

Pulsed Doppler systems allow the use of a single transducer in pulse-echo mode to estimate blood flow motion based on the time-of-flight shifts of echoes returned after consecutive pulsing events (see Figure 4.4). To construct the pulsed Doppler signal, the inter-pulse phase shift of echoes returned from a specific axial depth is evaluated based on the signal amplitude at that fixed axial depth sampled at the time of each successive pulse. The pulsed Doppler signal is sampled in time at an interval equal to the pulse repetition interval, T_{PRI}, that is referred to as slow time. The frequency spectrum of the pulsed Doppler signal is found from its discrete-time Fourier transform. Each frequency, f_D, in this spectrum can be related to a blood flow velocity, v, as described in the pulsed Doppler equation which very closely resembles the CW Doppler equation:

$$f_D = \frac{2v \cdot \cos\theta}{c_0} f_0 \qquad [1.50]$$

As for CW Doppler, a range of frequency shifts are detected and the relative proportion of flow at different speeds is related to the relative intensity of the spectrum at each frequency. There are, however, some very important differences. First, the pulsed Doppler estimate can be more tightly localized to a time-gated zone within the beam's focal zone. Furthermore, aliasing can occur if the movement to detect is insufficiently sampled in time. To evaluate rapid blood flow, this effect can be overcome by increasing the pulse repetition frequency, PRF. Recall, however (see section 1.5.8), that the PRF is the inverse of the time-to-echo from the deepest region of the image so that increasing the PRF will decrease the explorable depth.

The smallest Doppler frequency (smallest blood flow) that can be detected with pulsed Doppler is limited by the bin size of the spectrum calculated from the Doppler signal:

$$f_{D\_Min} = \frac{PRF}{Number\ of\ samples\ in\ the\ pulsed\ Doppler\ signal} \qquad [1.51]$$

so that to detect very slow flow, it may be necessary to reduce the PRF or detect echoes from a greater number of pulse-echo sequences. Much more extensive information on Doppler-related techniques, their display and advances enabled by high-frame-rate systems is provided in Chapter 4, and its use in echocardiography is presented in Chapter 5.

1.6.2. *Shear wave propagation speed and elastic properties*

The longitudinal compressional waves used for ultrasonic imaging are presented in section 1.3.1. A second kind of wave, shear waves, can also propagate in an elastic medium when a shearing force is applied. Shear waves do not propagate as readily in biological media as compressional waves, and their speed of propagation is much slower (~1–20 m/s) compared to compressional waves (~1,500 m/s). Since they propagate much more slowly than longitudinal compressional ultrasound, and since the propagation speed of these waves is related to the shear elastic modulus of the medium, it is possible to interrogate a medium with ultrafast, compressional pulses to track speckle decorrelation that occurs as a shear wave moves through a region. This can be used to assess the shear wave speed and thus to estimate medium elastic properties. Biological tissues are not perfectly elastic, but are rather viscoelastic. This means that there is a frequency-dependent delay in the strain response. This feature can be used to assess the viscosity of a medium. Shear wave propagation, the challenges of creating shear waves in biological media and their use for elasticity assessment are presented in Chapter 3.

1.6.3. *Ultrasound contrast imaging*

Ultrasound contrast imaging relies on the intravascular injection of exogenous microbubbles with a unique acoustic response (resonance, nonlinearity, destruction), which can be used to enhance the Doppler SNR, for tracer-perfusion modeling of the microvascular flow or for ultrasound localization microscopy. Microbubbles contain a gas and so, relative to the surrounding blood, they present a very strong acoustical impedance mismatch and scatter ultrasound very efficiently. Since they are micrometric in size, they remain within the vascular tree and are not spatially resolved on ultrasonic images. Once injected, microbubbles flow along with the red blood cells so they can be used as tracers of blood flow. After injection, the signal from the circulating bubbles is only visible for a few minutes because they are progressively taken up into the liver, and the gas that they contain is ultimately diffused through the lungs.

The acoustic impedance mismatch is not the only factor that favors the detectability of ultrasound contrast microbubbles. The radius and compressibility of microbubbles are also very important. When exposed to the pressure changes caused by ultrasound, these highly compressible microbubbles present resonant behavior and the bubble wall can oscillate nonlinearly about its equilibrium position. The resonance for microbubbles able to pass through the capillary bed happens to fall within the frequency range used in diagnostic ultrasound. When microbubbles oscillate in a nonlinear manner, they can be more sensitively detected relative to surrounding media due to the specific frequency content, amplitude or phase of their response. Thus, specific pulse-sequences can be used to highlight the nonlinear behavior of microbubbles. They can also be detected based on their acoustic disruption. To evaluate microvascular flow, even though tiny vessels and microbubbles are too small to resolve, the time-dependent modification of nonlinear echoes received from contrast agent microbubbles moving with very slow speeds can be related to blood flow and relative blood concentration within a region of interest. Ultrasound contrast agents and the methods enabling their use to assess the microvascularization are presented in detail in Chapter 6.

1.6.4. *Super-resolution imaging*

Tracer-based contrast imaging provides highly useful information, but it would be nice to map out the vessels within organs such as the brain, kidney and tumors. Increased resolution cannot be obtained by increasing the ultrasound frequency because the attenuation at high frequencies strongly limits the penetration depth. Although it is not possible to spatially resolve an individual microbubble because the image resolution is limited by beam diffraction, it is possible to detect a single microbubble. This is the key premise of ultrasound localization microscopy or super-resolution imaging that is presented in much greater detail in Chapter 7. Since each contrast microbubble is much smaller than the wavelengths used to image them, by localizing the center of an individual microbubble source on an ultrasound image, the diffraction resolution limit can be defied to image fine vascular structure. By using ultrafast imaging, it is further possible to track individual microbubbles to obtain information about the flow rate and direction on a scale down to about 10 microns.

1.6.5. *Photoacoustic imaging*

Photoacoustic imaging is based on the fact that acoustic signals can be detected when optical absorbers undergo thermoexpansion. Thus, by illuminating zones within tissue using a laser pulse, acoustic signals can be detected to map out structures with different optical absorption characteristics. Depths of a few centimeters can be imaged using this approach. The spatial resolution of the image depends on the resolution of the ultrasonic detection. A very complete description of photoacoustic imaging and its applications is provided in Chapter 9.

1.7. References

Chen, C. and Pertijs, M.A.P. (2021). Integrated transceivers for emerging medical ultrasound imaging devices: A review. *IEEE Open Journal of the Solid-State Circuits Society*, 104–114. doi: 10.1109/OJSSCS.2021.3115398.

Christensen-Jeffries, K., Couture, O., Dayton, P.A., Eldar, Y.C., Hynynen, K., Kiessling, F., O'Reilly, M., Pinton, G.F., Schmitz, G., Tang, M.X. et al. (2020). Super-resolution ultrasound imaging. *Ultrasound in Medicine & Biology*, 46, 865–891.

Cobbold, R.S.C. (2006). *Foundations of Biomedical Ultrasound*. Oxford University Press, Oxford.

Evans, D.H. and McDicken, W.N. (2000). *Doppler Ultrasound: Physics, Instrumentation and Signal Processing*, 2nd edition. Wiley, Chichester.

Hill, C.R., Bamber, G.R., ter Haar, G.R. (eds) (2004). *Physical Principles of Medical Ultrasonics*, 2nd edition. Wiley, Chichester.

Leighton, T. (1997). *The Acoustic Bubble*, 1st edition. Academic Press, London.

Lindner, J.R. (2004). Microbubbles in medical imaging: Current applications and future directions. *Nature Reviews Drug Discovery*, 6, 527–532. doi: 10.1038/nrd1417.

Montaldo, G., Tanter, M., Bercoff, J., Benech, N., Fink, M. (2009). Coherent plane-wave compounding for very high frame rate ultrasonography and transient elastography. *IEEE Transactions on Ultrasonics, Ferroelectrics and Frequency Control*, 56, 489–506. doi: 10.1109/TUFFC.2009.1067.

Szabo, T.L. (2013). *Diagnositic Ultrasound Imaging: Inside Out*. Academic Press, New York.

Tanter, M. and Fink, M. (2014). Ultrafast imaging in biomedical ultrasound. *IEEE Transactions on Ultrasonics, Ferroelectrics, and Frequency Control*, 61, 102–119. doi: 10.1109/TUFFC.2014.2882.

2

Transducers, Imaging Systems and Image Formation

Enrico BONI[1], Alessandro RAMALLI[1], Alessandro Stuart SAVOIA[2] and Piero TORTOLI[1]

[1] *Department of Information Engineering, University of Florence, Italy*

[2] *Department of Industrial, Electronic and Mechanical Engineering, Roma Tre University, Rome, Italy*

2.1. Ultrasonic transducers

Ultrasonic transducers are devices that can convert electrical energy into acoustic energy and vice versa. They operate at acoustic frequencies above the audible range. The transducer undoubtedly represents the component of modern ultrasound imaging systems with the strongest impact on the system's performance. In effect, their features limit the field of view and the resolving power that can be obtained. The majority of medical ultrasound imaging systems are equipped with several transducers, having different sizes and shapes, that operate within different frequency ranges. This allows the operator to select the transducer best adapted for each imaging application.

While focusing on medical imaging applications, this section will introduce the fundamental aspects of ultrasonic transducers such as the operating principles, the

For a color version of all the figures in this chapter, see www.iste.co.uk/bridal/innovative.zip.

Innovative Ultrasound Imaging Techniques,
coordinated by S. Lori BRIDAL.

most common transducer configurations and the main performance parameters. Well-established technologies currently used for medical transducer fabrication, as well as the emerging, cutting-edge technologies that are leading the way towards future generation imaging systems, will then be illustrated. Finally, novel transducer configurations that are enabling real-time volumetric imaging will be described.

2.1.1. *Transducer fundamentals*

A typical transducer array for medical imaging is based on a piezoelectric plate driven at a frequency near its fundamental thickness-mode resonance. The central frequency and bandwidth of the electro-acoustic response are determined by the thickness of the plate and by the way it is mechanically supported and acoustically coupled to the propagation medium.

2.1.1.1. *Main concepts and characteristics*

Figure 2.1(a) shows the elementary form of a thickness-mode transducer, i.e. a plate of piezoelectric material with thickness **t** sandwiched between two electrodes. When an alternating voltage is applied across the electrodes, an alternating electric field, E, is created in the material and, due to the inverse piezoelectric effect, opposing mechanical forces are generated across the plate that cause it to vibrate along its thickness. Conversely, if the plate is deformed by an external force, the charge is displaced in the material and, via the direct piezoelectric effect, an electric potential difference is produced across the electrodes. Electro-acoustic transduction by both direct and inverse piezoelectric effects can be achieved while coupling the transducer to a propagation medium. The methods used to achieve effective coupling heavily influence the overall performance of the transducer.

A simple yet effective way to describe a transducer's electro-acoustic behavior is by using an equivalent circuit model, as introduced in section 1.2.3. The simplest equivalent circuit model of a thickness-mode transducer, known as the Butterworth–Van Dyke (BVD) model (Butterworth 1914; Van Dyke 1925), is shown in Figure 2.1(b). This circuit can be used to model the electrical impedance of the transducer operating at a frequency close to its thickness-mode resonance frequency. More advanced models are based on an analogy between electrical and mechanical oscillators. Mason's model (Mason 1948) and the KLM (Krimholtz et al. 1970) model are among the most popular and are diagramed in Figure 2.1. These models treat the transducer as a three-port network, including a single electrical port and two mechanical ports representing the two faces of the transducer. Equations relating electrical and mechanical quantities are represented by equivalent networks coupled using an ideal transformer, where the electro-mechanical analogy is employed to represent forces and velocities (F, v) using voltages and currents (V, i), respectively.

In the Mason's and KLM models, a voltage V is applied to the piezoelectric plate to produce acoustic forces F_1 and F_2 on the faces of the transducer as well as particle velocities of v_1 and v_2 on these two faces, respectively. The speed of sound and the acoustic impedance of the piezoelectric plate are denoted as c and Z_0, respectively. The acoustic impedances of the media in contact with the transducer on its two faces can be denoted as Z_1 and Z_2. The models, as shown in the diagrams of Figure 2.1(c) and (d), also include a capacitor, C_0, where the capacitance is related to the dielectric properties of the piezoelectric material (it is polarized under an electric potential and has a dielectric permittivity, ε, characterizing its ability to hold an electrical charge). The negative capacitance, $-C_0$, in Mason's model, and similarly, the reactance, X_1, in the KLM model, account for the mechano-electric feedback. The multi-resonant mechanical behavior is modeled using lumped elements (Mason) and transmission lines (KLM). The term θ in Mason's model is directly proportional to the frequency and the thickness, and inversely proportional to the speed of sound. Intervening between the electrical and the mechanical domains, there is a transformer that converts between electrical and mechanical energy with a specified transformation ratio (1:n).

In the BVD model, the transducer behavior "seen" from the electrical port of the transducer is modeled using the two parallel branches. The electrical branch includes a purely electrical capacitance, C_0, while the mechanical branch consists of an RLC-series circuit, where L_m and C_m represent the equivalent mass and stiffness, and R_m identifies the losses. Note that R_m accounts for all possible losses, including the dissipation of energy inside the transducer and, more importantly, radiation of acoustic energy.

Even though these models only provide an approximate and linear description of the system, they are surprisingly accurate and are therefore often used to predict transducer behavior in system-level analysis frameworks such as estimation of the power conversion and wave propagation. For example, these models can be used to predict the pressure wave emanating from the surface of a piezoelectric transducer under different conditions for impedance matching.

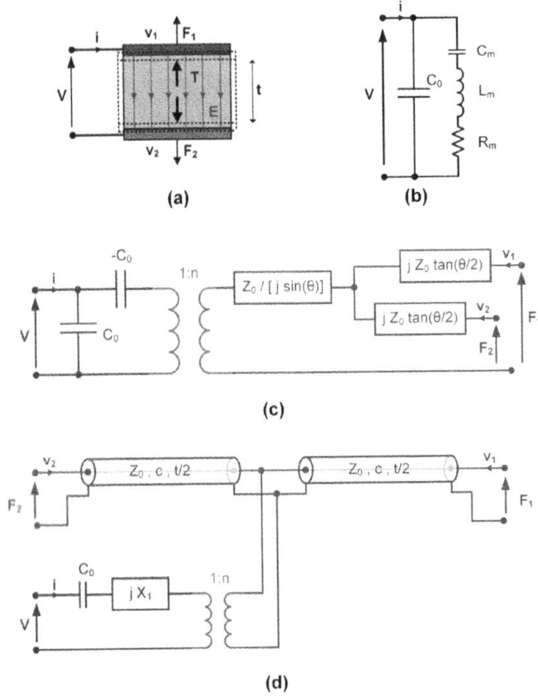

Figure 2.1. *(a) Thickness-mode transducer of thickness, **t**, with an electrode on each face (in red and blue). When a voltage (electrical potential), V, is applied across the piezoelectric plate, the faces of the transducer experience acoustic forces (F_1 and F_2) and particle velocities of v_1 and v_2, respectively. Diagrams of (b) BVD, (c) Mason's and (d) KLM equivalent circuit models. For (c) and (d), the electrical and mechanical domains (in red and blue, respectively) connect through an electro-mechanical transformer (in green)*

2.1.1.2. *Basic transducer array configurations*

Arrays are produced by dividing a piezoelectric plate into individual transducer elements, which are independently connected to the imaging system. This allows electronic control of the transmission and reception of acoustic beams for focusing or steering. As briefly described in Chapter 1 and extensively discussed in the next sections, traditional ultrasound image formation is achieved by scanning the medium under investigation using the acoustic beam produced by a transducer array. The shape of the acoustic beam is determined by the spatial and temporal characteristics of the acoustic waves generated by the transducer array elements as they propagate and diffract into the medium. These spatial and temporal characteristics are directly related to the transducer array geometry and its frequency response, and they have a direct effect on the imaging resolution.

The resolution along the propagation direction is referred to as the axial resolution. It is predominantly related to the frequency bandwidth of the transducer. A broadband frequency response centered at higher frequencies allows the generation of very short pressure pulses leading to a higher axial resolution. However, since a broadband response is generally achieved at the expense of gain (in analogy to the gain–bandwidth trade-off in an amplifier), and because tissue attenuation increases with frequency, the transducer's frequency response is typically determined after considering the trade-off between the desired axial resolution and penetration requirements. For thickness-mode transducers, the center frequency is determined by the thickness of the piezoelectric plate, while the bandwidth is adjusted by adding a suitable backing layer on the rear face of the plate to damp any back radiation and by integrating a matching layer on the front face to improve the acoustic matching between the piezoelectric material and biological tissues. The resulting structure, schematically represented in Figure 2.2(b), is often referred to as an acoustic stack. Typical design guidelines are described in McKeighen (1998).

The resolution in the direction perpendicular to the beam axis and along the lateral axis of a transducer array is referred to as lateral resolution. It depends on both the amplitude and phase distribution of the acoustic pressure at the transducer surface as well as on the frequency content of the acoustic pulses. Such pressure distribution is controlled by the imaging system, which activates and electrically drives a suitable number of adjacent array elements, i.e. the aperture. The electronic control of the amplitude and phase of the driving signals makes it possible to rapidly change the beam propagation direction, therefore allowing for focusing and steering.

The most common transducer configurations for medical imaging consist of one-dimensional (1D) arrays in which the elements are equally spaced along a linear or curvilinear path. As shown in Figure 2.2(c), the array elements are typically rectangular: the distance along the azimuth between the center of adjacent elements is referred to as the pitch, while their separation is called kerf. As described in detail in the next section, acoustic beam focusing and steering are performed electronically by the imaging system in the azimuth direction. The beam shape in the elevation direction is statically defined using an acoustic lens. This lens relies on a principle similar to that used in optical systems. Acoustic focusing with the lens is achieved by refracting ultrasound through a curved interface between two media with different wave propagation speeds. As shown in Figure 2.2(a), an acoustic lens for elevation focusing is obtained by applying a cylindrically shaped additional front layer made of a material characterized by a different speed of sound as compared to that in the biological medium.

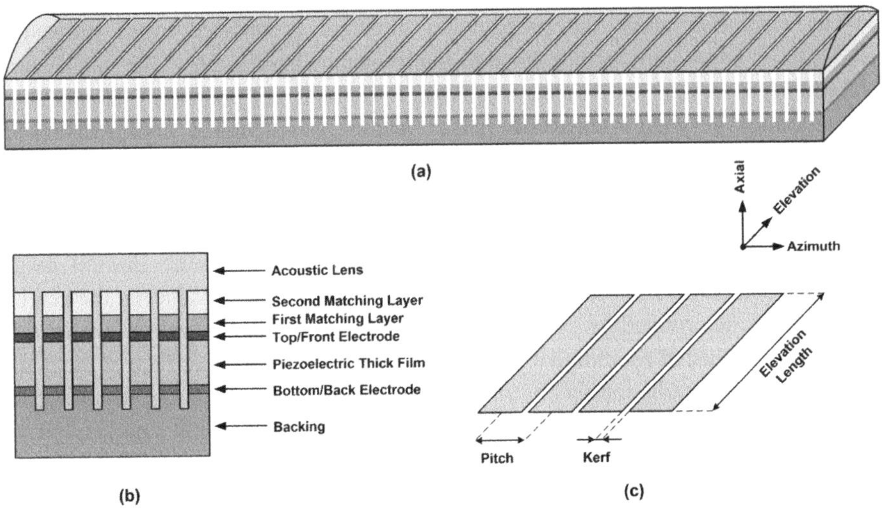

Figure 2.2. *(a) 1D piezoelectric transducer array. (b) Typical acoustic stack of a medical imaging transducer. (c) Geometrical array parameters*

Commercial imaging systems are equipped with a variety of ultrasound probes of different sizes, shapes and operating frequencies that have been designed for distinct clinical applications. The probe is connected to the imaging system through a multi-polar cable containing one micro-coaxial cable for each transducer array element. Each type of probe can be related to one of the three main classes of 1D arrays, i.e. linear, phased and convex, as represented in Figure 2.3.

Linear arrays are characterized by a large number of elements, in the range of 128–256, in which subgroups of adjacent elements are used to focus and sweep an acoustic beam orthogonally with respect to the transducer surface. The image is formed by parallel scan lines, and the typical field of view is rectangular. Since beam steering is normally not used, the array element width is relatively large, up to two acoustic wavelengths at the highest frequency in the transducer bandwidth, to laterally increase the field of view as much as possible. Linear arrays are typically designed in the mid- to high-frequency range, from 5 MHz to 15 MHz for high-resolution imaging and flow measurement applications, such as musculoskeletal and vascular ultrasound.

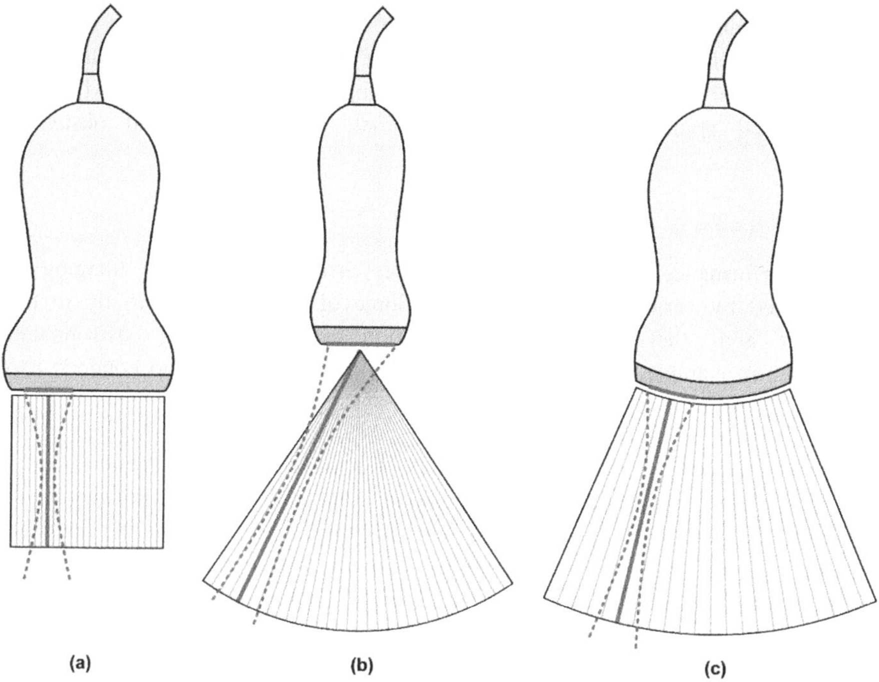

Figure 2.3. *(a) Linear array, (b) phased array and (c) convex array probes, and related typical fields of view*

Phased arrays use all the elements to focus and steer each acoustic beam. The resulting image is formed by a set of lines describing a circular sector of up to 90°. Given the large steering angles, the primary design criterion is that the element width and the array pitch must be on the order of or smaller than half a wavelength to achieve suitable element directivity and to avoid grating lobes in the field of view. Inter-element crosstalk needs to be kept as low as possible to preserve the field of view. Phased arrays typically have between 64 and 128 elements. The limited number of array elements together with their narrow width results in a relatively small transducer footprint. This limits the lateral resolution at large depths. Phased arrays are commonly designed in the low-frequency range, from 1.5 MHz to 4 MHz, and are often employed in cardiac applications where the small footprint allows scanning through the small acoustic windows defined by the intercostal spaces.

The disadvantages of linear arrays in terms of limited field of view and of phased arrays in terms of limited lateral resolution are overcome by the curvilinear (or convex) array, which is essentially a "linear" array arranged on an arc. As in the linear array, subgroups of elements are used to sweep the beam, but the resulting field of view is much larger in depth. Curvilinear arrays have large element counts and are designed in the low- to mid-frequency range, from 2.5 MHz to 6 MHz, for many clinical applications such as abdominal, gynecological and obstetrics ultrasound.

2.1.1.3. *Transducer and array performance*

The performance of ultrasonic transducer arrays for medical imaging is characterized by various figures of merit. Some of them pertain strictly to the transducer, and others refer to its integration in the operating environment, including, for example, the cables and electrical components used to connect it to the imaging system.

One of the most important characteristics of a transducer is its electro-acoustic response, which quantifies its ability to generate an acoustic pressure in response to an electrical excitation and vice versa. This is typically defined for the one-way (transmit-only and receive-only) or for the two-way (pulse-echo) electro-acoustic response, and it is characterized in the frequency domain by specifying the center frequency and the bandwidth at -3 dB and -6 dB, respectively, and the peak magnitude of the spectral sensitivity.

Another important characteristic of a transducer is the electrical impedance, which has to do with its electro-mechanical energy conversion capability when operating in conjunction with the electronic circuits of the imaging system. To understand the relation between the electrical impedance and the overall system performance, consider the case of a driving circuit, simplified as a voltage generator with its predominantly resistive source impedance, loaded with the transducer equivalent circuit of Figure 2.1(b) characterized by an impedance with a significant reactive component. During operation, the power transfer from the source to the load depends on how close the relative impedance values are. In practical cases, due to this electrical impedance mismatch, a significant amount of power may be wasted, leading to poor overall efficiency. Therefore, electrical impedance matching techniques, typically consisting of introducing passive-component circuits between the transducer and the imaging system circuits, are used to maximize the power transfer. Analogously, impedance matching also improves the performance in receive operation by minimizing the noise figure of the transducer in conjunction with an amplifier.

As the range of transducer parameters determining the overall performance is wide, computer-aided simulation tools have been developed based on the modeling approaches presented in this section. For example, the free-to-use online tool

BioSono KLM v2.0 (see: http://biosono.com/TrnsLgd20/TrnsLgd.php), based on the KLM model, allows the simulation of the behavior of a transducer provided with matching and backing layers of arbitrary size and material under typical electrical driving and loading conditions.

2.1.2. *Transducer technologies*

Most of today's medical imaging arrays use thickness-mode transducers made up of bulk piezoelectric materials, among which the most commonly used are polycrystalline ceramics, single crystals and composites. These piezoelectric materials have been the subject of considerable research. Their development throughout the 20th century has improved their properties and optimized their manufacturing processes. With the evolution of microelectronics, towards the end of the 20th century, a new class of silicon-based ultrasonic transducers was introduced: the micromachined ultrasonic transducer (MUT). These are micro-electro-mechanical-systems (MEMS), i.e. microscopic, movable structures fabricated on a silicon wafer using micromachining technologies, similar to the process used to fabricate microphones, accelerometers and many other sensors and actuators that are embedded in smartphones, cars and other everyday-use devices.

2.1.2.1. *Bulk piezoelectric transducers*

As introduced earlier in this chapter, arrays based on bulk piezoelectric materials are fabricated by stacking different material layers and by mechanically dicing them to define individual transducer elements. Due to their small size, high-precision mechanical processing is required to accurately control the lateral dimensions of the elements and the thicknesses of the different layers. The cost of such processing may be very high, especially for the manufacturing of high-frequency arrays, due to the small size of the elements (< 100 μm), and for 2D arrays, due to the large number (> 1,000) of elements.

Among the materials used in bulk piezoelectric transducers, the most common is lead zirconate titanate (PZT) polycrystalline ceramic, which, during manufacturing, organizes in domains, i.e. volumes of material with randomly oriented dipoles, and exhibits ferroelectric and piezoelectric properties. After fabrication, ceramic PZT may be poled along the thickness direction to enhance its electro-mechanical conversion capability. Poling is carried out by applying an electrical field and by heating it for a certain time in order to permanently align the domains. Ceramic PZT exists in several formulations with different characteristics and is used for a wide range of applications. Ceramic PZT exhibits outstanding properties, such as high piezoelectric coefficients (d_{33} = 450 pC/N) and coupling coefficients (k_t = 0.5), as well as high relative dielectric permittivity (ε_{33} = 1,000). Moreover, stability over time and low manufacturing costs make it one of the most preferred materials for medical imaging transducer array fabrication.

Another class of piezoelectric materials that are used in medical imaging transducer arrays are relaxor-ferroelectric single crystals. During manufacturing, domains of single crystals grow with a high level of alignment, resulting in superior piezoelectric properties as compared to ceramics. Examples of relaxor-ferroelectric single crystals are lead zinc niobate-lead titanate (PZN-PT) and lead magnesium niobate-lead titanate (PMN-PT), which can exhibit very high piezoelectric coefficients (d_{33} > 1,000 pC/N). These materials allow the fabrication of high-performance transducer arrays, but the increased fragility of single crystals as compared to ceramics generally makes manufacturing costs higher.

Both ceramic and single-crystal bulk piezoelectric transducer materials are characterized by a high specific acoustic impedance (Z_p = 35 MRayl), and therefore require the use of multiple matching layers to achieve efficient and broadband operation when coupled to biological tissue. A possible approach to lower the specific acoustic impedance of a transducer is to combine bulk piezoelectric material with a lower impedance material to obtain a piezocomposite. The most common piezocomposite structure, known as 1-3, consists of a grid of piezoelectric pillars, produced by mechanical dicing of a bulk PZT ceramic layer filled with a polymer, which is typically an epoxy resin. Many transducer manufacturers use PZT-based piezocomposites to make high-performance arrays used in high-end medical imaging systems.

2.1.2.2. *Micromachined transducers*

A MUT (Pappalardo et al. 2008) consists of a thin plate suspended over a cavity. Unlike a bulk piezoelectric thickness-mode transducer, a MUT vibrates in flexural mode, just like a drumhead. Its mechanical impedance is much lower than that of a thickness-mode transducer operating at the same frequency. Consequently, MUTs are generally well acoustically matched to biological tissue and do not require the use of the matching layers typically employed to achieve broadband operation for bulk piezoelectric transducers. A MUT plate designed to operate in the ultrasound imaging frequency range (from 1 MHz to 20 MHz) has lateral dimensions in the 30–300 μm range and a thickness in the 1–5 μm range. Therefore, array elements are created by tiling multiple MUT plates and by electrically connecting them in parallel. Figure 2.4(a) schematically shows an array of four rectangular elements, each composed of 16 plates.

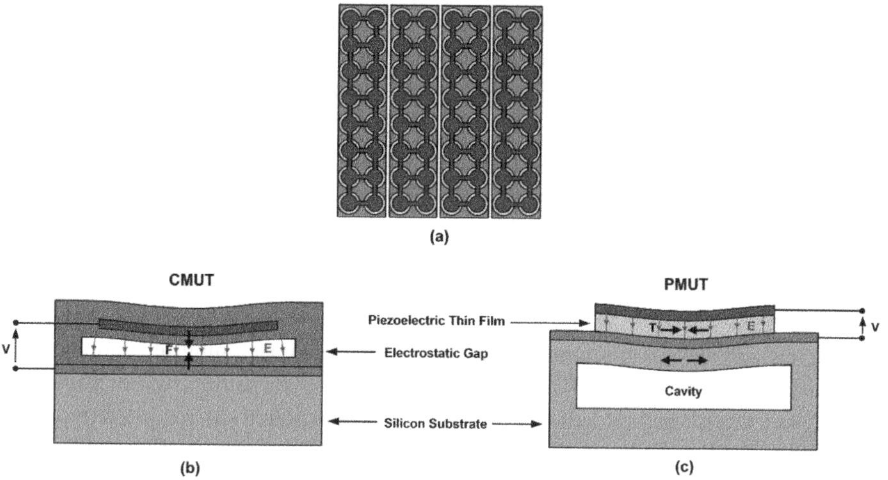

Figure 2.4. *(a) Schematic layout of a four-element MUT array. Each rectangular element (in blue) is composed of 16 circular plates connected in parallel. Diagram of a CMUT (b) and a PMUT (c): when a voltage (electrical potential), V, is applied across the two electrodes (in red and blue), electrostatic forces, F, and stresses, T, are generated in the CMUT and PMUT, respectively, which deflect the plate*

Two main types of MUTs are classified according to their operating principle: capacitive micromachined ultrasonic transducers (CMUT) (Khuri-Yakub and Oralkan 2011) are based on the electrostatic effect, while piezoelectric micromachined ultrasonic transducers (PMUT) (Qiu et al. 2015) rely on the piezoelectric effect.

A CMUT cell, shown in Figure 2.4(b), is basically a parallel plate capacitor in which one of the two electrodes is part of a movable plate. The cavity that separates the plate from the substrate is called the "gap". When a DC voltage (electrical potential), V, is applied across the two electrodes, electrostatic forces, F, generate and deflect the plate towards the substrate. Elastic forces opposed to the electrostatic forces maintain the plate in a stable position. If an AC voltage is superimposed on the DC voltage, the plate vibrates, and ultrasound waves are transmitted into the surrounding medium. Conversely, if an ultrasound wave impinges on the plate, the capacitance variation under a DC voltage biasing produces an electrical current.

In a PMUT cell, shown in Figure 2.4(c), the movable plate is composed of a piezoelectric thin-film layer, typically PZT or aluminum nitride, sandwiched between two electrodes and coupled to an elastic plate suspended over a cavity. If a DC voltage is applied across the electrodes, an electrical field is generated in the thin-film piezoelectric layer due to the inverse piezoelectric effect and induces a stress in the plate, which relaxes into a flexural deformation of the plate itself. If an AC voltage is applied, the plate vibrates and generates acoustic waves in the surrounding medium. Vice versa, the piezoelectric effect can be used to detect acoustic waves impinging on the plate.

Different microfabrication technologies have been developed to manufacture MUT arrays on silicon wafers. To define the cavities, the two most common approaches use surface micromachining and bulk micromachining techniques. The surface micromachining MUT microfabrication process relies on sacrificial release. The cavities are formed underneath the plates by depositing a sacrificial layer on the substrate which is then removed by selective chemical etching. In bulk micromachining processes, the cavities are formed by vertical etching of silicon. For CMUTs in particular, closed cavities are obtained by bonding two wafers after having formed the cavities on one of them. For PMUTs, the cavities are often formed by etching the backside of the wafer after having deposited the plate and the piezoelectric layers. Both surface and bulk micromachining have been successfully used to make CMUTs and PMUTs, and a variety of microfabrication technologies, often combining several of the described approaches, are available today.

Arrays for medical imaging have been developed and integrated into ultrasound imaging probes and systems using both CMUT and PMUT technologies, and they have been successfully demonstrated to be suitable for high-quality medical imaging (Savoia et al. 2012, 2021). Today, MUTs are playing a fundamental role in the development of novel applications such as ultra-portable medical imaging systems, where the enhanced compatibility between MEMS and standard integrated circuit technologies favors the integration of the transducer and the electronics in a single "smart" silicon chip provided with both electro-acoustic transduction and electrical signal processing capabilities.

2.1.2.3. *Advanced transducer array configurations for volumetric imaging*

As mentioned earlier, 1D arrays are capable of electronically steering the acoustic beam along the azimuth direction and are therefore used to scan planes and produce 2D images. On the contrary, 2D arrays can scan volumes and therefore generate 3D images. However, the number of elements needed to enable acoustic beam steering in the volume with reasonably low grating lobes is extremely high. As an example, considering that the minimum number of elements in a 1D phased array is N = 64, an equivalent fully sampled 2D array able to scan a volumetric sector with similar resolution and contrast requires NxN = 64x64 = 4,096 elements, as shown in Figure 2.5(a). Currently, high-end 1D arrays require at most 256 cables and system channels. Direct handling of 4,096 elements by the imaging system is impractical due to the large number of cables and system channels required. Therefore, different solutions to this challenge have been proposed. One solution is based on the use of complex, application-specific integrated circuits (ASIC) placed inside the probe, close to the fully sampled 2D transducer array, to partially process the signals and reduce their number so that they can be transferred and further processed by a standard imaging system. This solution provides the best performance at the expense of increased complexity and cost related to the design of the ASIC and its integration with the transducer.

Other solutions are based on the reduction of the number of physical elements of the 2D array. These include sparse arrays and crossed electrode arrays.

Sparse arrays

Simply speaking, sparse arrays are 2D phased arrays with a reduced number of small transducer elements distributed across a large area. An example of a sparse array of 256 elements randomly picked from a 4,096-element fully sampled 2D array is shown in Figure 2.5(a). In sparse arrays, the width of the single elements is determined using a criterion similar to that for 1D phased arrays. For example, a half wavelength element width may be selected to achieve suitable element directivity, but the pitch is much larger and, more importantly, is not constant. The non-constant pitch characteristic means that the array aperture is sampled aperiodically. As a result, the grating lobes are reduced by distributing the sidelobes to the entire sector. Due to the lower active surface, sparse arrays have limited performance in terms of maximum transmit pressure and signal-to-noise ratio (SNR). There are many approaches to define the position of the elements. Stochastic approaches have been extensively investigated in the past decades, and advanced optimization techniques have been proposed and experimentally tested (Roux et al. 2017). Alternative approaches in which the elements are positioned along aperiodic spiral patterns have been recently shown to provide performance comparable to optimized stochastic methods. These methods have the advantage of being deterministic and scalable with respect to frequency. An example of a 256-element sparse array design, based on Fermat's spiral pattern layout, is presented in Ramalli et al. (2015) and shown in Figure 2.5(c).

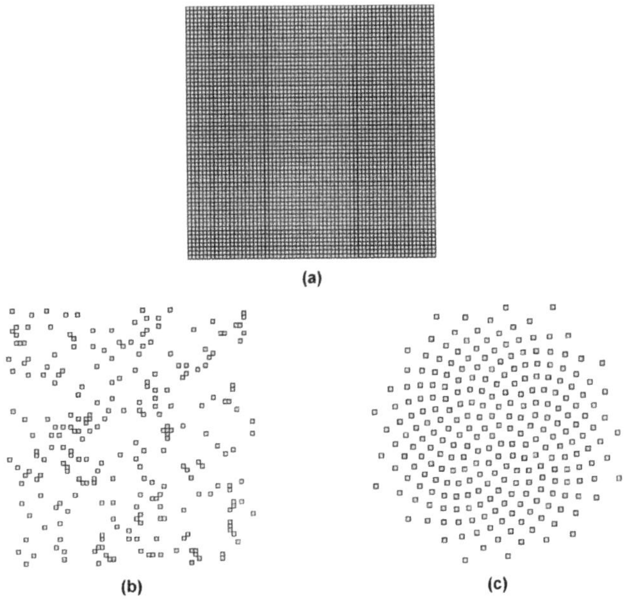

Figure 2.5. *(a) A fully sampled 2D array of 4,096 (64x64) elements. (b) A sparse array of 256 elements randomly picked from the fully sampled 2D array shown in (a). (c) 256-element sparse array based on Fermat's spiral pattern layout*

Crossed electrode arrays

Crossed electrode arrays are 2D arrays that behave as two overlapped, orthogonal 1D arrays (Morton and Lockwood 2003). A crossed electrode array can be obtained by configuring the top and bottom electrodes of a 2D array as two 1D arrays in orthogonal directions. Figure 2.5 schematically shows the concept: a 4+4-element crossed electrode array is obtained from a 16-element 2D array by shaping the top and bottom electrodes in vertical and horizontal 1D arrays. Crossed electrode arrays (see Figure 2.6) can scan volumes with a reduced number of elements (from NxN of fully sampled arrays to N+N), by combining the information acquired from 1D scans of orthogonal planes. The disadvantages are related to the higher sidelobes and reduced field of view compared to fully sampled 2D arrays and the presence of artifacts deriving from the absence of elevational focus for the two linear arrays.

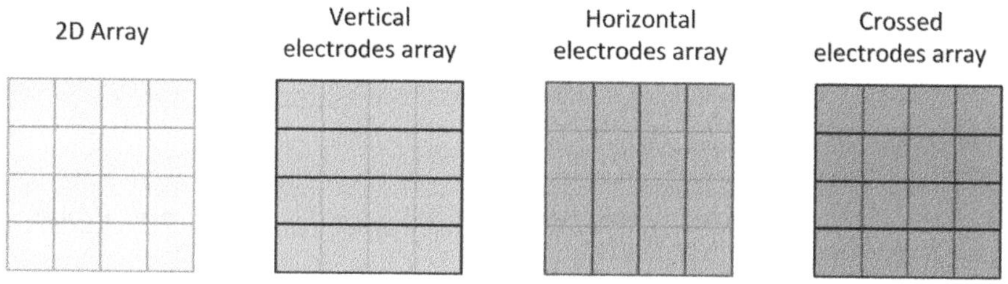

Figure 2.6. *A 4+4-element crossed electrode array is obtained by connecting the top and bottom electrodes of a 16-element 2D array along the vertical and horizontal directions*

Several CMUT crossed electrode implementations have been proposed with different names, i.e. crisscross (Savoia et al. 2007), row–column addressed (RCA) (Logan et al. 2011) and top-orthogonal–bottom electrode (TOBE) (Zemp et al. 2011) arrays. Improved crossed array configurations with integrated elevation apodization (Christiansen et al. 2013) and Fresnel focusing (Savoia et al. 2018) have been proposed for artifact reduction.

2.2. Image formation techniques

2.2.1. *Imaging system building blocks*

As explained in Chapter 1, ultrasound imaging systems are based on pulse-echo techniques, i.e. an ultrasound packet is transmitted, and the relevant echo signals are subsequently received and processed. With new strides in electronic technologies, the systems performing these tasks have shifted over the years from analog to digital circuits (Szabo 2004).

2.2.1.1. *Basic architecture*

Imaging systems are based on a multi-element ultrasound transducer array as described in section 2.1, connected to suitable transmission/reception electronic circuits. A system is said to be an “N-channel” scanner if N is the maximum number of elements that can be simultaneously connected to distinct transmitters and receivers during each transmission (TX) event.

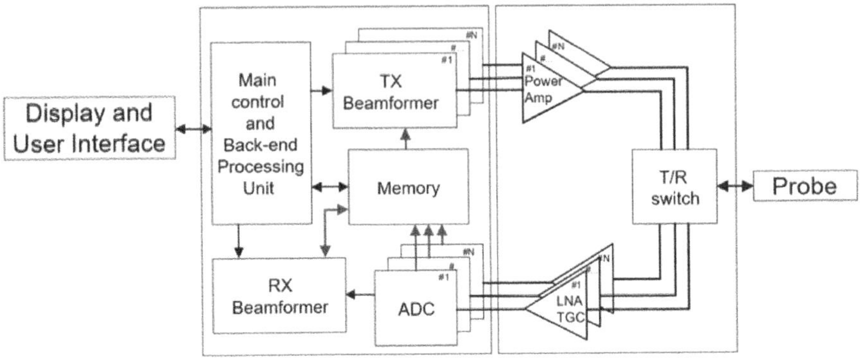

Figure 2.7. *Block diagram of a typical imaging system connected to an ultrasound transducer array (probe). The display and user interfaces are usually embedded in a PC. Digital and analog circuits are included in the left and right main blocks, respectively*

As shown in Figure 2.7, an imaging system includes the following key blocks:

– Transmit beamformer

For each active channel, the transmit beamformer delays the corresponding TX signal (usually a short tone burst) by the amount needed to focus the transmitted energy to the desired depth. The beamformer is usually implemented in the digital domain by field programmable gate arrays (FPGAs). For each TX event, the FPGA produces the delays and the possible pulse shaping needed to produce the desired focused beam. The transmit delays and pulse shapes are usually precomputed by the digital back-end and are stored, for each scanline, in the FPGA memory.

– Transmitter circuits

These circuits typically include power amplifiers (Power Amps), each one independently driven by the transmit beamformer to generate the signals to be delivered to the active transducer array elements. The number of transmitter channels in high-end, cart-based systems is usually the same as the total number of transducer elements. In this configuration, each transducer element has its own transmitter circuit and there is no need for high-voltage multiplexing circuits.

– Transmit-to-receive (T/R) electronics

Once the transmission has been completed, the transducer elements of the selected receiving aperture need to be connected to the reception (RX) chain. This task is performed by the transmit/receive (T/R) switches. A high-voltage switch connects each transducer element either to the transmit electronics (during TX) or to the receiving electronics (during RX) (Chen and Pertijs 2021).

– Receiver circuits

For each channel, the receiving chain following the T/R switches is typically composed of a low noise amplifier (LNA), time gain compensation (TGC) circuits and an analog-to-digital converter (ADC). The digital raw data are temporarily stored in buffer memories, typically inside a front-end FPGA.

– Receive beamformer

The front-end FPGA can also be used to "beamform" the digital raw radiofrequency (RF) data. A delay-and-sum (DAS) algorithm is typically applied to the RF channels to produce an echo scanline. The RX beamforming is dynamically operated (dynamic focusing), i.e. for each channel, the receive delays are continuously varied to keep the focal point consistent with the time-range equation (section 1.5.3) of pulse-echo systems. As for TX beamforming, all the DAS parameters can be precomputed by the back-end software for all the scanlines, and recalled by the beamforming FPGA on a per-line basis.

– Back-end imaging pipeline

- Downconversion and envelope extraction:

The envelope of the beamformed RF data is usually calculated through coherent demodulation followed by low-pass filtering and modulus extraction, or through Hilbert filtering of the RF data followed by modulus extraction.

- Scan conversion:

Depending on the scanning configuration (linear, convex or phased), the received scanlines are not necessarily oriented on a rectangular grid like that typical of a (PC) display. Scan conversion is thus necessary, i.e. the samples of each received scanline must be projected on a rectangular grid and eventually interpolated to match the video frame resolution. The resulting final image is then low-pass filtered to avoid artifacts (typically Moiré patterns) associated with this processing step.

- Filtering and display:

The scan-converted image can be further filtered and processed to enhance the details and/or to reduce the noise. For a brightness-mode (B-Mode) image, the amplitude information of each pixel is log-compressed. The pixels below a user-selected "reject" threshold are displayed as black, and the pixels above a "saturation" threshold are displayed as white. The pixel amplitudes between these two extremes are plotted as grayscale levels ranging from black to white where the mapping of different grayscale levels can be linear or, more commonly, a sigmoidal S-shaped curve.

2.2.2. *High-frame-rate imaging*

As previously described in section 1.5.3, the imaging frame rate is directly proportional to the pulse repetition frequency (PRF) and inversely proportional to the number of sequential TX events required to scan the region of interest. Hence, the frame rate can be increased either by increasing the PRF, which is, however, limited by the maximum depth to be imaged, or by decreasing the number of TX events. One way to achieve this goal is to reduce the number of scan lines per frame. However, doing so with conventional imaging techniques (beamforming along sequential scan lines) will limit either the spatial resolution or the width of the field of view of the image. Ultrafast or high-frame-rate (HFR) techniques based on the transmission of unfocused beams can overcome these restrictions by reconstructing one image per transmission event, without sacrificing the field of view. In such a case, advanced beamforming strategies such as parallel beamforming (Shattuck et al. 1984) or limited diffraction beams (Lu 1997a) must be implemented.

HFR is an ultrasound imaging innovation that has emerged over the last decade (Tanter and Fink 2014). The provided high temporal resolution opens up novel possibilities to study, with unprecedented detail, dynamic events in the human body. Just as modern high-speed cameras allow detailed slow-motion viewing of key moments during sporting events or the visualization of natural phenomena that are too rapid to observe with the naked eye, ultrasound HFR imaging allows the detection of the dynamics of fast physiological or acoustic events that could not be studied before. For example, HFR imaging allows better evaluation of blood flow (Udesen et al. 2008; Lenge et al. 2014), tissue motion (Joos et al. 2018; Orlowska et al. 2020) and shear wave propagation (Montaldo et al. 2009; Santos et al. 2019) in the body. Moreover, the thousands of frames per second that are available can be exploited to create new imaging modes such as tissue elastography (Montaldo et al. 2009), super-resolution tracking of microbubble displacements in the microvasculature (Errico et al. 2015; Harput et al. 2020) and functional ultrasound imaging reflecting hemodynamic changes due to neuronal activity (Mace et al. 2013).

2.2.2.1. *Parallel beamforming*

Unlike the classic imaging schemes, in which the image is formed line by line, parallel beamforming simultaneously reconstructs multiple lines after each TX event. For this reason, it is also referred to as multiline acquisition (MLA). Following the emission of a transmission pulse, the echo signals received by N elements of the transducer array are simultaneously processed with different sets of relative phase delays and apodization weights. The processing of the data is thus the same as if many beamformers operate in "parallel" on the same data to produce different scan lines.

In ultrasound imaging, the parallel beamforming technique was first introduced by Shattuck et al. (1984) who proposed the Explososcan processing scheme to reconstruct four receive lines per transmission event. The method was initially conceived to improve the image SNR by averaging independent frames. It could also be applied either to limit the patient's exposure to ultrasound radiation by reducing the transmit PRF or to increase the field of view. Mildly focused beams were transmitted and, on reception, four different sets of dynamic delay lines were used for each channel. The system was implemented using analog electronics, which makes the Explososcan an even more exceptional technological feat! Although programmable digital devices are available today, parallel beamforming is still technically challenging because it requires the management of input and output data rates on the order of Giga samples per second.

2.2.2.2. *De-focused beams*

As proposed for the Explososcan, a natural way to reduce the number of TX events is to use wide TX beams that cover a set of imaging lines. The same concept can be extended until the beam is as wide as the whole region of interest. This can be achieved by the transmission of either plane (Montaldo et al. 2009) or diverging waves (Hasegawa and Kanai 2011).

As shown in Figure 2.8(a), a limited number of elements (active aperture) can be used to produce a diverging wave similar to the (spherical) wave generated by a virtual source and gated by the active aperture. The position and size of the active aperture determine the steering angle (θ_{TX}), and the aperture angle (2ϕ). Specifically, considering a virtual source located at coordinates (x_s, z_s) behind the array, the position, x_i, of the i-th active element should be selected in the following range:

$$x_s - z_s\left(\theta_{TX} - \frac{2\phi}{2}\right) < x_i < \left(\theta_{TX} + \frac{2\phi}{2}\right) \quad [2.1]$$

The transmission delay to be applied to the i-th element of the aperture can be calculated as follows:

$$d_i = \frac{\sqrt{(x_i - x_s)^2 + (z_s)^2} - \sqrt{(x_s)^2 + (z_s)^2}}{c} \quad [2.2]$$

where c is the sound propagation speed. The same equations can be applied to plane waves, which, as mentioned above, are a particular case of diverging waves when z_s is very far from the array.

Even though diverging and plane waves can cover the whole region of interest with a single transmission event, thus achieving a frame rate equal to the PRF, a compounded frame given by the superposition of raw images obtained after the transmission of waves with different steering angles is frequently preferred (Berson et al. 1981; Montaldo et al. 2009; Hasegawa and Kanai 2011). Compounding allows a better image quality in terms of contrast, SNR and lateral spatial resolution, at the expense of the frame rate. Several compounding schemes have been proposed to set the virtual source positions, steering angles and aperture angles; still, there is no clear-cut reference method to define these parameters. Indeed, the effectiveness of compounding is the result of trade-offs, which are heavily application-dependent.

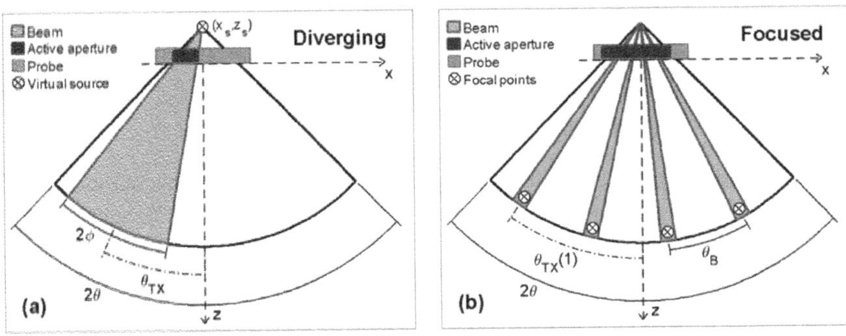

Figure 2.8. *Characteristic parameters of diverging (a) and focused wave (b) transmissions*

2.2.2.3. *Multiline focused beams*

As opposed to the previous strategies, the so-called multiline transmission (MLT) technique reduces the number of transmission events by simultaneously focusing a number, $nMLT$, of beams along different directions (Tong et al. 2013) so that they are spatially distributed over the region of interest, as shown in Figure 2.8(b). By exploiting the superposition principle, for a certain array element, the excitation pulse is obtained by the sum of the pulses which should be applied to the same element to generate, one by one, the desired beams. If each beam is suitably wide, more lines (e.g. $nMLA$) can be beamformed in parallel. The number of TX events required to reconstruct a whole frame, composed of nL lines, is therefore $nTX = \frac{nL}{nMLT \cdot nMLA}$.

As shown in the example of Figure 2.8(b), the MLT focusing directions can be computed as follows:

$$\theta_{TX}(i,j) = -\frac{2\theta}{2} + \frac{(nMLA-1)}{2} \cdot \theta_L + (i-1) \cdot \theta_B + (j-1) \cdot \theta_S \qquad [2.3]$$

where $i \in [1, nMLT]$ is the index of the simultaneous MLT beams and $j \in [1, nTX]$ is the index of the TX event, while $\theta_L = \frac{2\theta}{(nL-1)}$ is the step angle between image lines, $\theta_B = nTX \cdot nMLA \cdot \theta_L$ is the step angle between simultaneously transmitted beams and $\theta_S = nMLA \cdot \theta_L$ is the step angle between consecutive transmissions. Accordingly, the directions of the reconstructed lines are:

$$\theta_{RX}(i,j,k) = \theta_{TX}(i,j) + \left(k - 1 - \frac{(nMLA-1)}{2}\right)\theta_L \qquad [2.4]$$

where $k \in [1, nMLA]$ is the integer index of the MLA lines.

Although this technique has mainly been used in phased array cardiac imaging, it can also be applied to linear scan imaging (Demi et al. 2015). In this case, angular values in [2.3] and [2.4] can be changed to linear steps and dimensions.

2.2.2.4. *Limited diffraction beams*

Diffraction-free beams or non-diffracting beams (Durnin 1987; Durnin et al. 1987) are exact solutions of the scalar wave equation. In theory, they are propagation invariant and maintain their lateral profile, provided that they are generated by infinite apertures and with infinite bandwidths. In practice, since actual apertures and bandwidths are limited, they can only be approximated and, therefore, are referred to as *limited* diffraction beams (Lu 1997a).

The papers by Lu (1997b) and Cheng and Lu (2006) presented the so-called Fourier imaging method, showing that limited diffraction beams can be exploited, in both transmission and reception, to reconstruct the Fourier space of the region of interest. The final B-mode image is, in this case, computed through the inverse spatial transform. The production of limited diffraction beams requires amplitude weighting coefficients but no time or phase delays. Hence, their use could reduce the system's complexity. However, since current scanners still rely on the classic architecture based on a delay-and-sum beamformer, limited diffraction beam, Fourier imaging methods (Lu et al. 2006) are not yet widespread.

Although current clinical care is still mainly based on 2D ultrasound imaging, 3D ultrasound has recently experienced substantial growth. Three-dimensional imaging allows the evaluation of the morphology of the region of interest through the visualization of arbitrary scan planes or rendered volumes. It is widely used in abdominal applications for the examination of fetal development, colon and rectum diseases, prostate tumors and to examine breast lesions. Three-dimensional ultrasound provides several important advantages compared to 2D imaging (Fenster et al. 2001; Huang and Zeng 2017; Mozaffari and Lee 2017) such as:

– The volumetric morphological view facilitates optimal probe placement and rapid identification of the regions of interest. This makes the analysis less operator- and orientation-dependent.

– Quantitative parameters, such as dimensions or volumes, can be accurately estimated without the assumptions about structure geometry needed when the analysis is based on 2D images.

– Images acquired under different circumstances (time, patient's physical condition, operator, etc.) can be more reliably co-registered. This increases the capacity to monitor and follow up the progression of therapy or disease.

So far, 3D ultrasound imaging has mostly been performed using special probes that allow the reconstruction of a 3D volume through the acquisition of multiple 2D images. Those probes are often equipped with a stepper motor, which tilts, rotates or translates a 1D array (Helge Gilja et al. 1994; Smith and Fenster 2000; Iula et al. 2013; Huang et al. 2015). Depending on the motion, either linear, angular or rotational scanning can be performed, and consequently, the volume takes different shapes, for example, parallelepipedal, conical or pyramidal. However, the use of motors embedded in the probe, together with the moving array, makes the probes bulky, complex and expensive. An alternative is represented by 1D array probes adapted for 3D freehand scanning. In this case, a standard 1D probe is equipped with either acoustic, optical, magnetic or mechanical positioners that allow for the registration of the direction and the relative position of the main axis of the array relative to each acquired image (Barry et al. 1997; Gilja et al. 1998; Huang et al. 2013; Cenni et al. 2016; Matrone et al. 2017). The region of interest is manually scanned by the operator, who can choose the best views and adapt the scanning motion to the contours of the body's surface. Even though the design of freehand scanning probes is easier than that of mechanically scanned systems, the volume reconstruction process is complex and relatively inaccurate.

For all the above-mentioned scanning strategies, the achievable volumetric scanning rate is quite low (of the order of one volume per second). The growing interest in 3D ultrasound imaging has motivated the development of 2D matrix probes (see section 2.1.2), which can provide higher volumetric scanning rates by enabling electronic beam steering in both elevation and azimuthal directions. However, even with electronic steering, the conventional acquisition schemes based on line-by-line scanning do not provide the spatio-temporal resolution required for reproducible quantitative measurements of dynamic physiological events. Some manufacturers have introduced real-time, multi-plane modes (mainly bi- and tri-plane imaging) to provide an intermediate solution between 2D and full volumetric 3D imaging (Sugeng et al. 2003; Eroglu et al. 2006). Indeed, acquiring multiple planes of interest, rather than the whole volume, reduces the acquisition time, thus improving time resolution. On the other hand, as compared to full 3D imaging, multi-plane modes limit the field of view and do not allow full volumetric morphological views.

In recent studies mainly based on research scanners (Boni et al. 2018), HFR techniques have been applied to 3D imaging. As described in section 2.2.2, techniques based on plane/diverging waves or multiline transmissions have been extended to 3D and have shown great potential to obtain high temporal resolution and fully volumetric capabilities (Provost et al. 2014; Holbek et al. 2016; Ortega et al. 2016; Santos et al. 2016; Petrusca et al. 2018; Wigen et al. 2018; Rossi et al. 2020; Harput et al. 2020).

2.2.4. *Image quality enhancement by beamforming techniques*

Compared to other imaging modalities such as magnetic resonance or computed tomography, the quality of ultrasound images is typically poorer in terms of spatial resolution, SNR, contrast and level of artifacts. In the literature, several methods have been proposed to increase the visibility of anatomical structures, ease image interpretation and facilitate clinical parameter extraction for an increasingly effective diagnostic process. Here, we briefly review the methods for image quality enhancement based on the modification of the reception beamforming strategy.

The classic DAS beamforming is based only on geometrical assumptions, without considering the full information included in the received echo signals, i.e. it is said to be data-independent. Various beamforming algorithms have been proposed to enhance the information coming from the direction of interest and to attenuate, as much as possible, the contributions due to off-axis interferences, for example, generated by noise and side lobes. Data-adaptive beamformers aim at adapting the apodization weights to the echo signals. Minimum variance beamformers (Synnevag et al. 2007, 2009) find an optimal set of weights by minimizing the variance of the beamformed signal, which is linked to the presence of noise in the signal itself. Non-linear beamformers (Matrone et al. 2015; Polichetti et al. 2018) adopt inter-element multiplications and n-th root extraction to artificially generate higher harmonic components and thus improve resolution and clutter rejection. Alternatively, the so-called coherence-based beamforming methods (Mallart and Fink 1994; Li and Li 2003; Camacho et al. 2009) apodize the echo signals according to their spatial coherence. Finally, the short-lag spatial coherence imaging (Lediju et al. 2011) directly generates an image of the spatial coherence of backscattered echoes evaluated at short lags.

Of course, advanced beamforming algorithms increase the computational complexity, which is difficult to address with the currently available system architectures. This limitation is even more important for HFR techniques characterized by increased data rates. Deep learning beamforming approaches have recently been proposed (Bell et al. 2020; Sloun et al. 2020) to simultaneously improve the image quality and reduce the computational burden of HFR imaging.

2.3. Advanced imaging systems

2.3.1. *Advanced architectures and research platforms*

The basic architecture described in section 2.2.1, which is used in most commercial ultrasound instruments, is not able to support the above-mentioned advanced imaging schemes. Whenever these modalities need to be implemented or tested, a different class of ultrasound equipment has to be used. This class includes two categories of scanners: 1) the so-called high-end scanners, purposely designed to implement specific advanced imaging modalities; 2) the scanners designed to provide very high flexibility for programming any novel imaging scheme. The former ones usually embed custom-designed application-specific integrated circuits (ASICs) capable of performing demanding processing tasks in real time. For example, as mentioned in section 2.1.2.3, in commercial 3D systems, thousands of echo signals are received by the active elements of a 2D probe. Such signals are partially beamformed inside the probe itself by an ASIC, which makes the number of signals compatible with the dimensions of a standard probe cable. On the contrary, advanced programmable systems, which are widely used within ultrasound laboratories, are usually referred to as research platforms or open scanners

(Boni et al. 2018). An example of images and data from such a scanner are presented in Figure 2.9. The following sections highlight the main features of such systems.

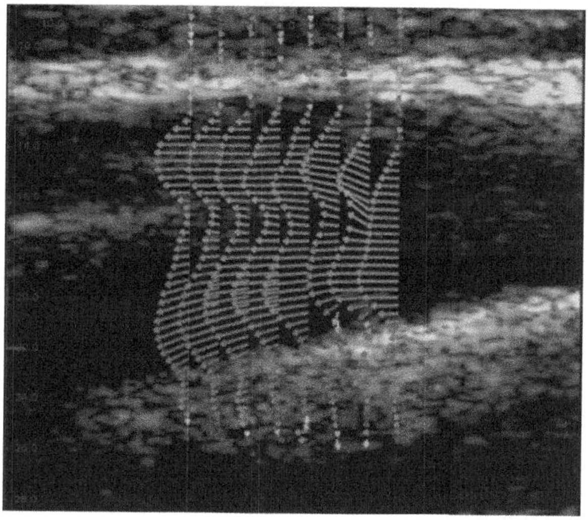

Figure 2.9. *Real-time multi-line vector Doppler imaging of the carotid artery bifurcation. During systole, non-symmetric profiles are visible both in the bulb (right-most Doppler line) and in the internal and external carotid branches (left-most Doppler lines)*

2.3.1.1. *Transmit architecture*

The most relevant requirement in advanced imaging schemes is the full flexibility in the transmit chain. Delay flexibility, element-by-element customized TX patterns and a cycle-by-cycle switching strategy can all be accomplished by the back-end software. This software pre-calculates all patterns, which must be stored in the memory of the TX beamforming circuits. The amount of memory typically available inside a mid-range FPGA (1–10 MB) is not sufficient to store all required details, so an additional external memory (usually a high-capacity double data rate: DDR memory) must be added to the FPGA beamformer.

The transmission circuits can include either linear amplifiers or square wave pulsers. Linear amplifiers provide maximum flexibility for waveform generation (Boni et al. 2016) and can produce arbitrary waveforms such as those used in coded imaging methods (Chiao and Hao 2005; Ramalli et al. 2016). The drawbacks of linear amplifiers are the high power consumption and reduced scalability of high-voltage/high-power/wide-bandwidth integrated circuits. This, in turn, limits the number of active linear transmitters that can be embedded in a system. Square wave signals, on the contrary, can be produced by complementary metal-oxide-semiconductor (CMOS) high-voltage switches commutated to high-voltage rails. The use of switches rather than linear output stages allows for reduction of the dissipated heat and the integration in chips driving up to 16 channels each (see, for example, STHV1600, STMicroelectronics SRL). This high integration, however, comes at the expense of flexibility, either for the waveform or for the ability to generate arbitrary sequences of pulses.

2.3.1.2. *Receive architecture*

The number of receive signals that can be addressed simultaneously is limited by the need to have a low noise preamplifier (LNA), a TGC stage and an analog-to-digital converter (ADC), for each channel (see Figure 2.7). With few exceptions (Jensen et al. 2013), in most systems, the number of active channels is limited to 256 (Smith et al. 2012; Boni et al. 2016).

Research platforms are frequently used for the experimental evaluation of innovative processing algorithms. In this case, it is convenient to preliminarily implement an offline version of the new algorithm, working on the raw channel data that are stored in the front-end memory. Let us consider a 256 channel system, based on ADCs sampling at 50 MHz, with 12-bit resolution (1.5 Byte per sample). In this example, the overall data rate will be:

$$D = 1.5 \times 50 \times 10^6 \times 256 = 19.2\ GB/s \qquad [2.5]$$

Even though the entire pulse repetition interval (PRI) is not dedicated to data acquisition, the embedded DDR memory must sustain such a peak data rate and have a capacity consistent with the acquisition of raw data over long intervals. The fast download of acquired data can be done by the controlling interface of the instrument, through either USB 3.0 or gigabit Ethernet connection, the former being more efficient (300 MB/s vs. 80 MB/s).

Some research platforms have an architecture suitable for real-time data processing. In this case, they typically contain several devices such as FPGAs, digital signal processors (DSPs) and/or embedded graphic processing units (GPUs) (Yiu et al. 2011; Jensen et al. 2013; Boni et al. 2016). One of the most demanding real-time processing tasks is parallel beamforming (see section 2.2.2.1). Although many beamforming units can be instantiated to work independently, the overall number is limited by the system hardware complexity. Furthermore, parallel beamforming considerably stresses the data rate bandwidth. Advanced research systems need to be designed with high-capacity interconnections such as Serial Rapid IO (SRIO) and PCI-Express.

2.3.1.3. *Conclusion*

Ultrasound research has made amazing strides in the last two decades due to several concurring factors. Firstly, the quality of transducer arrays has considerably improved. New technologies like CMUT and PMUT have been established, and 2D arrays have finally become mature for clinical use. Outstanding new approaches like HFR imaging have been proposed, and their utility has been demonstrated in new applications such as shear wave elastography and super-resolution imaging. HFR breakthroughs have been made possible by the introduction of research platforms that have enabled any research laboratory to experimentally test, mainly offline, their new methods. Finally, the availability of powerful parallel processing engines from FPGA and GPU technologies has enabled the real-time implementation of computationally intensive methods that would have been impossible a few years ago.

2.4. References

Barry, C.D., Allott, C.P., John, N.W., Mellor, P.M., Arundel, P.A., Thomson, D.S., Waterton, J.C. (1997). Three-dimensional freehand ultrasound: Image reconstruction and volume analysis. *Ultrasound in Medicine & Biology*, 23, 1209–1224. https://doi.org/10.1016/S0301-5629(97)00123-3.

Bell, M.A.L., Huang, J., Hyun, D., Eldar, Y.C., van Sloun, R., Mischi, M. (2020). Challenge on ultrasound beamforming with deep learning (CUBDL). In *2020 IEEE International Ultrasonics Symposium (IUS)*, 1–5. https://doi.org/10.1109/IUS46767.2020.9251434.

Berson, M., Roncin, A., Pourcelot, L. (1981). Compound scanning with an electrically steered beam. *Ultrasonic Imaging*, 3, 303–308. https://doi.org/10.1016/0161-7346(81)90162-0.

Bonacina, L., Froio, A., Conti, D., Marcolin, F., Vezzetti, E. (2016). Automatic 3D foetal face model extraction from ultrasonography through histogram processing. *Journal of Medical Ultrasound*, 24(4), 142–149. https://doi.org/10.1016/j.jmu.2016.08.003.

Boni, E., Bassi, L., Dallai, A., Guidi, F., Meacci, V., Ramalli, A., Ricci, S., Tortoli, P. (2016). ULA-OP 256: A 256-channel open scanner for development and real-time implementation of new ultrasound methods. *IEEE Transactions on Ultrasonics, Ferroelectrics, and Frequency Control*, 63, 1488–1495. https://doi.org/10.1109/TUFFC.2016.2566920.

Boni, E., Yu, A.C.H., Freear, S., Jensen, J.A., Tortoli, P. (2018). Ultrasound open platforms for next-generation imaging technique development. *IEEE Transactions on Ultrasonics, Ferroelectrics, and Frequency Control*, 65, 1078–1092. https://doi.org/10.1109/TUFFC.2018.2844560.

Butterworth, S. (1914). On a null method of testing vibration galvanometers. *Proceedings of the Physical Society of London*, 26, 264–273.

Camacho, J., Parrilla, M., Fritsch, C. (2009). Phase coherence imaging. *IEEE Transactions on Ultrasonics, Ferroelectrics, and Frequency Control*, 56, 958–974. https://doi.org/10.1109/TUFFC.2009.1128.

Cenni, F., Monari, D., Desloovere, K., Aertbeliën, E., Schless, S.-H., Bruyninckx, H. (2016). The reliability and validity of a clinical 3D freehand ultrasound system. *Computer Methods and Programs in Biomedicine*, 136, 179–187. https://doi.org/10.1016/j.cmpb.2016.09.001.

Chen, C. and Pertijs, M.A.P. (2021). Integrated transceivers for emerging medical ultrasound imaging devices: A review. *IEEE Open Journal of the Solid-State Circuits Society*, 1, 104–114. https://doi.org/10.1109/OJSSCS.2021.3115398.

Cheng, J. and Lu, J.-Y. (2006). Extended high-frame rate imaging method with limited-diffraction beams. *IEEE Transactions on Ultrasonics, Ferroelectrics and Frequency Control*, 53, 880–899. https://doi.org/10.1109/TUFFC.2006.1632680.

Chiao, R.Y. and Hao, X. (2005). Coded excitation for diagnostic ultrasound: A system developer's perspective. *IEEE Transactions on Ultrasonics, Ferroelectrics, and Frequency Control*, 52, 160–170. https://doi.org/10.1109/TUFFC.2005.1406543.

Christiansen, T.L., Dahl-Petersen, C., Jensen, J.A., Thomsen, E.V. (2013). 2-D row-column CMUT arrays with an open-grid support structure. In *2013 IEEE International Ultrasonics Symposium (IUS)*, 1712–1715. https://doi.org/10.1109/ULTSYM.2013.0436.

Demi, L., Ramalli, A., Giannini, G., Mischi, M. (2015). In Vitro and in Vivo tissue harmonic images obtained with parallel transmit beamforming by means of orthogonal frequency division multiplexing. *IEEE Transactions on Ultrasonics, Ferroelectrics, and Frequency Control*, 62, 230–235. https://doi.org/10.1109/TUFFC.2014.006599.

Durnin, J. (1987). Exact solutions for nondiffracting beams I. The scalar theory. *Journal of the Optical Society of America A*, 4, 651. https://doi.org/10.1364/JOSAA.4.000651.

Durnin, J., Miceli, J.J., Eberly, J.H. (1987). Diffraction-free beams. *Physical Review Letters*, 58, 1499–1501. https://doi.org/10.1103/PhysRevLett.58.1499.

Eroglu, E., D'hooge, J., Herbots, L., Thijs, D., Dubois, C., Sinnaeve, P., Dens, J., Vanhaecke, J., Rademakers, F. (2006). Comparison of real-time tri-plane and conventional 2D dobutamine stress echocardiography for the assessment of coronary artery disease. *European Heart Journal*, 27, 1719–1724. https://doi.org/10.1093/eurheartj/ehl023.

Errico, C., Pierre, J., Pezet, S., Desailly, Y., Lenkei, Z., Couture, O., Tanter, M. (2015). Ultrafast ultrasound localization microscopy for deep super-resolution vascular imaging. *Nature*, 527, 499–502. https://doi.org/10.1038/nature16066.

Fenster, A., Downey, D.B., Cardinal, H.N. (2001). Three-dimensional ultrasound imaging. *Physics in Medicine and Biology*, 46, R67. https://doi.org/10.1088/0031-9155/46/5/201.

Gilja, O.H., Hausken, T., Olafsson, S., Matre, K., Ødegaard, S. (1998). In vitro evaluation of three-dimensional ultrasonography based on magnetic scanhead tracking. *Ultrasound in Medicine & Biology*, 24, 1161–1167. https://doi.org/10.1016/S0301-5629(98)00098-2.

Harput, S., Christensen-Jeffries, K., Ramalli, A., Brown, J., Zhu, J., Zhang, G., Leow, C.H., Toulemonde, M., Boni, E., Tortoli, P. et al. (2020). 3-D super-resolution ultrasound imaging with a 2-D sparse array. *IEEE Transactions on Ultrasonics, Ferroelectrics, and Frequency Control*, 67, 269–277. https://doi.org/10.1109/TUFFC.2019.2943646.

Hasegawa, H. and Kanai, H. (2011). High-frame-rate echocardiography using diverging transmit beams and parallel receive beamforming. *Journal of Medical Ultrasonics*, 38, 129–140. https://doi.org/10.1007/s10396-011-0304-0.

Helge Gilja, O., Thune, N., Matre, K., Hausken, T., Ødegaard, S., Berstad, A. (1994). In vitro evaluation of three-dimensional ultrasonography in volume estimation of abdominal organs. *Ultrasound in Medicine & Biology*, 20, 157–165. https://doi.org/10.1016/0301-5629(94)90080-9.

Holbek, S., Christiansen, T.L., Stuart, M.B., Beers, C., Thomsen, E.V., Jensen, J.A. (2016). 3-D vector flow estimation with row–column-addressed arrays. *IEEE Transactions on Ultrasonics, Ferroelectrics, and Frequency Control*, 63, 1799–1814. https://doi.org/10.1109/TUFFC.2016.2582536.

Huang, Q. and Zeng, Z. (2017). A review on real-time 3D ultrasound imaging technology. *BioMed Research International*, 6027029. https://doi.org/10.1155/2017/6027029.

Huang, Q., Yang, Z., Hu, W., Jin, L., Wei, G., Li, X. (2013). Linear tracking for 3-D medical ultrasound imaging. *IEEE Transactions on Cybernetics*, 43, 1747–1754. https://doi.org/10.1109/TSMCC.2012.2229270.

Huang, Q., Xie, B., Ye, P., Chen, Z. (2015). Correspondence – 3-D ultrasonic strain imaging based on a linear scanning system. *IEEE Transactions on Ultrasonics, Ferroelectrics, and Frequency Control*, 62, 392–400. https://doi.org/10.1109/TUFFC.2014.006665.

Iula, A., Hine, G.E., Ramalli, A., Guidi, F., Boni, E., Savoia, A.S., Caliano, G. (2013). An enhanced ultrasound technique for 3D palmprint recognition. In *Ultrasonics Symposium (IUS), 2013 IEEE International*, 978–981. https://doi.org/10.1109/ULTSYM.2013.0251.

Jensen, J.A., Holten-Lund, H., Nilsson, R.T., Hansen, M., Larsen, U.D., Domsten, R.P., Tomov, B.G., Stuart, M.B., Nikolov, S.I., Pihl, M.J. et al. (2013). SARUS: A synthetic aperture real-time ultrasound system. *IEEE Transactions on Ultrasonics, Ferroelectrics, and Frequency Control*, 60, 1838–1852. https://doi.org/10.1109/TUFFC.2013.2770.

Joos, P., Porée, J., Liebgott, H., Vray, D., Baudet, M., Faurie, J., Tournoux, F., Cloutier, G., Nicolas, B., Garcia, D. (2018). High-frame-rate speckle-tracking echocardiography. *IEEE Transactions on Ultrasonics, Ferroelectrics, and Frequency Control*, 65, 720–728. https://doi.org/10.1109/TUFFC.2018.2809553.

Khuri-Yakub, B.T. and Oralkan, Ö. (2011). Capacitive micromachined ultrasonic transducers for medical imaging and therapy. *Journal of Micromechanics and Microengineering*, 21, 054004. https://doi.org/10.1088/0960-1317/21/5/054004.

Krimholtz, R., Leedom, D.A., Matthaei, G.L. (1970). New equivalent circuits for elementary piezoelectric transducers. *Electronics Letters*, 6(13), 398–399. https://doi.org/: 10.1049/el:19700280.

Lediju, M.A., Trahey, G.E., Byram, B.C., Dahl, J.J. (2011). Short-lag spatial coherence of backscattered echoes: Imaging characteristics. *IEEE Transactions on Ultrasonics, Ferroelectrics, and Frequency Control*, 58, 1377–1388. https://doi.org/10.1109/TUFFC.2011.1957.

Lenge, M., Ramalli, A., Boni, E., Liebgott, H., Cachard, C., Tortoli, P. (2014). High-frame-rate 2-D vector blood flow imaging in the frequency domain. *IEEE Transactions on Ultrasonics, Ferroelectrics, and Frequency Control*, 61, 1504–1514. https://doi.org/10.1109/TUFFC.2014.3064.

Li, P.-C. and Li, M.-L. (2003). Adaptive imaging using the generalized coherence factor. *IEEE Transactions on Ultrasonics, Ferroelectrics, and Frequency Control*, 50, 128–141. https://doi.org/10.1109/TUFFC.2003.1182117.

Logan, A.S., Wong, L.L.P., Chen, A.I.H., Yeow, J.T.W. (2011). A 32 x 32 element row-column addressed capacitive micromachined ultrasonic transducer. *IEEE Transactions on Ultrasonics, Ferroelectrics, and Frequency Control*, 58, 1266–1271. https://doi.org/10.1109/TUFFC.2011.1937.

Lu, J.-Y. (1997a). Designing limited diffraction beams. *IEEE Transactions on Ultrasonics, Ferroelectrics, and Frequency Control*, 44, 181–193. https://doi.org/10.1109/58.585215.

Lu, J.-Y. (1997b). 2D and 3D high frame rate imaging with limited diffraction beams. *IEEE Transactions on Ultrasonics, Ferroelectrics and Frequency Control*, 44, 839–856. https://doi.org/10.1109/58.655200.

Lu, J.-Y., Cheng, J., Wang, J. (2006). High frame rate imaging system for limited diffraction array beam imaging with square-wave aperture weightings. *IEEE Transactions on Ultrasonics, Ferroelectrics and Frequency Control*, 53, 1796–1812. https://doi.org/10.1109/TUFFC.2006.112.

Mace, E., Montaldo, G., Osmanski, B.F., Cohen, I., Fink, M., Tanter, M. (2013). Functional ultrasound imaging of the brain: Theory and basic principles. *IEEE Transactions on Ultrasonics, Ferroelectrics, and Frequency Control*, 60, 492–506. https://doi.org/10.1109/TUFFC.2013.2592.

Mallart, R. and Fink, M. (1994). Adaptive focusing in scattering media through sound–speed inhomogeneities: The van Cittert Zernike approach and focusing criterion. *The Journal of the Acoustical Society of America*, 96, 3721–3732. https://doi.org/10.1121/1.410562.

Matrone, G., Savoia, A.S., Caliano, G., Magenes, G. (2015). The delay multiply and sum beamforming algorithm in ultrasound B-mode medical imaging. *IEEE Transactions on Medical Imaging*, 34, 940–949. https://doi.org/10.1109/TMI.2014.2371235.

Matrone, G., Ramalli, A., Savoia, A.S., Quaglia, F., Castellazzi, G., Morbini, P., Piastra, M. (2017). An experimental protocol for assessing the performance of new ultrasound probes based on CMUT technology in application to brain imaging. *Journal of Visualized Experiments*, 127, e55798. https://doi.org/10.3791/55798.

Mazierli, D., Ramalli, A., Boni, E., Guidi, F., Tortoli, P. (2021). Architecture for an ultrasound advanced open platform with an arbitrary number of independent channels. *IEEE Transactions on Biomedical Circuits and Systems*, 15(3), 486–496. https://doi.org/10.1109/TBCAS.2021.3077664.

Montaldo, G., Tanter, M., Bercoff, J., Benech, N., Fink, M. (2009). Coherent plane-wave compounding for very high frame rate ultrasonography and transient elastography. *IEEE Transactions on Ultrasonics, Ferroelectrics and Frequency Control*, 56, 489–506. https://doi.org/10.1109/TUFFC.2009.1067.

Morton, C.E. and Lockwood, G.R. (2003). Theoretical assessment of a crossed electrode 2-D array for 3-D imaging. In *IEEE Symposium on Ultrasonics, 2003*, 1, 968–971. https://doi.org/10.1109/ULTSYM.2003.1293560.

Mozaffari, M.H. and Lee, W.-S. (2017). Freehand 3-D ultrasound imaging: A systematic review. *Ultrasound in Medicine and Biology*, 43, 2099–2124. https://doi.org/10.1016/j.ultrasmedbio.2017.06.009.

Orlowska, M., Ramalli, A., Petrescu, A., Cvijic, M., Bézy, S., Santos, P., Pedrosa, J., Voigt, J.-U., D'hooge, J. (2020). A novel 2-D speckle tracking method for high-frame-rate echocardiography. *IEEE Transactions on Ultrasonics, Ferroelectrics, and Frequency Control*, 67, 1764–1775. https://doi.org/10.1109/TUFFC.2020.2985451.

Ortega, A., Provost, J., Tong, L., Santos, P., Heyde, B., Pernot, M., D'hooge, J. (2016). A comparison of the performance of different multiline transmit setups for fast volumetric cardiac ultrasound. *IEEE Transactions on Ultrasonics, Ferroelectrics, and Frequency Control*, 63, 2082–2091. https://doi.org/10.1109/TUFFC.2016.2614652.

Pappalardo, M., Caliano, G., Savoia, A.S., Caronti, A. (2008). Micromachined ultrasonic transducers. In *Piezoelectric and Acoustic Materials for Transducer Applications*, Safari, A. and Akdoğan, E.K. (eds). Springer US, Boston. https://doi.org/10.1007/978-0-387-76540-2_22.

Petrusca, L., Varray, F., Souchon, R., Bernard, A., Chapelon, J.-Y., Liebgott, H., N'Djin, W.A., Viallon, M. (2018). Fast volumetric ultrasound B-mode and Doppler imaging with a new high-channels density platform for advanced 4D cardiac imaging/therapy. *Applied Sciences*, 8, 200. https://doi.org/10.3390/app8020200.

Polichetti, M., Varray, F., Béra, J.-C., Cachard, C., Nicolas, B. (2018). A nonlinear beamformer based on p-th root compression–application to plane wave ultrasound imaging. *Applied Sciences*, 8, 599. https://doi.org/10.3390/app8040599.

Provost, J., Papadacci, C., Arango, J.E., Imbault, M., Fink, M., Gennisson, J.-L., Tanter, M., Pernot, M. (2014). 3D ultrafast ultrasound imaging in vivo. *Physics in Medicine and Biology*, 59, L1–L13. https://doi.org/10.1088/0031-9155/59/19/L1.

Qiu, Y., Gigliotti, J.V., Wallace, M., Griggio, F., Demore, C.E.M., Cochran, S., Trolier-McKinstry, S. (2015). Piezoelectric micromachined ultrasound transducer (PMUT) arrays for integrated sensing, actuation and imaging. *Sensors*, 15, 8020–8041. https://doi.org/10.3390/s150408020.

Ramalli, A., Boni, E., Savoia, A.S., Tortoli, P. (2015). Density-tapered spiral arrays for ultrasound 3-D imaging. *IEEE Transactions on Ultrasonics, Ferroelectrics, and Frequency Control*, 62, 1580–1588. https://doi.org/10.1109/TUFFC.2015.007035.

Ramalli, A., Boni, E., Dallai, A., Guidi, F., Ricci, S., Tortoli, P. (2016). Coded spectral Doppler imaging: From simulation to real-time processing. *IEEE Transactions on Ultrasonics, Ferroelectrics, and Frequency Control*, 63, 1815–1824. https://doi.org/10.1109/TUFFC.2016.2573720.

Rossi, S., Ramalli, A., Fool, F., Tortoli, P. (2020). High-frame-rate 3-D vector flow imaging in the frequency domain. *Applied Sciences*, 10, 5365. https://doi.org/10.3390/app10155365.

Roux, E., Ramalli, A., Liebgott, H., Cachard, C., Robini, M.C., Tortoli, P. (2017). Wideband 2-D array design optimization with fabrication constraints for 3-D US imaging. *IEEE Transactions on Ultrasonics, Ferroelectrics, and Frequency Control*, 64, 108–125. https://doi.org/10.1109/TUFFC.2016.2614776.

Santos, P., Haugen, G.U., Lovstakken, L., Samset, E., D'hooge, J. (2016). Diverging wave volumetric imaging using subaperture beamforming. *IEEE Transactions on Ultrasonics, Ferroelectrics, and Frequency Control*, 63, 2114–2124. https://doi.org/10.1109/TUFFC.2016.2616172.

Santos, P., Petrescu, A., Pedrosa, J., Orlowska, M., Komini, V., Voigt, J., D'hooge, J. (2019). Natural shear wave imaging in the human heart: Normal values, feasibility and reproducibility. *IEEE Transactions on Ultrasonics, Ferroelectrics, and Frequency Control*, 66, 442–452. https://doi.org/10.1109/TUFFC.2018.2881493.

Savoia, A.S., Bavaro, V., Caliano, G., Caronti, A., Carotenuto, R., Gatta, P., Longo, C., Pappalardo, M. (2007). Crisscross 2D cMUT array: Beamforming strategy and synthetic 3D imaging results. In *2007 IEEE Ultrasonics Symposium Proceedings*, 1514–1517. https://doi.org/10.1109/ULTSYM.2007.381.

Savoia, A.S., Caliano, G., Pappalardo, M. (2012). A CMUT probe for medical ultrasonography: From microfabrication to system integration. In *IEEE Transactions on Ultrasonics, Ferroelectrics, and Frequency Control*, 59, 1127–1138. https://doi.org/10.1109/TUFFC.2012.2303.

Savoia, A.S., Mauti, B., Fanni, L., Caliano, G., Boni, E., Mattesini, P., Scaringella, M., Tortoli, P. (2018). A 120+ 120- element crisscross CMUT probe's with real-time switchable electronic and Fresnel focusing capabilities. *2018 IEEE International Ultrasonics Symposium (IUS)*, 1–4. https://doi.org/10.1109/ULTSYM.2018.8580084.

Savoia, A.S., Casavola, M., Boni, E., Ferrera, M., Prelini, C., Tortoli, P., Giusti, D., Quaglia, F. (2021). Design, fabrication, characterization, and system integration of a 1-D PMUT array for medical ultrasound imaging. In *2021 IEEE International Ultrasonics Symposium (IUS)*, 1–3. https://doi.org/10.1109/IUS52206.2021.9593751.

Shattuck, D.P., Weinshenker, M.D., Smith, S.W., von Ramm, O.T. (1984). Explososcan: A parallel processing technique for high speed ultrasound imaging with linear phased arrays. *The Journal of the Acoustical Society of America*, 75, 1273–1282. https://doi.org/10.1121/1.390734.

von Sloun, R.J.G., Cohen, R., Eldar, Y.C. (2020). Deep learning in ultrasound imaging. *Proceedings of the IEEE*, 108, 11–29. https://doi.org/10.1109/JPROC.2019.2932116.

Smith, W.L. and Fenster, A. (2000). Optimum scan spacing for three-dimensional ultrasound by speckle statistics. *Ultrasound in Medicine & Biology*, 26, 551–562. https://doi.org/10.1016/S0301-5629(99)00162-3.

Smith, P.R., Cowell, D.M.J., Raiton, B., Ky, C.V., Freear, S. (2012). Ultrasound array transmitter architecture with high timing resolution using embedded phase-locked loops. *IEEE Transactions on Ultrasonics, Ferroelectrics, and Frequency Control*, 59, 40–49. https://doi.org/10.1109/TUFFC.2012.2154.

Sugeng, L., Kirkpatrick, J., Lang, R.M., Bednarz, J.E., DeCara, J.M., Lammertin, G., Spencer, K.T. (2003). Biplane stress echocardiography using a prototype matrix-array transducer. *Journal of the American Society of Echocardiography*, 16, 937–941. https://doi.org/10.1016/S0894-7317(03)00469-3.

Synnevag, J.F., Austeng, A., Holm, S. (2007). Adaptive beamforming applied to medical ultrasound imaging. *IEEE Transactions on Ultrasonics, Ferroelectrics and Frequency Control*, 54, 1606–1613. https://doi.org/10.1109/TUFFC.2007.431.

Synnevag, J.F., Austeng, A., Holm, S. (2009). Benefits of minimum-variance beamforming in medical ultrasound imaging. *IEEE Transactions on Ultrasonics, Ferroelectrics, and Frequency Control*, 56, 1868–1879. https://doi.org/10.1109/TUFFC.2009.1263.

Szabo, T.L. (2004). *Diagnostic Ultrasound Imaging: Inside Out*, 1st edition. Academic Press, Cambridge, MA.

Tanter, M. and Fink, M. (2014). Ultrafast imaging in biomedical ultrasound. *IEEE Transactions on Ultrasonics, Ferroelectrics, and Frequency Control*, 61, 102–119. https://doi.org/10.1109/TUFFC.2014.2882.

Tong, L., Gao, H., D'hooge, J. (2013). Multi-transmit beam forming for fast cardiac imaging – A simulation study. *IEEE Transactions on Ultrasonics, Ferroelectrics, and Frequency Control*, 60, 1719–1731. https://doi.org/10.1109/TUFFC.2013.2753.

Udesen, J., Gran, F., Hansen, K.L., Jensen, J.A., Thomsen, C., Nielsen, M.B. (2008). High frame-rate blood vector velocity imaging using plane waves: Simulations and preliminary experiments. *IEEE Transactions on Ultrasonics, Ferroelectrics, and Frequency Control*, 55, 1729–1743. https://doi.org/10.1109/TUFFC.2008.858.

Van Dyke, K.S. (1925). The electric network equivalent of a piezoelectric resonator. *Physical Review*, 25(6), 895.

Wigen, M.S., Fadnes, S., Rodriguez-Molares, A., Bjåstad, T., Eriksen, M., Stensæth, K.H., Støylen, A., Lovstakken, L. (2018). 4-D intracardiac ultrasound vector flow imaging – Feasibility and comparison to phase-contrast MRI. *IEEE Transactions on Medical Imaging*, 37, 2619–2629. https://doi.org/10.1109/TMI.2018.2844552.

Yiu, B.Y.S., Tsang, I.K.H., Yu, A.C.H. (2011). GPU-based beamformer: Fast realization of plane wave compounding and synthetic aperture imaging. In *IEEE Transactions on Ultrasonics, Ferroelectrics, and Frequency Control*, 58, 1698–1705. https://doi.org/10.1109/TUFFC.2011.1999.

Zemp, R.J., Zheng, W., Zhang, P. (2011). Feasibility of top-orthogonal-to-bottom electrode (TOBE) 2D CMUT arrays for low-channel-count 3D imaging. *2011 IEEE International Ultrasonics Symposium*, 498–502. https://doi.org/10.1109/ULTSYM.2011.0120.

3

Shear Wave Propagation and Probing Tissue Mechanical Properties

Stefan CATHELINE and Bruno GIAMMARINARO
Laboratory of Therapeutic Applications of Ultrasound (LabTAU), INSERM, University of Lyon, France

3.1. Introduction: a historical perspective of palpation

The oldest known written medical procedures, discovered by Eber and Smith, were recorded on papyrus between 1,500 and 1,600 BC. Several passages describe the diagnostic practice of palpation. Placing the "hand on the chest" and the use of "touch" were probably common for the evaluation of temperature, as well as for probing tissue elasticity in the early history of humanity (see Figure 3.1). This concept of palpation using the fingers is very close to the diagnostic principle behind static elastography, an ultrasonic technique developed by Jonathan Ophir in the early 1990s to visualize internal tissue movement during the application of an external force. A second very simple diagnostic test consists of listening (with or without a stethoscope) to sounds produced within the body, such as those due to the heart beat, breathing or coughing. This second approach uses sound waves to probe the inner workings of the body's systems. Both of these methods can be related to modern modalities of elastography that have been integrated into clinical ultrasound imaging devices. Manual palpation senses change based on static stress–strain properties under compression, such as those visualized with ultrasonic elastography. Detection

For a color version of all the figures in this chapter, see www.iste.co.uk/bridal/innovative.zip.

Innovative Ultrasound Imaging Techniques,
coordinated by S. Lori BRIDAL.

of elastic acoustic waves emitted during biological processes is somewhat akin to passive elastography techniques of today that use cardiac activity and other acoustic sources within the body to consider internal displacements resulting from the vibrations.

In 1987, the initial aim of the elastography field was to detect innate elastic waves within the body. During the 1990s, however, static elastography became more popular than the passive detection approach. Since the turn of the century in 2000, the central interest of elastography research has reoriented towards approaches able to follow waves propagating within the body, and the majority of research and clinical elastography acts today privilege wave propagation-based elastography. In this chapter, we will retrace the history of the field to explain the basis for the success of wave propagation elastography.

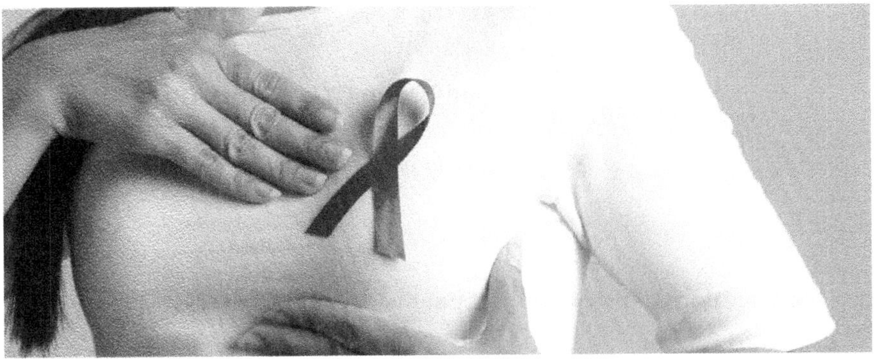

Figure 3.1. *Palpation of the breast is routinely used to screen for tumors. Image reproduced under the under the Creative Commons licence CC-BY-SA-4.0: https://commons.wikimedia.org/wiki/File:Breast-Cancer-Treatment-in-Lucknow.jpg*

3.1.1. *What is elasticity?*

Courses on elasticity begin with the simplest form of Hooke's law, which states that stress is proportional to strain through a constant that is called the elastic modulus. Things are a little bit more complex in elastic bodies since these quantities (stress, strain and elastic modulus) are tensors. As a result, the shape and axes of the propagation medium and the relative directions of wave propagation must be defined. The quantity referred to as Young's modulus is the elasticity that is measured along a cylinder of a homogeneous, isotropic material when a uniaxial loading is applied (see Figure 3.2).

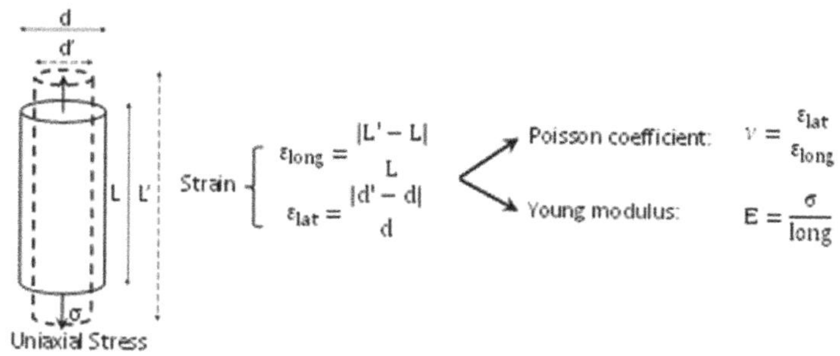

Figure 3.2. *Uniaxial stress is applied to a cylinder of homogeneous, isotropic material based on changes in the cylinder's length, L, and diameter, d. The parameters obtained are the Poisson coefficient, v, and Young's modulus, E. In wave physics, the Lamé coefficients, λ and μ, are used to describe a material's elasticity*

Young's modulus alone does not completely describe the elasticity of the cylinder. A second, independent measurement is required to assess the lateral strain that characterizes the change of the cylinder's cross-sectional diameter. This component of the cylinder's elastic properties is indicated by a second normalized coefficient called Poisson's ratio. The need for a pair of independent elastic moduli finds its roots within elasticity theory: only two independent eigenvalues are associated with the strain tensor. In other words, there are only two ways to apply a strain to a solid: with or without a change of volume. Therefore, only two associated independent elasticity constants are needed to describe elastic phenomena. However, there is a huge lexical field (stiffness, elasticity, rigidity, flexibility, compliance, etc.) for describing elasticity. The choice of the proper terms and parameters to use depends on the problem's specific geometry. For example, the Young's modulus definition is only valid for a cylinder. If a rod with a square cross-section is tested under the same conditions of uniaxial stress, the measured modulus is no longer Young's modulus. The choice of the pair of elasticity constants to use for a specific problem is, therefore, not universal. For wave physicists, the chosen natural elastic moduli are the Lamé coefficients, λ and μ, because they are involved in the description of the propagation of the two different elastic waves that travel in any solid: the compressional wave and the shear wave.

To summarize, there are only two independent ways to apply a strain to a solid (with or without a change of volume), and therefore there are two independent moduli and two types of elastic waves.

The values of elastic moduli in different materials that have been gathered in handbooks have been obtained through the estimation of the ultrasonic speed of propagation for compressional and shear waves. As far as elastography is concerned, in the audible frequency range, the shear Lamé coefficient μ, also called the shear modulus, is extracted from the shear wave speed. In soft tissues, the shear modulus is exactly the elasticity that a doctor would feel with their fingers during a palpation exam. This shear modulus happens to be one-third of the value of Young's modulus for the same isotropic solid. Due to the strength of linguistic habits, ultrasound companies present the parameter assessed by ultrasound elastography as Young's modulus, although, of course, the configuration considered is far from the cylindrical geometry characterized by Young's modulus, and it would be more appropriate to refer to the shear elastic modulus. It is worth mentioning another common confusion related to Young's modulus. Although descriptions of ultrasonic elastographic techniques often refer to things like "hand compression" for palpation or "compression" instead of uniaxial stress on a cylinder, it should not be concluded that a compressional modulus is being evaluated. In soft, quasi-incompressible tissues, the elastic modulus (abusively often called Young's modulus) has nothing to do with compression elasticity $\boldsymbol{\lambda}$ and is only related to the shear elasticity $\boldsymbol{\mu}$ of the material.

3.1.2. *Clinical elastography and emergent applications*

Today, elastography has been applied most successfully in the liver. It has become a gold standard for hepatic screening that avoids thousands of biopsies a year. Nearly all the major organs have been the subject of elastography clinical trials: the breast, the prostate, the kidney, the heart, the blood vessels and the cornea, for example. The list of potential diagnostic applications is continuously growing. Although it was first developed in the field of ultrasound, elastography is now used in conjunction with MRI, optical and, probably very soon, X-ray modalities. Indeed, shear waves can be detected in many different ways by many different medical imaging modalities. Regardless of what type of imaging is being used, the common aim of most current techniques is to precisely measure the propagation speed of shear waves traveling through the body.

3.1.3. *Chapter overview*

This chapter roughly follows the history of discoveries in the field of elastography. Section 3.2 describes the state-of-the-art for early ultrasound elastography – when the human body was considered to be a fluid-like propagation material (the liquid man). Section 3.3 describes how understanding changed when the "solid-man" point of view began to spread. Inspired by seismology, shear wave physics made big progress during this stage to better evaluate soft tissues. In section 3.4, the recurrent problem related to shear wave sources or how to best generate shear waves is considered. Section 3.5 describes how elastography can be evaluated using medical imaging modalities other than ultrasound and the interest and specificities of these other approaches.

3.2. Sound waves in human tissue: the liquid man

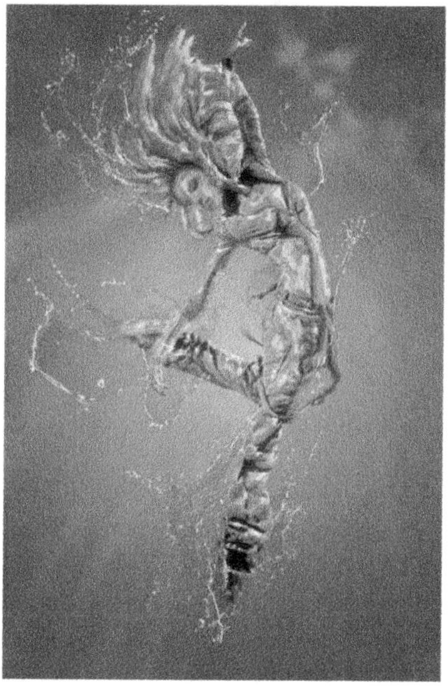

Figure 3.3. *The physics of ultrasound in soft tissues: the liquid man (or woman) model. Public Domain image CC Copyright-Only Dedication*or Public Domain Certification: https://pixabay.com/illustrations/young-girl-person-female-woman-1861716/*

In soft tissues, ultrasonic waves are associated with compressional waves. Approximately 70% of the human body is composed of water, and the concentration of water in soft tissues can be even higher than 70%. It is, therefore, not surprising that, in soft tissues, properties like the compressibility (~1) and the sound speed (~1,500 m/s) are nearly the same as for water. Since ultrasonic shear waves cannot propagate far in soft tissue due to their strong dissipation at megahertz frequencies, the field of sonography has long considered the human body (except for bones) to be a liquid-filled medium (see Figure 3.3). Due to the predominance of this model, it took considerable time for the ultrasonic community to correctly interpret early signs that shear waves were indeed propagating within the body under certain conditions. Nevertheless, the well-established fluid-filled-body point of view ultimately did not prevent the development of tools at the heart of elastography.

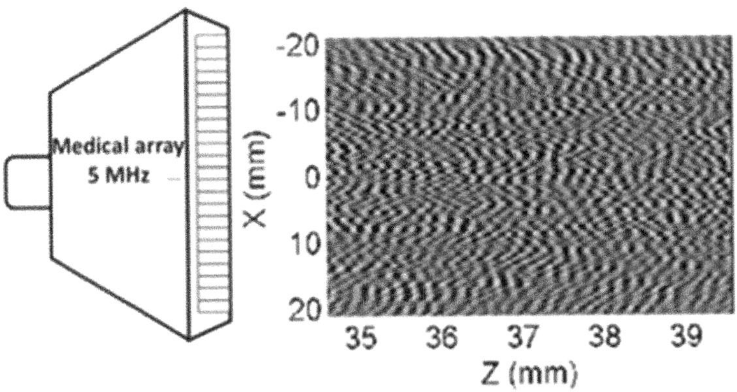

Figure 3.4. *The ultrasound speckle at the origin of motion detection*

The breakthrough that moved the model away from the fluid-filled body emerged from fundamental studies that were focused on an entirely different problem – how to improve images by getting rid of ultrasonic speckle. The term speckle has been carried over from the domain of optics where it is used to describe the random fluctuation of intensity due to constructive or destructive interferences observed when laser light is scattered by a rough surface. As explained in section 1.4.8, the same phenomenon results in ultrasonic speckle when echoes return from a random distribution of scatterers in soft tissues (see Figure 3.4). Ultrasonic speckle is thus considered to be a source of noise for standard imaging, but it has proven to be of great importance for motion detection. Speckle-tracking algorithms are at the heart of many Doppler techniques used to characterize fluid or tissue motion. In the early 1980s, Dickinson et al. (1982) used ultrasonic speckle to measure the natural vibrations in organs. Later, Eisenscher developed a similar approach, but replaced the natural vibrations of living tissues by motions induced using an external mechanical shaker (Eisenscher et al. 1983). Building on these innovations and using an external shaker with Doppler detection, Kroutskop et al. (1987) first described shear wave speed estimation as a potential proxy for palpation elasticity. Modern elastography was born! Soft tissues were finally recognized as a propagative medium for both compressional and shear waves – a property associated with solids but not with liquids.

3.3. Beyond ultrasound imaging: the solid man

As stated in section 3.1.1, the existence of two elastic waves, a compression wave and a shear wave in a medium, is a direct consequence of the fact that two possible, independent types of strain can be applied to a solid. As a result, once the propagation of shear waves in the body had been recognized within the emerging field of elastography, the liquid man model was slowly abandoned and elastography developed as a sort of human-body seismology. The representation used to consider ultrasonic waves in the human body had to be replaced by the solid man model or, more realistically, the soft, viscoelastic man model. Indeed, the first (compressional) wave is "curl free", meaning that no rotation occurs during propagation and there is only volumic change. The second one (shear wave) is "divergent free" which characterizes any shape change except volumic change. The associated pair of elasticities differ by several orders of magnitude. Compression elasticity is typically 10^6 times bigger than shear elasticity, and it is this compressional dominance that conveys soft properties to human tissues. As a further result, the shear wave speed is thousands of times slower than compressional wave speed. Since Poisson's ratio for biological tissue is very close to 0.5, soft tissues are said to be (almost) incompressible. Consider some typical wave speed values. The compressional wave travels like in water at a velocity close to 1,500 $m.s^{-1}$, whereas the shear wave speed is in the range of 1–20 $m.s^{-1}$. To compare with seismology within the Earth's crust, shear wave speed through rock is typically half as fast as compressional wave speed.

The properties of shear waves in biological tissue are familiar now, but this understanding did not emerge immediately following the discovery of sonoelasticity by Krouskop (1987). Initially, the ultrasound community was skeptical concerning the feasibility of shear wave propagation in soft tissues. It is important to note that sonoelasticity was still facing enormous theoretical difficulties and remained unable to explain the dispersion of shear waves in soft tissues (the differences in the propagation speed as a function of frequency) or the polarization of the observed shear waves (Yamakoshi et al. 1996). A breakthrough was made by replacing the monochromatic vibrations of early sonoelasticity by a pulsed method called transient elastography. This overcame several technical obstacles and resolved two paradoxal observations: a strange infinite phase velocity observed at low frequencies and the apparent longitudinal polarization of shear waves. Indeed, transient elastography allowed the observation of both types of elastic waves for the first time in 1999 (see

Figure 3.5). After emission of a pulse by a piston at the surface of the tissue, two waves became apparent on the experimental displacement map as a function of depth. Following the naming convention usually applied in seismology, since compressional waves are the fastest, they are called P-waves for primary waves. The shear waves are referred to as S-waves, for secondary waves. This clear separation of the two waves elucidated the physics of shear wave propagation in soft tissues. As seen in the figure, and taking the velocities into account, the P-wave propagation in soft tissues seems instantaneous compared to the S-wave propagation. Thus, the strange infinite phase velocity observed at low frequency was due to the much more rapid compressional wave. As for the longitudinal polarization of a shear wave, it is now clearly established that a transverse wave represents a special case of a shear wave, just like a longitudinal wave is a special case of a compressional wave. It is not the longitudinal or transverse polarization that defines the kind of wave propagating in a medium. Rather, elastodynamic physics explains that the wave kind is defined based on the volumic change or volumic invariance produced during propagation. Therefore, a shear wave can have a longitudinal polarization and a compressional wave can be transversally polarized (Catheline and Benech 2015).

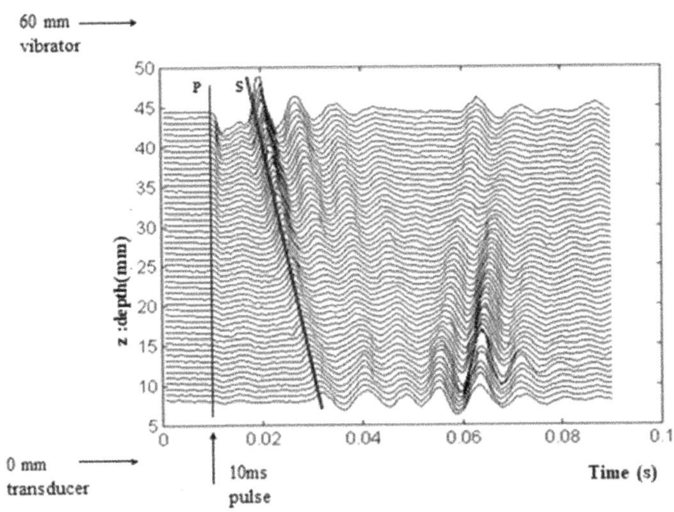

Figure 3.5. *Experimental detection of elastic waves in a soft solid reveals evidence of a compressional wave (P) and, at a later time, the shear wave (S)*

Ultrafast ultrasonic sequencing, also called high-frame-rate ultrasound imaging, is another very important development contributing to the emergence of transient elastography. Although the displacements shown in Figure 3.5 were detected using a single transducer that allowed data acquisition along a single line of sight at a rate of 1,000 ultrasound backscattered signals per second, it soon became clear that more rapid data acquisition was necessary to evaluate elastic properties in an image plane for elastography. Fortunately, new ultrasound devices that would be called ultrafast scanners were on the horizon.

3.4. The shear wave source problem

In order to study the elastic properties of the human body, many methods now use ultrasonic shear wave propagation to extract the shear wave velocity. Generating shear waves is no secret in the fields of optics and acoustics due to our technological control of both light and sound sources. However, the attenuation in soft tissues is much higher for shear waves than for the longitudinal compressional waves that are typically used for ultrasonic imaging. This limits the usable frequency bandwidth. Fluid-filled media within the body can also prevent effective shear wave propagation. So, how can we generate a shear wave in the human body that can propagate over a significant distance? This question is known as the shear wave source problem, and several of the solutions that have been applied to solve this problem are presented in the following sections.

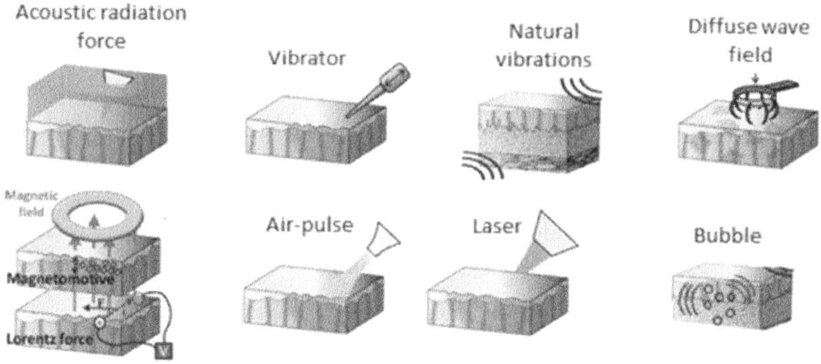

Figure 3.6. *Shear wave sources. Most clinical devices use a vibrator or acoustic radiation force*

3.4.1. *External vibrating piston source*

Eisenscher et al. (1983), presented an ultrasonic method to produce shear waves for use in soft tissues that was called "echosonography". This method was based on a mechanical piston, vibrated against the skin's surface to create low-frequency mechanical shear waves within the body. These waves were then detected using ultrasound. This was the first study to mix ultrasound and low-frequency mechanical vibrations. However, this method only provided qualitative information about the interrogated tissues.

Krouskop et al. (1987) proposed a method for quantitative measurements of shear wave propagation in tissue through the measurement of the shear wave velocity. In this study, an external vibrating source was placed in contact with in vivo human limb tissue. This induced shear wave displacements which were estimated using an ultrasonic Doppler method. The authors showed that this technique can detect the local displacement field of shear waves and that it can be used to quantify the elastic properties of soft tissues.

In parallel, Lerner et al. (1998) proposed another method based on an external shear wave source. However, contrary to the technique proposed by Krouskop et al. (1987), this technique was only a qualitative imaging method. It used a color-flow map imaging system that had been designed for real-time display of blood flow. With this method, the frequency of the vibrations had to be limited to a few Hz because of the low frame rate of the imaging device. This method became known as "sonoelasticity".

Yamakoshi et al. (1990) modified this method. An external vibrating source was still used, but the measuring device was replaced by an ultrasonic phased-array transducer to obtain two-dimensional images. This allowed the acquisition of amplitude and phase maps from the Doppler frequency. Using this method, shear waves with higher frequencies of several hundred Hz could be obtained through synchronization with the vibrator. This technique with a transducer array and synchronization yielded shear wave amplitude and phase maps, and, therefore, provided an estimate of wavelengths at known frequencies. This made it feasible to create quantitative images of the shear wavelengths.

The first methods for sonoelasticity were thus based on harmonic imaging. However, this approach presented a problem because the measured shear wave speeds did not correspond to theoretical models, as observed in Fujii et al. (1995). The authors tried to apply different models to consider the nature of the shear wave source, but, for harmonic sources, theoretical and experimental correspondence remained elusive. The issue was finally resolved in 1999 by the development of transient elastography (Catheline et al. 1999a, 1999b; Sandrin et al. 1999). For this method, the vibrating source emits a pulse instead of a harmonic signal. The correct description of shear wave propagation in soft solids based on transient pulse emission was made possible by the exact solution of the wave equation: the elastic Green's function. Transient elastography was then developed in 1D for hepatic fibrosis characterization (Sandrin et al. 2002, 2003) and in 2D for the evaluation of breast tumors (Bercoff et al. 2003). These techniques were based on the measurement of the longitudinal component of shear waves, which has been precisely described in Catheline and Benech (2015).

3.4.2. *Radiation pressure*

In the previous section, the history of the development of external shear wave sources was described. However, external vibrating sources have practical limitations. They are not "user-friendly" for clinical application due to the size and weight of the mechanical vibrating systems. A new method based on the acoustic radiation force was proposed in 1990 (Sugimoto et al. 1990). Acoustic radiation force is a unidirectional force that can be applied to absorbing and reflecting targets (Torr 1984). This force results from the transfer of momentum from the acoustic wave to the target to create a displacement in the medium. This principle can be applied to produce a shearing effect by using compressional ultrasonic waves to apply local acoustic radiation force. In the study presented by Sugimoto et al. (1990) the acoustic radiation force was created using a transducer that was geometrically focused on a position within the body to create radiation pressure. The resulting shear strain was measured by an ultrasonic transducer over time. Authors wanted to investigate the different possible parameters that could be assessed based on the shear strain to measure the tissue hardness. They showed a correlation between the spring coefficient of the different materials studied and the relative deformation.

The earliest studies using acoustic radiation force impulses (ARFI) sought to use it in order to mimic the palpation by a physician. One such approach aimed to directly measure the elastic modulus in the medium based on the relation between the applied force and the observed deformation, which is known as the spring ratio. It was also possible to observe the corresponding relaxation time with this method. Nightingale et al. (2001) applied this idea using ultrasonic transducer arrays. This method provided two-dimensional stiffness maps by controlling the location of multiple acoustic radiation force pushes and then tracking the resulting displacements using the same transducer array. Feasibility was first shown in gels with calibrated stiffness before an in vivo clinical feasibility study (Nightingale et al. 2002). However, this method has some limitations. It is a qualitative method which requires the application of many focused pushes to map the relative stiffness of the medium. Furthermore, the number of ultrasonic pushes that can be applied per unit time must be limited to remain below the US Food and Drugs Administration recommendations for high intensity acoustic pulse exposure.

In the studies cited above by Nightingale et al. (2001), acoustic radiation force was used to create palpation within tissues through a quasi-static method. In parallel, some studies began to consider the interest of shear wave propagation speed. Sarvazyan et al. (1998) proposed the evaluation of the elasticity through the response in time of the tissue at the focal spot. This was based on the analytical scalar solution for shear wave propagation in the near field of a source beam. Thus, they still used an acoustic radiation force to produce the shear waves locally, but they also derived the equations for shear wave propagation by considering the ultrasonic focal spot as a source. The initial idea was to measure the local displacement at the spot, but it was also found to be possible to estimate the wave front position near the focal spot as a function of time and radial distance. Thus, it became possible to obtain an estimate of the local velocity of the shear wave. It should be noted, however, that in the study presented by Sarvazyan et al. (1998), MRI was used to detect the shear wave propagation after application of each acoustic radiation force impulse. This detection method is expensive and can only provide a low frame rate. Different elastography methods that use MRI are described in greater detail in section 3.5.

Later, Bercoff et al. (2004) presented a method based entirely on ultrasound. Ultrasound provided both the acoustic radiation force and the imaging technique needed to follow the shear wave propagation. The main idea consisted of focusing ultrasound on multiple points at successively deeper regions to generate a shear wave front as a Mach cone. This required the displacement of the ultrasonic focal spot at a faster rate than the shear wave propagation velocity in the medium. This novel shear wave source was detected with an ultrafast ultrasound imaging system (Sandrin et al. 1999) at more than 1,000 frames per second to measure the local shear wave velocity, and thus the tissue stiffness. This imaging technique is very different from the former methods because it is based on the characterization of the propagation of the transient shear wave front and not on the local displacement induced by the shearing radiation force impulses. Since propagation characteristics must be precisely tracked, this method is strongly dependent on the frame rate of the ultrafast scanner. Furthermore, this method improved the practicality of the method initially developed in Sandrin et al. (1999) because it did not require a vibrating source to be held by the physician, as in Bercoff et al. (2003). This technique is now usually referred to as shear wave elastography (SWE).

Acoustic radiation force has been used to study many different organs and is now widely used in shear wave elastography. For liver fibrosis, a clinical study based on the ARFI method was reported by Takahashi et al. (2010). More recently, Urban et al. (2015) studied myocardial anisotropy using a harmonic, shear wave imaging method, and Pernot et al. (2016) measured diastolic myocardial stiffness with the SWE method. Acoustic radiation force imaging has also allowed the combination of novel push methods. For example, several shear waves can be created and allowed to interfere with each other, to create crawling waves (Hah et al. 2010).

3.4.3. *Electromagnetic source*

Another very recent method developed to create shear waves in a medium is based on the Lorentz force. The principle is that an electrical current in a magnetic field induces a displacement due to the Lorentz force (Jackson 1962). The first methods in the literature to generate shear waves using electromagnetic sources were based on external coils (Muthupillai et al. 1996), which provided another way to create an external vibrating source. This method was modified by Basford et al. (2005), who performed experiments by passing an electrical current through conductive gel phantoms, while using an MRI system to create the magnetic field, as well as to estimate the induced tissue displacements. They illustrated the generation of shear waves using displacement maps. This idea was also used by Grasland-Mongrain et al. (2013a, 2013b), by applying low-frequency electrical currents (10–1,000 Hz) in soft solids made of polyvinyl alcohol gels containing graphite powder and salt that were placed in a constant magnetic field. However, in this study, the imaging device was an ultrafast ultrasound scanner that used the speckle pattern scattered from the graphite inclusions to measure the displacement, and the magnetic field was created by magnets instead of an MRI system. Shear waves were observed in the medium. Since no MRI system is required for this technique, it can be applied much more readily, more widely and with strongly reduced expense. Grasland-Mongrain et al. (2016b) presented a contactless experiment, performed with a commercial transcranial magnetic stimulator, allowing the creation of shear waves without any electrode in contact with the medium.

3.4.4. *Bubbles and laser sources*

Montalescot et al. (2016) also used electrical currents to create shear waves through a different mechanism based on the production of water electrolysis in soft solids to induce bubbling. Bubble growth induces both compression waves and shear waves. However, the difference in the time scale for wave propagation allows the separation of the two wave types. This technique still requires refinement, however, because it would require relatively high electrical currents for application in human subjects. Bubbles do not necessarily have to be created with electrical currents, however, and this study provides a basis that may ultimately be extended to the use of bubbles from other sources to create waves in different media.

In a subsequent study, they presented the use of another electromagnetic wave: light produced by laser beams (Grasland-Mongrain et al. 2016a) to generate shear waves. The optical energy of the laser is converted into heat and creates a small local increase in temperature that leads to dilatation of the tissue. This induces a displacement that can generate shear waves. This method can then be extended to create waves in small, highly localized zones or to create surface waves. The technique is well adapted to perform elastography of media like the cornea.

The methods using bubbles and lasers usually create waves near the electrodes or near a surface point targeted by the laser. Both of these methods can be considered as similar to the use of vibrating sources to create shear waves, because they create shear wave sources at the surface of the sample.

3.4.5. *Natural sources*

The previously described imaging and characterization techniques are based on shear wave generation using an active source. However, a medium can also be analyzed using the innate, natural waves that can be observed with ultrasound, as shown by Dickinson and Hill (1982). For example, in the human body, shear waves can be produced through muscular activity, cardiac activity (Vos et al. 2015) or arterial pulsatility. The first passive elastography methods used vibrations created by the heart. This concept has been studied since 1996 when Kanai et al. demonstrated the possibility of measuring tissue displacement due to cardiac motion based on Doppler effects (Kanai et al. 1996). Later, they used their method to characterize cardiac tissue (Kanai et al. 1996, 1997; Kanai 2005). Another example of passive elastography of the heart was reported by Konofagou et al. (2000), who measured the displacement and strain created by cardiac activity.

Other studies have used noise correlation, a method that can be used to retrieve the wave's Green's function in a medium (Cassereau and Fink 1992; Derode et al. 2002; Karim et al. 2005; Sánchez-Sesma and Campillo 2006). In other words, this method extracts the shear wave speed properties from any complex field. The technique shares the same physical background as time-reversal techniques. This method was used for the first time by Sabra et al. (2007) to characterize muscle stiffness. Their first experiment consisted of using 15 accelerometers placed along a line on the surface of the leg. To measure the shear wave phase velocity, the cross-correlation between the signals measured by each of these accelerometers was performed. This allowed retrieval of Green's function along the line and the extraction of the shear wave velocity.

At about the same time, Catheline et al. (2008) presented a time-reversal experiment in a gel that improved on Sabra et al. (2007) because, by using an ultrafast scanner with a transducer array, Green's function could be retrieved in a two-dimensional plane within a medium. Soon after, one-dimensional measurements were performed with a single transducer, to investigate the feasibility of measuring the elasticity with this method (Benech et al. 2009). This study showed that, even if Green's function is not isotropic, the width of the focal spot along the direction of propagation of the ultrasound is approximately equal to the wavelength of the shear waves, which thus allows the elasticity to be measured. Gallot et al. (2011) combined both of these more recent ideas to estimate the elasticity of the liver. They directly measured a two-dimensional wave field induced by cardiac motion with a transducer array and determined the shear wave displacement using a speckle-tracking method. Determination of the shear wave velocity was then based on the space–time representation of Green's function, as in the one-dimensional case with a calculation along the depth. This study thus proposed a method to obtain elasticity maps that, contrary to Benech et al. (2009), were based on global elasticity estimation.

Catheline et al. (2013) presented a new algorithm in 2013 that was based on a plane-wave approximation near the focal spot of Green's function. This consisted of comparing the time-reversed wave field in the strain and in the particle velocity, to obtain an approximate group velocity. An interesting part of their study was the demonstration of the feasibility to apply this technique with the use of a conventional ultrasound imaging system (frame rates < 100 Hz). The pulse repetition frequency was too low to obtain any time information related to the propagation of the shear wave, but the spatial resolution was high enough to obtain an estimate of the central wavelength of the shear wave displacements. This method is thus only based on spatial information. The possibility of performing measurements with very low frame rates allows this technique to be used with MRI, for example. This type of approach was thus used by Zorgani et al. (2015) to measure the elasticity of the brain. Since this method is based only on the spatial information of displacements between successive frames, it would also be possible to use a non-constant frame rate.

3.5. Elastography beyond ultrasound

It would be naive to believe that, before the 1980s, no one was interested in low-frequency propagation in soft tissues. Using optics, electrical impedance or piezo-detectors, researchers started to investigate elastic waves in soft material before this period to characterize propagative media (Kazakov et al. 1989;

Oestreicher 1951; Truong 1974). Efforts towards elastography imaging emerged upon the ultrasonic landscape towards the end of the 1980s (Krouskop et al. 1987; Parker et al. 1990). Shear wave elastography shares common limitations with conventional ultrasound imaging that are due to physical acoustics and currently available technologies. The organs of the lung and the brain are hardly accessible to ultrasound. Images remain bidimensional and centimeter sized.

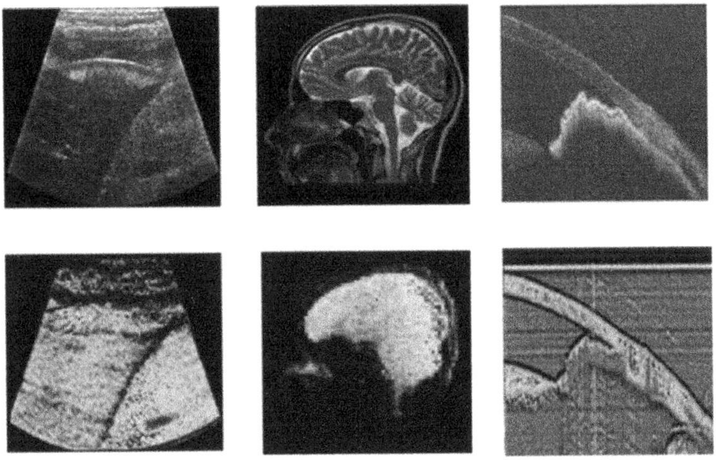

Figure 3.7. *Top: standard ultrasound, MRI and OCT images of the liver, the brain and the eye, respectively, from left to right. Bottom: associated shear wave elastography images*

In the field of MRI, researchers have developed a 3D method that is able to provide elastography maps in any soft tissue, including the brain and the lungs (Muthupillai et al. 1996). The main drawback of magnetic resonance elastography (MRE) is its relative slowness. Its frame rate is limited by the collective spin dynamics, which are roughly on the order of a second. Therefore, an elastography MRE sequence has to be synchronized with monochromatic vibrations. As a result, a few minutes of data acquisition can provide only a single frequency shear wave movie. Although MRI is nicely adapted to provide a more global view of volumes within the human body, anatomical details cannot be probed with MRE with the same precision as with ultrasound.

From the point of view of spatial resolution, the best results can be obtained using optical elastography (Li et al. 2012; Grasland-Mongrain et al. 2018). Elasticity maps of objects as small as a single cell are possible. Nevertheless, it is highly probable that shear wavelength techniques reach their limit for these experiments due to the strong dissipation that takes place in soft tissues. The highest shear wave frequencies propagating within soft tissues are approximately 20 kHz. Thus, ultrasound shear wave elastography is likely to be able to provide spatial resolution that is adequate to characterize wavelengths within the range of the available shear wave frequencies. Furthermore, only transparent media can be characterized to significant depths with optical elastography. For turbid media, optical coherent tomography (OCT) can barely reach depths on the order of a millimeter. In conclusion, optical elastography provides a useful solution for elastography in soft tissue structures with tiny dimensions such as cornea, lens, sclera or skin.

From a historical perspective, it can be concluded that, just as seismology made its first modern steps around 1830 and is still an important field of investigation today, the study of elastic waves in soft biological tissues, which was first considered about 160 years after the genesis of seismology, is only at an early stage of development. This new field of human-body seismology, called elastography, no doubt holds many discoveries, for example, in the fields of viscosity, rheology, nonlinearity and anisotropy, and with the definition of new, unique mechanical biomarkers.

3.6. References

Basford, A.T.T., Basford, J.R., Kugel, J., Ehman, R.L. (2005). Lorentz-force-induced motion in conductive media. *Magnetic Resonance Imaging*, 23(5), 647–651. https://doi.org/10.1016/j.mri.2005.02.014.

Benech, N., Catheline, S., Brum, J., Gallot, T., Negreira, C. (2009). 1-D elasticity assessment in soft solids from shear wave correlation: The time-reversal approach. *IEEE Transactions on Ultrasonics, Ferroelectrics and Frequency Control*, 56(11), 2400–2410. https://doi.org/10.1109/TUFFC.2009.1328.

Bercoff, J., Muller, M., Tanter, M., Fink, M. (2003). Study of viscous and elastic properties of soft tissues using supersonic shear imaging. *IEEE Symposium on Ultrasonics*, 1(2000), 135–142. https://doi.org/10.1109/ULTSYM.2003.1293551.

Bercoff, J., Tanter, M., Muller, M., Fink, M. (2004). The role of viscosity in the impulse diffraction field of elastic waves induced by the acoustic radiation force. *IEEE Transactions on Ultrasonics, Ferroelectrics, and Frequency Control*, 51(11), 1523–1536. https://doi.org/10.1109/TUFFC.2004.1367494.

Cassereau, D. and Fink, M. (1992). Time-reversal of ultrasonic fields. Part III: Theory of the closed time-reversal cavity. *IEEE Transactions on Ultrasonics, Ferroelectrics, and Frequency Control*, 39(5), 579–592. https://doi.org/10.1109/58.156176.

Catheline, S. and Benech, N. (2015). Longitudinal shear wave and transverse dilatational wave in solids. *Journal of the Acoustical Society of America*, 137(2), El200-5. https://doi.org/10.1007/s10597-015-9836-x\r10.1121/1.4907742.

Catheline, S., Thomas, J.L.L., Wu, F., Fink, M. (1999a). Diffraction field of a low frequency vibrator in soft tissues using transient elastography. *IEEE Transactions on Ultrasonics, Ferroelectrics, and Frequency Control*, 46(4), 1013–1019.

Catheline, S., Wu, F., Fink, M. (1999b). A solution to diffraction biases in sonoelasticity: The acoustic impulse technique. *The Journal of the Acoustical Society of America*, 105(5), 2941–2950. https://doi.org/10.1121/1.426907.

Catheline, S., Benech, N., Brum, J., Negreira, C. (2008). Time reversal of elastic waves in soft solids. *Physical Review Letters*, 100(6), 1–4. https://doi.org/10.1103/PhysRevLett.100.064301.

Catheline, S., Souchon, R., Rupin, M., Brum, J., Dinh, A.H., Chapelon, J.-Y. (2013). Tomography from diffuse waves: Passive shear wave imaging using low frame rate scanners. *Applied Physics Letters*, 103(1). https://doi.org/10.1063/1.4812515.

Derode, A., Larose, E., Tanter, M., de Rosny, J. (2002). Recovering the Green's function from field-field correlations in an open scattering medium (L). *The Journal of the Acoustical Society of America*, 113(6), 2973. https://doi.org/10.1121/1.1570436.

Dickinson, R.J. and Hill, C.R. (1982). Measurement of soft tissue motion using correlation between A-scans. *Ultrasound in Medicine & Biology*, 8(3), 263–271. https://doi.org/10.1016/0301-5629(82)90032-1.

Eisenscher, A., Schweg-Toffler, E., Pelletier, G., Jacquemard, P. (1983). Rhythmic echographic palpation. Echosismography. A new technic of differentiating benign and malignant tumors by ultrasonic study of tissue elasticity. *Journal de Radiologie*, 64(4), 255–261.

Fujii, K., Sato, T., Kameyama, K., Inoue, T., Yokoyama, K., Kobayashi, K. (1995). Imaging system of precise hardness distribution in soft tissue in vivo using forced vibration and ultrasonic detection. In *Acoustical Imaging*, Jones, J.P. (ed.). Springer, New York. https://doi.org/10.1007/978-1-4615-1943-0_25.

Gallot, T., Catheline, S., Roux, P., Brum, J., Benech, N., Negreira, C. (2011). Passive elastography: Shear-wave tomography from physiological-noise correlation in soft tissues. *IEEE Transactions on Ultrasonics, Ferroelectrics, and Frequency Control*, 58(6), 1122–1126. https://doi.org/10.1109/TUFFC.2011.1920.

Grasland-Mongrain, P., Catheline, S., Souchon, R., Cartellier, F., Zorgani, A., Montalescot, S., Chapelon, J.-Y., Lafon, C. (2013a). Imaging of shear waves induced by Lorentz force in soft solids. *IEEE International Ultrasonics Symposium (IUS)*, 038101(July), 1158–1161. https://doi.org/10.1109/ULTSYM.2013.0296.

Grasland-Mongrain, P., Mari, J.M., Chapelon, J.-Y., Lafon, C. (2013b). Lorentz force electrical impedance tomography. *IRBM*, 34(4–5), 357–360. https://doi.org/10.1016/j.irbm.2013.08.002.

Grasland-Mongrain, P., Lu, Y., Lesage, F., Catheline, S., Cloutier, G. (2016a). Generation of shear waves by laser in soft media in the ablative and thermoelastic regimes. *Applied Physics Letters*, 109(22). https://doi.org/10.1063/1.4968538.

Grasland-Mongrain, P., Miller-Jolicoeur, E., Tang, A., Catheline, S., Cloutier, G. (2016b). Contactless remote induction of shear waves in soft tissues using a transcranial magnetic stimulation device. *Physics in Medicine and Biology*, 61(6), 2582–2593. https://doi.org/10.1088/0031-9155/61/6/2582.

Grasland-Mongrain, P., Zorgani, A., Nakagawa, S., Bernard, S., Paim, L.G., Fitzharris, G., Catheline, S., Cloutier, G. (2018). Ultrafast imaging of cell elasticity with optical microelastography. *Proceedings of the National Academy of Sciences*, 115(5), 861–866. https://doi.org/10.1073/pnas.1713395115.

Hah, Z., Hazard, C., Cho, Y.T., Rubens, D.J., Parker, K.J. (2010). Crawling waves from radiation force excitation. *Ultrasonic Imaging*, 32(3), 177–189 [Online]. Available at: http://www.ncbi.nlm.nih.gov/pubmed/20718246.

Jackson, J.D. (1962). *Classical Electrodynamics*. John Wiley & Sons, New York.

Kanai, H. (2005). Propagation of spontaneously actuated pulsive vibration in human heart wall and in vivo viscoelasticity estimation. *IEEE Transactions on Ultrasonics, Ferroelectrics and Frequency Control*, 52(11), 1931–1942. https://doi.org/10.1109/TUFFC.2005.1561662.

Kanai, H., Sato, M., Koiwa, Y., Chubachi, N. (1996). Transcutaneous measurement and spectrum analysis of heart wall vibrations. *IEEE Transactions on Ultrasonics, Ferroelectrics, and Frequency Control*, 43(5), 791–810. https://doi.org/10.1109/58.535480.

Kanai, H., Hasegawa, H., Chubachi, N., Koiwa, Y., Tanaka, M. (1997). Noninvasive evaluation of local myocardial thickening and its color-coded imaging. *IEEE Transactions on Ultrasonics, Ferroelectrics and Frequency Control*, 44(4), 752–768. https://doi.org/10.1109/58.655190.

Kazakov, V.V., Klochkov, B.N., Chichagov, P.K. (1989). The study of dispersive characteristics of a wave on a human body. In *Methods of Vibrational Diagnostics of Rheological Properties of Soft Materials and Biological Tissue*, Antonets, V.A. (ed.). Institute of Applied Physics Publications, Gorky.

Konofagou, E., D'hooge, J., Ophir, J. (2000). Cardiac elastography: A feasibility study. *IEEE Ultrasonics Symposium. Proceedings, An International Symposium (Cat. No. 00CH37121)*, 2, 1273–1276. https://doi.org/10.1109/ULTSYM.2000.921555.

Krouskop, T.A., Dougherty, D.R., Vinson, F.S. (1987). A pulsed Doppler ultrasonic system for making noninvasive measurements of the mechanical properties of soft tissue. *Journal of Rehabilitation Research and Development*, 24(2), 1–8.

Lerner, R.M., Parker, K.J., Holen, J., Gramiak, R., Waag, R.C. (1988). Sono-elasticity: Medical elasticity images derived from ultrasound signals in mechanically vibrated targets. *Acoustical Imaging*, 16, 317–327. https://doi.org/10.1007/978-1-4613-0725-9_31.

Li, C., Guan, G., Cheng, X., Huang, Z., Wang, R.K. (2012). Quantitative elastography provided by surface acoustic waves measured by phase-sensitive optical coherence tomography. *Optics Letters*, 37(4), 722. https://doi.org/10.1364/OL.37.000722.

Montalescot, S., Roger, B., Zorgani, A., Souchon, R., Grasland-Mongrain, P., Ben Haj Slama, R., Bera, J.-C., Catheline, S. (2016). Electrolysis-induced bubbling in soft solids for elastic-wave generation. *Applied Physics Letters*, 108(9). https://doi.org/10.1063/1.4942610.

Muthupillai, R., Rossman, P.J., Lomas, D.J., Greenleaf, J.F., Riederer, S.J., Ehman, R.L. (1996). Magnetic resonance imaging of transverse acoustic strain waves. *Magnetic Resonance in Medicine: Official Journal of the Society of Magnetic Resonance in Medicine/Society of Magnetic Resonance in Medicine*, 36(2), 266–274. https://doi.org/10.1002/mrm.1910360214.

Nightingale, K., Palmeri, M.L., Nightingale, R.W., Trahey, G.E. (2001). On the feasibility of remote palpation using acoustic radiation force. *The Journal of the Acoustical Society of America*, 110(1), 625–634. https://doi.org/10.1121/1.1378344.

Nightingale, K., Soo, M.S., Nightingale, R.W., Trahey, G.E. (2002). Acoustic radiation force impulse imaging: In vivo demonstration of clinical feasibility. *Ultrasound in Medicine & Biology*, 28(2), 227–235 [Online]. Available at: http://www.sciencedirect.com/science/article/pii/S0301562901004999.

Oestreicher, H.L. (1951). Field and impedance of an oscillating sphere in a viscoelastic medium with an application to biophysics. *The Journal of the Acoustical Society of America*, 23(6), 707–714. https://doi.org/10.1121/1.1906828.

Parker, K.J., Huang, S.R., Musulin, R.A., Lerner, R.M. (1990). Tissue response to mechanical vibrations for "sonoelasticity imaging". *Ultrasound in Medicine & Biology*, 16(3), 241–246. https://doi.org/10.1016/0301-5629(90)90003-U.

Pernot, M., Lee, W.N., Bel, A., Mateo, P., Couade, M., Tanter, M., Crozatier, B., Messas, E. (2016). Shear wave imaging of passive diastolic myocardial stiffness: Stunned versus infarcted myocardium. *JACC: Cardiovascular Imaging*, 9(9), 1023–1030. https://doi.org/10.1016/j.jcmg.2016.01.022.

Sabra, K.G., Gerstoft, P., Roux, P., Kuperman, W.A., Fehler, M.C. (2005). Extracting time-domain Green's function estimates from ambient seismic noise. *Geophysical Research Letters*, 32(3), 1–5. https://doi.org/10.1029/2004GL021862.

Sabra, K.G., Conti, S., Roux, P., Kuperman, W.A. (2007). Passive in vivo elastography from skeletal muscle noise. *Applied Physics Letters*, 90(19), 10–12. https://doi.org/10.1063/1.2737358.

Sánchez-Sesma, F.J. and Campillo, M. (2006). Retrieval of the Green's function from cross correlation: The canonical elastic problem. *Bulletin of the Seismological Society of America*, 96(3), 1182–1191. https://doi.org/10.1785/0120050181.

Sandrin, L., Catheline, S., Tanter, M., Hennequin, X., Fink, M. (1999). Time-resolved pulsed elastography with ultrafast ultrasonic imaging. *Ultrasonic Imaging*, 21(4), 259–272. https://doi.org/10.1177/016173469902100402.

Sandrin, L., Tanter, M., Gennisson, J.-L., Catheline, S., Fink, M. (2002). Shear elasticity probe for soft tissues with 1-D transient elastography. *IEEE Transactions on Ultrasonics, Ferroelectrics, and Frequency Control*, 49(4), 436–446. https://doi.org/10.1109/58.996561.

Sandrin, L., Fourquet, B., Hasquenoph, J.-M., Yon, S., Fournier, C., Mal, F., Christidis, C., Ziol, M., Poulet, B., Kazemi, F. et al. (2003). Transient elastography: A new noninvasive method for assessment of hepatic fibrosis. *Ultrasound in Medicine & Biology*, 29(12), 1705–1713. https://doi.org/10.1016/j.ultrasmedbio.2003.07.001.

Sarvazyan, A.P., Rudenko, O.V.O.V., Swanson, S.D., Fowlkes, J.B.B., Emelianov, S.Y. (1998). Shear wave elasticity imaging: A new ultrasonic technology of medical diagnostics. *Ultrasound in Medicine and Biology*, 24(9), 1419–1435. https://doi.org/10.1016/S0301-5629(98)00110-0.

Sugimoto, T., Ueha, S., Itoh, K. (1990). Tissue hardness measurement using the radiation force of focused ultrasound. *Ultrasonics Symposium, 1990. Proceedings., IEEE*, 1377–1380. https://doi.org/10.1109/ULTSYM.1990.171591.

Takahashi, H., Ono, N., Eguchi, Y., Eguchi, T., Kitajima, Y., Kawaguchi, Y., Nakashita, S., Ozaki, I., Mizuta, T., Toda, S. et al. (2010). Evaluation of acoustic radiation force impulse elastography for fibrosis staging of chronic liver disease: A pilot study. *Liver International*, 30(4), 538–545. https://doi.org/10.1111/j.1478-3231.2009.02130.x.

Torr, G.R. (1984). The acoustic radiation force. *American Journal of Physics*, 52(5), 402–408. https://doi.org/10.1119/1.13625.

Truong, X. (1974). Viscoelastic wave propagation and rheologic properties of skeletal muscle. *American Journal of Physiology-Legacy Content*, 226(2), 256–264. https://doi.org/10.1152/ajplegacy.1974.226.2.256.

Urban, M.W., Qiang, B., Song, P., Nenadic, I.Z., Chen, S., Greenleaf, J.F. (2015). Investigation of the effects of myocardial anisotropy for shear wave elastography using acoustic radiation force and harmonic vibration. *2015 IEEE International Ultrasonics Symposium (IUS 2015)*. https://doi.org/10.1109/ULTSYM.2015.0154.

Vos, H.J., Van Dalen, B.M., Bosch, J.G., Van Der Steen, A.F.W., De Jong, N. (2015). Myocardial passive shear wave detection. *IEEE International Ultrasonics Symposium (IUS 2015)*, 1–4. https://doi.org/10.1109/ULTSYM.2015.0152.

Yamakoshi, Y., Sato, J., Sato, T. (1990). Ultrasonic-imaging of internal vibration of soft-tissue under forced vibration. *IEEE Transactions on Ultrasonics Ferroelectrics and Frequency Control*, 37(2), 45–53. https://doi.org/10.1109/58.46969.

Yamakoshi, Y., Otaki, H., Shinozuka, N., Masuda, H. (1996). Internal tissue displacement measurement based on ultrasonic wave Doppler signal digital detection and its application to fetal movement monitoring. *Ultrasonics*, 34(8), 769–775. https://doi.org/10.1016/S0041-624X(96)00080-7.

Zorgani, A., Souchon, R., Dinh, A.-H.H., Chapelon, J.-Y.Y., Ménager, J.-M., Lounis, S., Rouvière, O., Catheline, S. (2015). Brain palpation from physiological vibrations using MRI. *Proceedings of the National Academy of Sciences*, 112(42), 12917–12921. https://doi.org/10.1073/pnas.1509895112.

4

Doppler Ultrasound and Flow Mapping

Alfred C.H. YU

Schlegel-UW Research Institute for Aging, University of Waterloo, Ontario, Canada

As first demonstrated in vivo in the 1950s (Kaneko 1986), Doppler ultrasound can non-invasively provide information about the flow velocity distribution within a blood vessel. Such information has long been recognized to be of high clinical value in cardiovascular diagnostics. For example, in atherosclerosis diagnostics, Doppler ultrasound may be applied to measure the peak flow velocity within a specific region in a patient's arteries (Johnston et al. 1985). In turn, the measured flow velocity value may be used as a quantitative indicator of the degree of occlusion in a specific region in a patient's arteries (Arbeille et al. 1995). From this information, clinicians can assess the severity of vascular occlusion and determine whether intervention should be made.

In terms of its operation, Doppler ultrasound generally works by transmitting ultrasound waves (at frequencies higher than the human audible range) into the blood vessel and receiving the echoes backscattered from red blood cell (RBC) scatterers flowing inside the blood vessel. Subsequently, by processing the received echoes, the flow velocity distribution and the peak flow velocity can be extracted. There are two modes of operation in Doppler ultrasound: continuous-wave (CW) mode and pulsed-wave (PW) mode. As revealed by its name, the CW mode involves the transmission of continuous ultrasound waves into the blood vessel and the reception of the backscattered echoes. In contrast, the PW mode involves the

For a color version of all the figures in this chapter, see www.iste.co.uk/bridal/innovative.zip.

Innovative Ultrasound Imaging Techniques,
coordinated by S. Lori BRIDAL.

periodic transmission of ultrasound pulses into the blood vessel and the reception of the pulse echoes.

This chapter provides a pedagogical walkthrough of the technical principles of Doppler ultrasound to guide readers who are new to ultrasound-based flow measurements. It will cover the fundamental physics and derivations in both the CW and PW Doppler modes. Also, it will introduce readers to ultrasound color flow imaging (CFI), which is a Doppler-based flow mapping mode. Emerging trends in ultrasound-based flow measurements and mapping will be highlighted.

4.1. Continuous-wave (CW) Doppler

CW Doppler ultrasound represents the first demonstration of the feasibility of using ultrasound for blood flow measurement applications. It is based upon the physics of the classical Doppler effect, which refers to a shift in the acoustic frequency perceived by a target due to the motion of either the source or the target (or both). As will be explained later in this section, through leveraging the classical Doppler effect, CW Doppler ultrasound can examine time-varying, pulsatile flow dynamics inside the vasculature.

4.1.1. *Origin of signals in blood*

In the blood, RBCs are the main Doppler targets of interest. These scatterers, each of which is an oval-shaped biconcave disc with a major diameter between 5 and 8 μm, constitute on average 40% of blood contents for a nominal hematocrit of 40% in humans. There are typically about 5–8 million RBCs in a 5 L human blood volume (Burton 2000). Because the size of individual RBCs is relatively small compared to the size of the tissue (which is composed of a group of cells), RBCs generally have a smaller backscattering strength in the clinical ultrasound frequency range (i.e. <20 MHz) (Foster et al. 2000). Accordingly, the strength of echoes from the blood is weaker than that from tissue parenchyma. Hence, in a B-mode image, blood vessel lumens are relatively echolucent with respect to the arterial wall and nearby tissue.

Although RBCs have a relatively weak backscattering strength, this issue does not stymie efforts to measure flow velocities from the detected blood echoes. This is because flow velocities are derived based on the extent of Doppler shifts detected from the ultrasound echoes, and as shown by the derivation in the next section, the Doppler shift magnitude is independent of the blood signal strength. As such, CW Doppler ultrasound can generally produce quantitative estimates of flow velocities, as long as the backscattered RBC echoes have an intensity above the system's noise floor and are, thus, detectable.

4.1.2. *Doppler equation in the context of blood flow measurements*

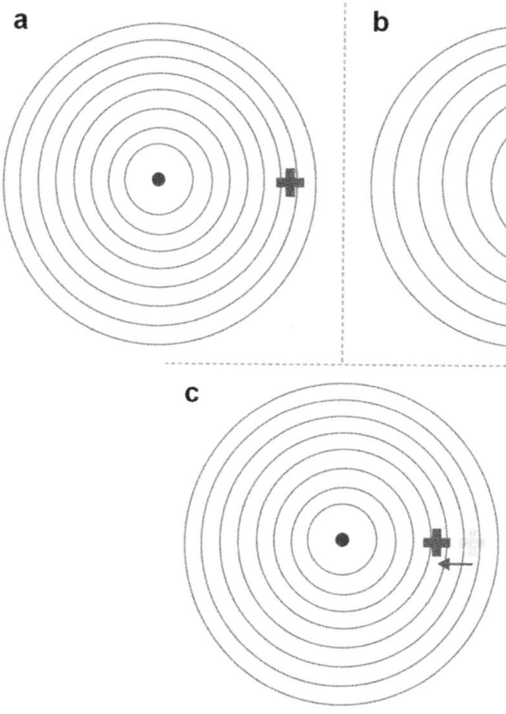

Figure 4.1. *The Doppler effect. (a) When both the source (red dot) and the target (blue cross) are stationary, the perceived frequency (with acoustic wavefronts represented by gray circles) is the same as that emitted by the source. (b) When the source is moving towards the stationary target, the frequency perceived by the target is higher than the emitted frequency because perceived acoustic wavelength is shortened. (c) When the target is moving towards the stationary source, the perceived frequency is also higher because the effective wave propagation speed is increased for the same acoustic wavelength*

The Doppler effect is named after Christian Doppler, who first discovered the phenomenon in 1842 (White 1982). In general, this effect refers to a motion-induced change in the perceived wave frequency. For the case of a source moving towards a stationary target, the perceived acoustic frequency at the target is shifted up from the frequency emitted by the source. Fundamentally, as illustrated in Figure 4.1(b), this frequency upshift is attributed to a change in the perceived wavelength as acoustic wavefronts propagate to the target over a shorter period due to the source's motion. For a single source moving directly towards the target with a speed of v_s, the frequency perceived by the target (f_{new}) is given by:

$$f_{new} = \frac{c_o}{\lambda_{new}} = \frac{c_o}{\lambda_o - v_s T_o} = \frac{c_o}{c_o / f_o - v_s / f_o} = \frac{c_o}{c_o - v_s} f_o \quad [4.1]$$

where c_o is the ultrasound wave propagation speed, f_o is the original ultrasound frequency of the source, λ_{new} is the new wavelength perceived by the target, λ_o is the original wavelength and T_o is the wave period, which equals $1/f_o$. Note that if the source is moving away from the target, the signage of v_s would become negative, thus resulting in a lower perceived frequency according to [4.1]. In the more general case where the source is moving at an angle ϑ with respect to the target, the new frequency can be expressed as follows because only the component of the source velocity directly towards or away from the target will result in a change of the frequency perceived by the target:

$$f_{new} = \frac{c_o}{c_o - v_s \cos\theta} f_o \quad [4.2]$$

In relation to the Doppler effect, a similar frequency shift phenomenon also occurs for a moving target and a stationary source. As illustrated in Figure 4.1(c) for a target moving towards a stationary source, the target would intersect with acoustic wavefronts more frequently, because the target's motion corresponds to an additive factor that changes the effective wave propagation speed. In this case, for a single target speed v_t, the frequency perceived by the target is given by:

$$f_{new} = \frac{c_{new}}{\lambda_o} = \frac{c_o + v_t}{c_o / f_o} = \frac{c_o + v_t}{c_o} f_o \quad [4.3]$$

where c_{new} is the ultrasound wave speed perceived by the moving target. If the target is moving at an angle φ with respect to the source, then the new frequency would become:

$$f_{new} = \frac{c_o + v_t \cos\phi}{c_o} f_o \quad [4.4]$$

Let us now consider the typical scenario in CW Doppler ultrasound measurements, where a pair of transducers (one for transmission and one for reception) are both stationary, but RBC scatterers are moving within the vasculature. This scenario is illustrated in Figure 4.2. In this case, two separate Doppler events arise. The first corresponds to the shift perceived by an RBC moving with a velocity of v in response to the incident ultrasound wave emitted by the stationary transmitting transducer. For the first Doppler event, the new frequency (f_1) can be found from [4.4]. The second Doppler event arises from the fact that the moving RBC scatterer effectively acts as a moving source when it backscatters incident ultrasound waves to the stationary receiving transducer. For this second Doppler event, the source frequency is equal to f_1 (i.e. the frequency perceived by the RBC scatterer from the first Doppler event); the resulting frequency detected at the stationary receiver (f_2), which is due to the motion of the RBC scatterer source moving with a velocity v, can be found from [4.2], wherein f_o is set to be equal to f_1. Mathematically, f_2 can be derived to be equal to:

$$f_2 = \frac{c_o}{c_o - v\cos\theta} f_1 = \frac{c_o + v\cos\phi}{c_o - v\cos\theta} f_o \qquad [4.5]$$

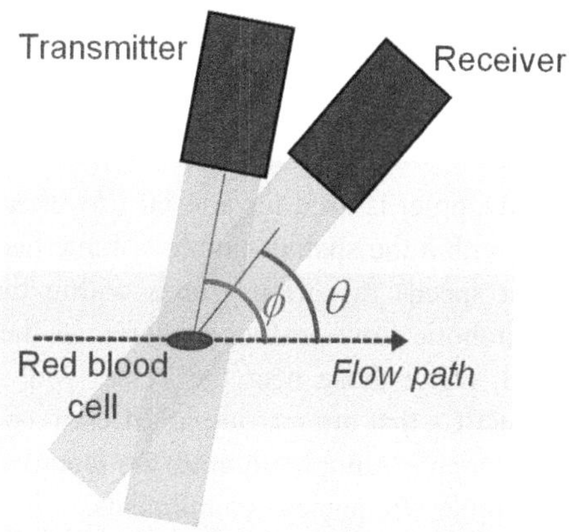

Figure 4.2. *General configuration for CW Doppler ultrasound measurements. Two transducers are used: 1) transmitter with a beam-to-flow angle of φ and 2) receiver with a beam-to-flow angle of ϑ. The RBC moves along the flow path with velocity v*

From [4.5], we can proceed to derive the Doppler equation that describes the total extent of frequency change (often referred to as the Doppler shift, f_D) resulting from the two Doppler events in the typical CW Doppler ultrasound measurement scenario. Specifically, the Doppler equation can be found to be equal to:

$$f_D = f_2 - f_o = \frac{v(\cos\theta + \cos\phi)}{c_o - v\cos\theta} f_o \qquad [4.6]$$

In practice, the ultrasound wave speed (approximately 1,500 m/s) is much greater than the RBC scatterer's speed within the vasculature (typically less than 2 m/s). As such, the denominator of [4.6] can be approximated as c_o, and we arrive at the more common form of the CW Doppler equation:

$$f_D \approx \frac{v(\cos\theta + \cos\phi)}{c_o} f_o \qquad [4.7]$$

4.1.3. *Practical implementations and considerations*

From an instrumentation standpoint, two transducers are needed to realize CW Doppler ultrasound. They are usually housed in a single probe, within which the transmitting and receiving transducers are positioned at an angle with respect to each other, as illustrated in Figure 4.2. The angled transducer pair is positioned to create a crossover region that corresponds to the device's spatial sample volume (Whittingham 2007). Such a crossover region tends to span at least a few mm in each spatial direction, and it can be even wider if unfocused transducers are used for ultrasound transmission and reception.

In practice, when CW Doppler is used for arterial flow measurement, a range of Doppler shifts is detected within the spatial sample volume because RBC scatterers typically flow at different speeds in various zones within the vessel lumen. For example, for a laminar parabolic flow profile, scatterers at the center of the artery move at the fastest speed, while those near the vessel wall advance much more slowly. Thus, when these RBCs that are moving at different speeds are interrogated simultaneously within the Doppler sample volume, the Doppler frequency spectrum contains a range of Doppler frequency components. The maximum Doppler frequency in this range corresponds to the fastest flow velocity which, for parabolic flow, represents the speed of the RBCs that are flowing the most swiftly along the central axis of the artery. Note that, in addition to spatial variations, Doppler frequency may vary temporally in pulsatile flow scenarios where the flow velocity at different spatial locations within the vessel lumen changes over time. As such, for different temporal measurement windows, the range of detected Doppler shifts may vary according to the temporal phase of the pulsatile flow profile.

One important issue that arises in practical CW Doppler measurements is that the acquired Doppler echoes can be contaminated by movement detected from tissue scatterers outside of the vessel lumen that are within the spatial sample volume of the transducer pair. Since tissue scatterers typically yield stronger echoes than RBC scatterers (as stated in section 4.1.1), tissue echoes tend to dominate the acquired Doppler echoes in magnitude, thus inevitably masking out the RBC echoes. Tissue echoes are often referred to as Doppler clutter, because they are generally undesired from a CW Doppler-based blood flow measurement standpoint. Fortunately, given that tissue motion is generally limited and is comparatively much slower than blood flow, tissue clutter tends to yield low Doppler frequency characteristics. Therefore, RBC signals may still be extracted for Doppler shift estimation purposes by suppressing tissue echoes via high-pass filtering (Evans and McDicken 2000). Note that, when CW Doppler ultrasound is applied specifically to track cardiac motion dynamics, no clutter filtering operation is performed in order to preserve the cardiac tissue echoes.

4.1.4. *Output format and applications*

Diagnostic information derived from CW Doppler ultrasound is typically presented in the form of a spectrogram. A spectrogram is a frequency–time plot that shows the measured Doppler shifts along the vertical axis and time along the horizontal axis. An example of a CW Doppler spectrogram is shown in Figure 4.3 for a scenario with pulsatile flow dynamics sampled over five cardiac cycles.

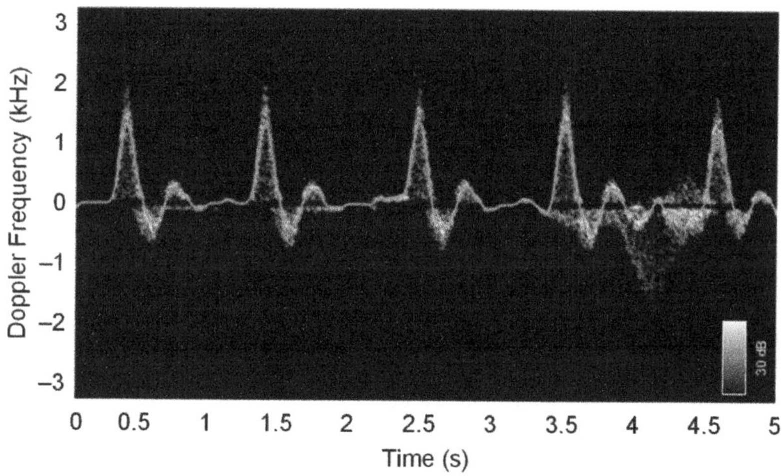

Figure 4.3. *Doppler spectrogram of blood flow in the femoral artery of a human subject over five cardiac cycles. At each time point, the range of detected Doppler shifts is depicted as grayscale pixels (with a 30 dB dynamic range in this example). The mean Doppler frequency time trace is also shown in green*

As shown in this figure, the range of detected Doppler shifts varies over different observation time windows. For each cardiac cycle, larger Doppler shift magnitudes are detected during systole when flow is fastest, while smaller Doppler shifts are detected during diastole when flow is slower. As such, for pulsatile flow, the appearance of a Doppler spectrogram would show periodic fluctuations between high and low Doppler frequency contents. Note that the Doppler frequency axis can be readily converted into a flow velocity axis via the Doppler equation shown in [4.7] if the ultrasound wave speed (c_o), the ultrasound frequency (f_o) and the beam-to-flow angles (θ and φ) are known or are presumed to have nominal values.

On CW Doppler devices, the Doppler shift information can be played on speakers in the form of stereo audio since the detected Doppler shifts tend to fall within the human audible range (i.e. between 20 and 20,000 Hz). Consider a numerical example. Suppose the speed of sound is 1,500 m/s, and we are using a pair of 5 MHz ultrasound transducers for CW transmission and reception (angled at 90° and 75°, respectively, relative to the flow direction). If blood flow velocity ranges from 0 to 2 m/s in the artery of interest, with flow moving towards the transducer, then the corresponding maximum Doppler frequency would be equal to 1,725 Hz according to [4.7]. Note that negative Doppler shifts may be detected if blood is flowing away from the transducer pair's beam axes. Accordingly, the positive and negative Doppler frequency contents may be separately broadcasted through the left and right channels of a stereo audio stream.

Perhaps, the most representative clinical application of CW Doppler ultrasound is fetal monitoring. Here, the operational goal is to non-invasively search for, and subsequently monitor, a fetus' beating heart using Doppler ultrasound principles. This diagnostic task is not at all straightforward, because the fetal heart's position inside the mother's womb is unknown. Thus, it is hard to ensure that the beam crossover region of a CW Doppler transducer pair encompasses the fetal heart. To help overcome this challenge, the CW Doppler device used for fetal monitoring may be specially designed so that the CW Doppler transducers have unfocused, diverging beams (Whittingham 2007). This configuration provides a very broad crossover region for the transducer pair to provide a large spatial sample volume. In addition to using unfocused transducers, multiple receiving transducers may be used so that multiple beam crossover regions can be generated to further increase the chance of detecting the cardiac dynamics of the fetus.

4.2. Pulsed Doppler

Instead of using continuous ultrasound waves, ultrasound pulses may be used to perform blood flow measurements. This second approach, commonly referred to as pulsed Doppler ultrasound, works via a multi-pulse-echo-sensing mechanism in which blood flow velocities are estimated from time-of-flight changes between consecutive pulse echoes. It is of interest to note that pulsed Doppler ultrasound does not make use of the classical Doppler effect during its operation (to be discussed further in section 4.2.4). Therefore, the name of this technique is, strictly speaking, a misnomer, although some consider the motion-induced inter-pulse time-of-flight change phenomenon to be an alternate form of the Doppler effect in the broad sense (Cobbold 2007; Chapter 10).

4.2.1. *Principles of pulse-echo sensing of blood flow*

Let us consider further why ultrasound pulse-echo sensing can be used to derive blood flow velocity estimates. Figure 4.4(a) shows a diagram of a single RBC scatterer traveling along the blood vessel at a velocity v that is being interrogated by an ultrasound beam positioned at a beam-to-flow angle ϑ. The ultrasound pulses are repeatedly emitted from the transducer at a pulse repetition interval T_{PRI}. Between two pulsing events, the scatterer has an inter-pulse displacement z_D towards the transducer. From the basic kinematics relation between velocity, displacement and time, z_D is equal to the following:

$$z_D = (v\cos\theta)T_{PRI} = vT_{PRI}\cos\theta \qquad [4.8]$$

The inter-pulse displacement in [4.8] would consequently yield an inter-pulse difference in the two-way time of flight. Note that, for a given speed of sound c_o, the two-way time of flight of pulse echoes is given by the well-known relation $2z/c_o$ (Yu 2018), so the inter-pulse time-of-flight change induced by a moving scatterer can be mathematically expressed as:

$$\Delta t = \frac{2z_D}{c_o} = \frac{2vT_{PRI}}{c_o}\cos\theta \qquad [4.9]$$

This time shift phenomenon between sequential pulse echoes is illustrated in Figure 4.4(b). Since each ultrasound pulse can essentially be considered as a time-windowed sinusoidal pulse with wave frequency f_o, the inter-pulse time-of-flight change shown in [4.9] naturally gives rise to an inter-echo phase change at the same time of reference on the echo time axis. Specifically, in each subsequent pulsing event, the scatterer's pulse echo (with frequency f_o) arrives at a time that is Δt earlier compared to the previous pulse echo. Hence, for the same time of reference (marked by the vertical dashed line in Figure 4.4(b)), the echo's phase changes slightly between pulses.

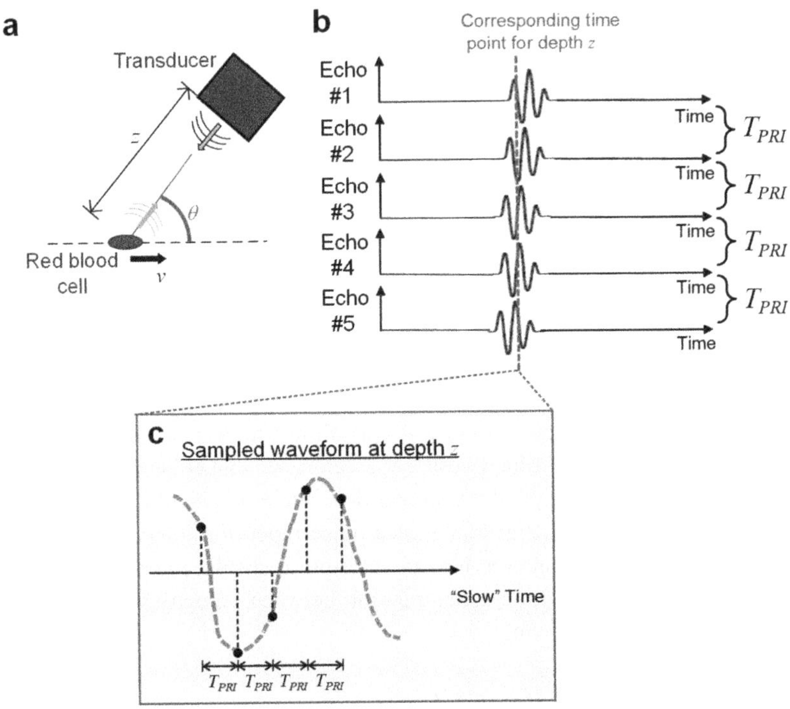

Figure 4.4. *Principles of pulsed Doppler ultrasound. (a) The pulse-echo sensing scenario for an RBC located at a depth z moving at a velocity v with a beam-to-flow angle of ϑ. (b) Due to the RBC's inter-pulse displacement, its echo undergoes a time shift between pulses. (c) Sampling each pulse echo at the same time of reference corresponding to depth z yields a sampled waveform that is known as the pulsed Doppler signal*

In interpreting the multi-pulse, moving scatterer echo-sensing scenario shown in Figure 4.4(a), one important point worth emphasizing is that the relative start time of each echo is synchronized to be identical, such that the pulse-echo time axis is temporally aligned for all echoes, as shown in Figure 4.4(b). In between each instance of the pulse-echo time axis in Figure 4.4(b), there is a lapsed time of one pulse repetition period, i.e. T_{PRI}. In this context, the pulse-echo time axis (i.e. the intra-pulse time axis) is typically referred to as the fast-time axis. The rationale of indicating this time axis as fast time is that the nominal duration of an ultrasound pulse, for typical ultrasound frequencies used for Doppler applications (e.g. 5 MHz), is usually at most on the order of a few μs, which is characteristically shorter than the pulse repetition period (typically hundreds of μs).

4.2.2. *The concept of slow-time sampling*

In pulsed Doppler ultrasound, blood flow velocity is derived by measuring the inter-pulse phase change at a desired fast-time point that corresponds to the axial depth of interest (based on the $z = c_o t_{echo}/2$ two-way time-of-flight relation). To realize this task, as illustrated in Figure 4.4(c), an alternative, sampled time axis is formed by extracting each echo's desired fast-time point of interest t_{echo} and remapping them in absolute time, such that the adjacent sampled time points differ in absolute time by T_{PRI}. This sampled time axis is referred to as the slow-time axis, since T_{PRI} is much longer than the ultrasound pulse duration. Slow-time sampling is then performed to obtain one sample from each pulse echo at the corresponding fast-time point. Accordingly, an ensemble of extracted pulse-echo samples is collected from multiple pulse-echo sensing events (one sample for each event). This ensemble is commonly known as the pulsed Doppler signal. Its sampling period is equal to T_{PRI}. As shown in Figure 4.4(c), the pulsed Doppler signal exhibits oscillatory characteristics as a result of the inter-pulse phase change induced by the RBC scatterer's inter-pulse displacement.

Flow velocity information can be obtained from analyzing the frequency of the pulsed Doppler signal, i.e. the slow-time frequency, or the pulsed Doppler frequency. This frequency entity emerges because of the motion-induced, inter-pulse phase change. To derive a mathematical expression for slow-time frequency based on inter-pulse phase change, let us first recall that, for each sinusoidal pulse echo, the analytic form is essentially an amplitude-modulated complex sinusoid, in which the echo's phase corresponds to the phase of the complex sinusoid term $\exp(2\pi f_o t_{echo})$. If, in between two pulse firings, the RBC scatterer has moved by z_D, the two corresponding adjacent pulsed Doppler signal samples will carry a phase difference equal to:

$$\Delta\phi = 2\pi f_o \Delta t = 2\pi f_o \left(\frac{2z_D}{c_o} \right) = 2\pi f_o \left(\frac{2vT_{PRI}}{c_o} \cos\theta \right) \qquad [4.10]$$

where the expression in [4.9] has been substituted into the above for $\frac{2z_D}{c_0}$.

Since it is well known that frequency is defined as the time rate of phase change divided by 2π, the frequency that corresponds to this inter-pulse phase change is equal to the following:

$$f_D = \frac{1}{2\pi}\frac{\Delta\phi}{T_{PRI}} = \frac{f_o}{T_{PRI}}\left(\frac{2vT_{PRI}}{c_o}\cos\theta\right) = \frac{2vf_o}{c_o}\cos\theta \qquad [4.11]$$

which is commonly known as the pulsed Doppler equation. Note that, in [4.11], the time rate of phase change is equal to $\Delta\varphi/T_{PRI}$ because inter-pulse phase change ($\Delta\varphi$) happens over a period of T_{PRI}. Also, f_D is essentially the pulsed Doppler frequency, and it is directly proportional to RBC scatterer velocity v.

4.2.3. *Practical implementation*

Pulsed Doppler ultrasound presents flow velocity information in the form of a Doppler spectrogram, as already described for CW Doppler's output format in section 4.1.4. In many clinical ultrasound systems that use array transducers for scanning, the pulsed Doppler mode is implemented as a feature that is displayed together with brightness-mode (B-mode) ultrasound imaging. To obtain this duplex mode, both pulsed Doppler and B-mode imaging are performed in sequence. For this process, the same array transducer can be used because the two modes are both based on pulse-echo sensing (Whittingham 2007). Note that, unlike CW Doppler, pulsed Doppler estimations can be made using a single transducer that serves as both the transmit-pulsing transducer and the echo-receiving transducer.

During the duplex mode's operation, real-time B-mode imaging is performed to allow the sonographer to navigate within the field of view and define the range gate position (i.e. the lateral and axial positions of interest in the field of view where Doppler information is to be acquired). The B-mode imaging process is essentially a multi-scanline pulse-echo sensing process in which one instance of pulse-echo sensing is performed over each scanline (Yu 2018). Once the range gate has been set with the help of B-mode imaging, the system switches to a pulsed Doppler mode to perform multi-pulse-echo-sensing at the position of a single scanline at the range gate's lateral position. For this process, slow-time sampling is performed at the range gate's axial position to derive the pulsed Doppler signal used to calculate spectrograms that show pulsed Doppler frequencies (or flow velocities) measured over different time points. Note that, for each time instant in the spectrogram, the Doppler frequencies are computed over an observational time window that spans multiple pulse-echo sensing events (e.g. 128 events).

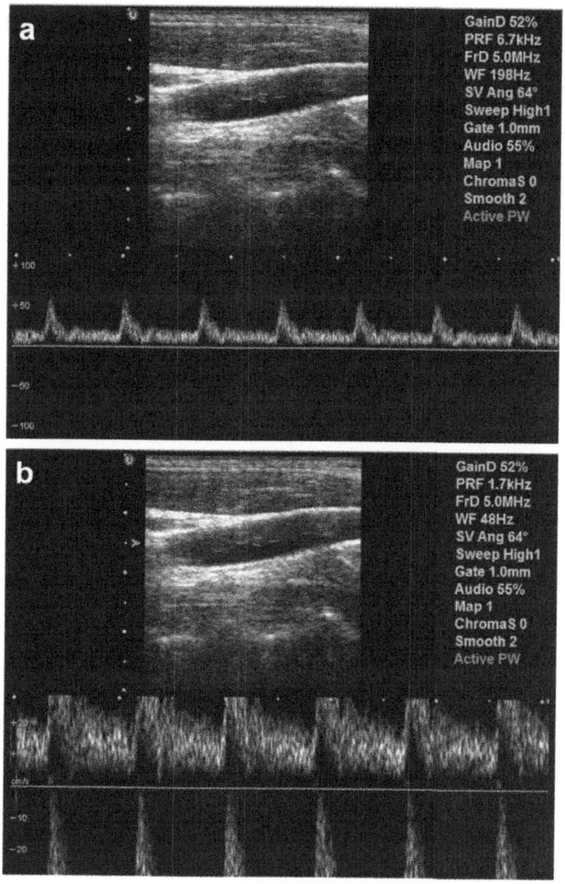

Figure 4.5. *Duplex display of the B-mode image and pulsed Doppler spectrogram obtained from a clinical scanner (SonixTouch). This example shows pulsatile flow in a human common carotid artery over seven cardiac cycles. Images are shown for two pulse repetition frequencies: (a) 6.7 kHz and (b) 1.7 kHz (for which aliasing occurred)*

Figure 4.5 shows an example of the output from a clinical scanner's duplex mode with both ultrasound image guidance in B-mode and the Doppler spectrogram. As can be observed, the duplex mode's spectrogram appearance is essentially the same as that shown in Figure 4.3. On clinical ultrasound scanners, pulsed Doppler information is concurrently played back as an audio output since Doppler frequencies are within the human audible range. The rationale for such an audio rendering is similar to the one for CW Doppler ultrasound (see section 4.1.4 for a numerical example).

4.2.4. Technical considerations: aliasing and Doppler resolution

From a signal processing perspective, pulsed Doppler ultrasound involves slow-time sampling to derive the pulsed Doppler signal. The slow-time sampling frequency (f_{PRF}) is equal to the reciprocal of the pulse repetition period (i.e. $1/T_{PRI}$). It is well known from the Nyquist theorem in signal processing that aliasing occurs if a signal is insufficiently sampled. Specifically, aliasing arises when the sampling rate is lower than twice the maximum frequency of the signal to detect. Due to aliasing, high-frequency components in the signal's original frequency spectrum would emerge spuriously as low-frequency components.

In the context of pulsed Doppler, aliasing occurs when f_{PRF} is too low or when flow is too fast. The minimum f_{PRF} can be found from the Nyquist theorem to be equal to:

$$f_{PRF(\min)} = 2 f_{D(\max)} \quad \Rightarrow \quad f_{PRF} \geq \frac{4 v_{\max} f_o}{c_o} \cos\theta \qquad [4.12]$$

where $f_{D(\max)}$ is the maximum Doppler frequency induced by blood flow, and the pulsed Doppler equation in [4.11] has been used to obtain the expression on the right hand side of [4.12]. As a numerical example, consider a pulsed Doppler scenario with a 5 MHz ultrasound frequency, a 70° beam-flow angle, a 1,500 m/s ultrasound wave speed and a 60 cm/s peak systolic flow speed. Applying [4.11], $f_{D(\max)}$ in this case is equal to 1.368 kHz. According to [4.12], f_{PRF} must be set to be greater than 2.736 kHz in order to avoid Doppler aliasing. As shown in Figure 4.5(a), for a case with an f_{PRF} of 6.7 kHz, the Doppler spectrogram can depict the artery's pulsatile flow pattern as expected. On the other hand, as shown in Figure 4.5(b), when the f_{PRF} is reduced to 1.7 kHz, the resulting Doppler spectrogram becomes unintuitive because aliasing occurs during systole (in general, the part of the cardiac cycle resulting in the fastest blood flow speeds). Flow during the systolic phase of the cardiac cycle has been incorrectly rendered as slow flow moving in the reversed direction. This issue can make it inherently more difficult for sonographers to properly interpret Doppler spectrograms derived from pulsed Doppler ultrasound.

Doppler resolution is another important consideration that is related to the sampled nature of the pulsed Doppler signal. Well-established in digital signal processing, the frequency bin size of a sampled signal's discrete-time Fourier transform essentially corresponds to the uncertainty range of the signal's frequency spectrum. In the context of pulsed Doppler, the frequency bin size defines the minimum detectable slow-time frequency and, in turn, governs whether slow flow can be detected. Note that a signal spectrum's frequency bin size is simply equal to the sampling rate divided by the number of samples in the signal ensemble. As such, the Doppler resolution can be mathematically expressed as:

$$f_{D(res)} = \frac{f_{PRF}}{N} \qquad [4.13]$$

where N is the number of samples in the pulsed Doppler signal ensemble.

Based on [4.13], a finer Doppler resolution (i.e. a lower detectable pulsed Doppler frequency) can be achieved either by using a smaller f_{PRF} or by acquiring more data samples. A numerical example is provided here to illustrate this relation. Suppose f_{PRF} is set to 5 kHz and 200 samples are available in each pulsed Doppler ensemble. The corresponding Doppler resolution is 25 Hz according to [4.13]. By substituting this value into [4.11], we can find that the minimum detectable flow velocity is equal to 1.1 cm/s, which may not be sufficient to detect micro-vascular flow. In contrast, if f_{PRF} is reduced to 3 kHz and each pulsed Doppler ensemble comprises 500 samples, then the Doppler resolution improves to 6 Hz and the minimum detectable flow velocity is 2.6 mm/s. This latter combination of f_{PRF} and N has improved slow flow detection capability.

4.2.5. *CW Doppler versus pulsed Doppler*

When comparing the principles of pulsed Doppler and CW Doppler, some similarities and differences can be readily noted. One obvious similarity is that both Doppler modes have an almost identical governing equation – i.e. [4.11] versus [4.7] – that relates Doppler frequency f_D to flow velocity v. The two equations become identical when $\vartheta = \varphi$ in [4.7]. Physically, the condition of $\vartheta = \varphi$ denotes that the beam-flow angle remains the same during both transmission and reception. It indeed corresponds well to the situation in pulsed Doppler ultrasound, given that the same transducer which yields a single beam-flow angle is used for both transmission and reception. Pulsed Doppler and CW Doppler also have similarities at the output level. Specifically, both use spectrograms as the main form of display to depict time-varying frequency shifts (or flow velocities) as a function of time (see sections 4.1.4 and 4.2.3). Furthermore, as supplementary output, the two Doppler ultrasound modes can audibly play the detected frequency shifts as stereo audio.

In terms of differences, from a theoretical standpoint, pulsed Doppler and CW Doppler rely on fundamentally different physical phenomena. The classical Doppler effect is at the core of the CW Doppler estimation (section 4.1.2), while pulsed Doppler is based on multi-pulse-echo-sensing (section 4.2.1) and slow-time sampling (section 4.2.2). Another salient point worth noting about pulsed Doppler estimation is that it is susceptible to aliasing (section 4.2.4) that can obscure the appearance of high-flow data in the resulting Doppler spectrogram. This is the biggest disadvantage of pulsed Doppler. In contrast, aliasing generally does not arise in CW Doppler.

One operational advantage of pulsed Doppler is its ability to specify the range gate position. In contrast, CW Doppler has limited spatial resolvability because it can only passively discern the spatial origin of Doppler echoes based on the nominal sample volume created from the beam crossover region of the transmitting and receiving transducers (section 4.1.3). If unfocused beams are used, as is often the case in practical CW Doppler applications (section 4.1.4), the sample volume can span across a broad spatial range. Under such conditions, it becomes difficult to specifically distinguish where Doppler echoes emerge, since the acquired CW Doppler signal is simply a superposition of Doppler echoes from all scatterers within the sample volume. Pulsed Doppler can effectively avoid this issue by allowing the sonographer to select the range gate's lateral and axial positions (section 4.2.3). On a signal processing level, this position-localization task works by forming the pulsed Doppler signal from multi-pulse-echo data that includes only the fast-time points that match the axial depth of interest and then performing slow-time frequency analysis on the pulsed Doppler signal (section 4.2.2).

From an instrumentation standpoint, pulsed Doppler is easier to implement in that it does not require application-specific transducer design. Indeed, it is possible to integrate pulsed Doppler with B-mode imaging on the same system since no separate transducer design is needed (section 4.2.3). In contrast, CW Doppler must use a pair of angled transducers for transmission and reception. Accordingly, the transducer design approach for CW Doppler is different from that used for ultrasound imaging based on pulse-echo sensing (section 4.1.3).

4.3. Color flow imaging (CFI)

Since CW Doppler and pulsed Doppler only measure blood flow velocities at a single spatial location, they inherently cannot depict flow information over the entire field of view. While we can argue that, with pulsed Doppler, flow dynamics in different parts of the field of view may be measured by manually moving the range gate position, this strategy is inefficient from a clinical workflow perspective since the spatial flow profile throughout the entire field of view cannot be visualized within a single image snapshot. There is, therefore, a practical need for a high-level flow visualization tool that allows sonographers to obtain an overall picture of blood flow pattern within a field of view, in real time. This need prompted the development of CFI: an ultrasound-based flow mapping modality that makes use of pulsed Doppler principles.

4.3.1. *An extension from single-gate pulsed Doppler*

In principle, CFI can be regarded as an extension of pulsed Doppler ultrasound at a single range gate. Specifically, this flow mapping modality seeks to perform multi-pulse-echo sensing over all the scanlines in the field of view. For each scanline, slow-time sampling is performed individually at different axial depth positions. In turn, pulsed Doppler data acquisition is performed over a spatial grid of range gates to form a spatial map of flow information. The pulsed Doppler signal obtained for each range gate is reduced to one color pixel depicting local flow in the CFI frame. This drastically reduces the level of flow information displayed relative to single-gate pulsed Doppler spectrograms, which provide the detected Doppler frequencies (or flow velocities) as a function of time over a single range gate.

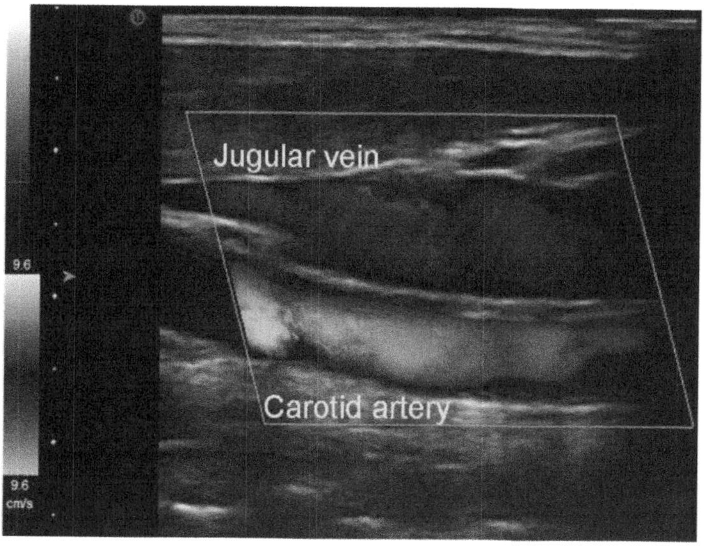

Figure 4.6. *Color flow image of a human carotid artery and jugular vein during cardiac diastole. The red–blue color codes, which depict bidirectional flow in blood vessels, are overlaid onto the B-mode image that renders anatomical information*

CFI can be implemented as a duplex feature together with B-mode imaging. Figure 4.6 shows an example of a duplex CFI frame presenting the common carotid artery and the jugular vein. Here, the color pixels of the CFI frame are overlaid on top of the B-mode image background that depicts anatomical information. In clinical ultrasound scanners, CFI frames are shown via the use of a hot–cold color map, in which the hot (red) and cold (blue) hues, respectively, depict flow in different directions. This bicolored flow visualization strategy is useful for identifying arteries and veins when arterial and venous flow moves in opposite directions within the same field of view.

4.3.2. *Principles of color pixel estimation*

From a signal processing perspective, a core operation in CFI is the derivation of one color pixel for each range gate in the map grid. The pulsed Doppler signal ensemble for each range gate has frequency characteristics that vary in time and that are related to flow velocities according to the pulsed Doppler equation in [4.11]. To reduce this time-varying range of Doppler frequency contents to one representative value describing the local flow pattern, one popular solution is to extract the mean Doppler frequency which is considered to be a quantitative indicator of local flow. From the mean Doppler frequency estimate, the mean flow velocity for each range gate can be derived by applying the pulsed Doppler equation in [4.11]. This estimation procedure is performed individually for each range gate to derive mean flow velocity values over the entire spatial grid of range gates. Note that, before the mean Doppler frequency estimation, clutter filtering (Yu et al. 2007) needs to be applied to each pulsed Doppler ensemble to suppress unwanted tissue echoes that may emerge locally at each individual range gate (akin to what has been described in section 4.1.3).

The mean Doppler frequency for CFI can be found by dividing the first-order Doppler spectral moment by the zeroth-order Doppler spectral moment (Jensen 2007). This computation theoretically requires the calculation of the Fourier transform of the pulsed Doppler signal. However, in practice, it is not necessary to explicitly carry out frequency-domain calculations. As first demonstrated for CFI in the 1980s (Kasai et al. 1985), the mean Doppler frequency can be found by calculating the lag-one autocorrelation phase of the pulsed Doppler signal. This principle is rooted in the Wiener–Khinchin relation, which states that the autocorrelation function of a signal is equivalent to the inverse Fourier transform of the signal's power spectral density (Moon and Stirling 2000). Using this relation, and by recognizing certain properties of the autocorrelation function in its analytic form, the mean Doppler frequency can be presented in analytic form for a pulsed Doppler signal ensemble with N samples (Evans and McDicken 2000) as:

$$\bar{f}_D = \frac{f_{PRF}}{2\pi}\arg\{R(1)\} \quad \text{for } R(1) = \sum_{k=1}^{N-1} s^*(k)s(k+1) \qquad [4.14]$$

where $R(1)$ denotes the pulsed Doppler signal's autocorrelation value with a one-sample lag, $s(k)$ refers to the kth Doppler signal sample in the ensemble and the superscript * denotes the complex conjugate. An illustration of this mean frequency estimation algorithm is shown in Figure 4.7. By inspection of [4.14], each mean Doppler frequency estimate mainly requires the calculation of the phase of the sum of the product between the conjugated Doppler signal ensemble and its lag-one form. This calculation is quite straightforward to implement, and thus the lag-one autocorrelation phase algorithm is highly popular for CFI implementation.

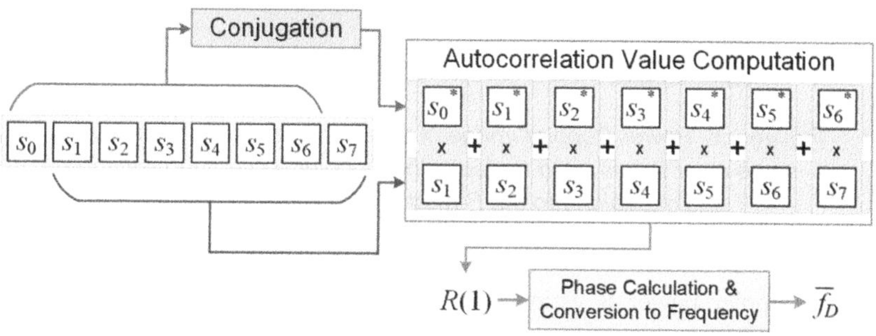

Figure 4.7. *Illustration of the lag-one autocorrelation phase algorithm for mean frequency estimation for a Doppler signal ensemble with N=8 samples* $\{s_0, s_1, \ldots, s_7\}$. *The algorithm computes the lag-one autocorrelation value* $R(1)$ *as the scalar product between the first N-1 samples (complex conjugate form) and the last N-1 samples. Mean frequency is then calculated as the phase of* $R(1)$ *multiplied by* $f_{PRF}/2\pi$

4.3.3. *Doppler power estimation and mapping*

For the CFI frame shown in Figure 4.6, a color pixel is shown only if the flow is deemed to be present locally within the corresponding range gate. Otherwise, only the B-mode grayscale image pixel is depicted for the location. This thresholding strategy, known as the color gain, is typically based on each range gate's detected Doppler power, which is mathematically defined as follows:

$$P_D = \frac{1}{N}\sum_{k=1}^{N}|s(k)|^2 \quad [4.15]$$

The calculation in [4.15] presumes that tissue clutter has been suppressed beforehand, because, to detect flow accurately, it is critical to perform clutter filtering on the pulsed Doppler signal ensemble before performing the power estimation calculations. Note that Doppler power is largely independent of the beam-flow angle and the pulsed Doppler equation, so this quantity is not correlated with flow velocity.

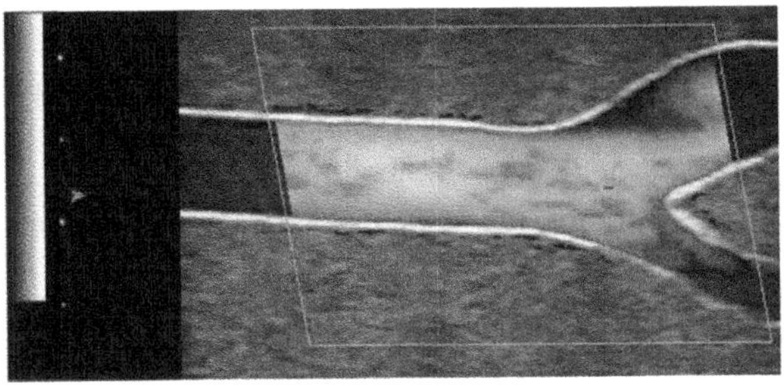

Figure 4.8. *Power Doppler image of a carotid bifurcation model. The same color hue is used to depict the Doppler power map, which is overlaid onto the B-mode background image*

Since Doppler power is estimated for color gain thresholding purposes, it is readily available for mapping in an alternate CFI modality displaying the Doppler power estimates instead of the mean Doppler frequency (or mean flow velocity). An example of a Doppler power map is shown in Figure 4.8. In this map, only one color hue is used since Doppler power does not give directional flow information. At large beam-flow angles, the Doppler power map has a sensitivity advantage over the mean Doppler frequency (or mean flow velocity) map because the echo power returned from RBC scatterers is less dependent on the beam-flow angle, whereas the pulsed Doppler frequency is angle-dependent. On the other hand, the mean Doppler frequency map has the advantage of being able to provide directional flow information that is clinically important for the identification of arteries and veins. It should be emphasized that, since Doppler power is not influenced by flow velocity, the flow information rendered in a Doppler power map is only qualitative in nature. As such, Doppler power maps are mostly used for visualization purposes only.

4.3.4. *Imaging considerations*

Since CFI is intended to be a real-time imaging modality akin to B-mode imaging, it is expected to satisfy real-time imaging constraints. Accordingly, one question that can be asked is: "How many pulse-echo sensing events can be performed over each scanline whilst meeting the real-time requirement of at least 5–10 frames per second (fps)?" The need to maintain real-time frame rates is in competition with the objective to perform a large number of pulse-echo sensing events for the Doppler signal from each range gate in order to improve Doppler resolution according to [4.13].

Let us denote the number of pulse-echo sensing events per scanline as N (i.e. the same as the pulsed Doppler ensemble size) and the number of scanlines as L. The CFI frame acquisition time T_{CFI} can be written in terms of the transducer's pulse repetition interval T_{PRI} as follows:

$$T_{CFI} = T_{PRI} NL \quad \Rightarrow N = \frac{T_{CFI}}{T_{PRI} L} = \frac{f_{PRF}}{f_{CFI} L} \qquad [4.16]$$

This expression can be rewritten as on the right to express the number of Doppler signal samples in terms of the CFI frame rate, f_{CFI}, and the pulse repetition frequency, f_{PRF}. In practice, in order to obtain an f_{CFI} of at least 5–10 fps for real-time imaging, N in [4.16] is often forced to be fewer than 20 samples for an image with 30–60 scanlines (i.e. value of L between 30 and 60) and f_{PRF} in the kHz range. Consequently, the Doppler resolution is severely limited. Note that N is even smaller when imaging slow flow, since a smaller f_{PRF} must be used according to [4.13]. The use of interleaved scanline firing strategies can partly alleviate the Doppler resolution constraint by allowing a larger N to be used when using small f_{PRF} values (Ferrara and DeAngelis 1997), but it remains impossible for N to be larger than 20 in conventional CFI for typical fields of view if real-time imaging requirements are to be met.

As a numerical example, consider a carotid imaging scenario with 10 fps, 5 kHz pulse repetition frequency, and 50 scanlines. Substituting these parameters into [4.16], we get N to be equal to 10 (i.e. 10 pulse-echo sensing events for each scanline). Based on [4.13], the corresponding Doppler resolution is 500 Hz; it is much worse than the numerical examples presented for pulsed Doppler (section 4.2.4), which showed that a Doppler resolution of a few Hz was necessary to detect flow on the order of a few millimeters per second. To facilitate slow flow imaging in the abdomen, suppose the CFI frame rate and the pulse repetition frequency are, respectively, reduced to 5 MHz and 2 kHz. In this case, N would be equal to only 8 (i.e. 8 pulse-echo sensing events for each scanline), and the Doppler resolution would still be 250 Hz, which is not sufficient for the detection of mm/s flow rates. These examples show why CFI does not, in general, favor slow-flow detection for typical imaging parameters.

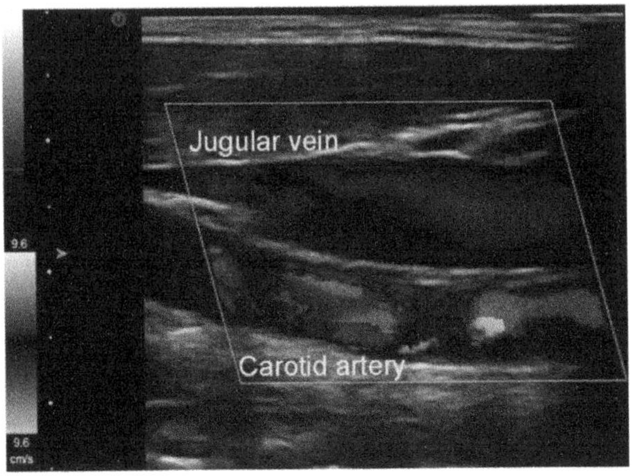

Figure 4.9. *An aliased color flow image of a human carotid artery and jugular vein during cardiac systole. In both the artery and the vein, red and blue color codes are present, which obscures flow visualization*

Since CFI uses a slow-time sampling process that is similar to that of pulsed Doppler, its mean Doppler frequency estimation operation is prone to aliasing, as described in section 4.2.4. Therefore, the value of f_{PRF} needs to be carefully chosen otherwise aliasing may occur. Figure 4.9 shows an example of a CFI frame (mean velocity map) with aliasing artifacts. As can be observed, in the presence of aliasing, fast flow beyond the Nyquist limit is spuriously depicted as a color pixel with the wrong color for the hot–cold bicolor hue mapping. Such aliasing significantly complexifies the image interpretation process for sonographers.

4.4. New flow mapping techniques

Aside from CW Doppler, pulsed Doppler and CFI, the ultrasound research community has continued to develop new flow measurement and mapping techniques. Four representative flow mapping innovations are briefly introduced here to highlight important research and development trends within this theme.

4.4.1. *B-flow imaging*

An alternative way for ultrasound to be used to derive flow information without using Doppler principles is to extract the acoustic speckle scattered from the blood in the field of view to track how RBC scatterers transit through the image over a stack of frames. This approach, commonly known as B-flow imaging (Chiao et al. 2000), relies on high frame refreshment rates to visualize RBC scatterer motion through the associated speckle. The image format, an example of which is shown in Figure 4.10, is based on grayscale rendering of Doppler signal power. Similar to CFI, it is possible to overlay B-flow speckle onto a B-mode background image for duplex display. B-flow speckle can even be overlaid onto CFI maps (Lovstakken et al. 2006). Note that B-flow imaging is a flow visualization tool and not a quantitative flow mapping technique.

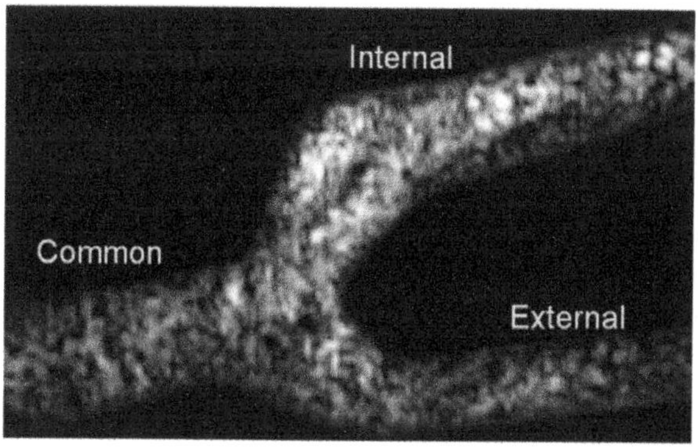

Figure 4.10. *B-flow image of a human carotid bifurcation phantom. The brightness displayed for grayscale speckles represents the Doppler signal power. Flow in the common carotid artery is bifurcated into the internal and external carotid artery branches*

B-flow speckle can be derived at each range gate by performing inter-frame high-pass filtering, which serves to suppress unwanted tissue echoes while preserving flow echoes. A simple example of such a high-pass filter is the first-order difference filter (i.e. the filter output is equal to the difference between two adjacent data samples in an ensemble). When this filter is applied to a range gate in the tissue region that remains stationary in between two pulse-echo sensing events, a zero filter output value is obtained since there are no inter-pulse phase changes (and thus consecutive Doppler echo samples remain constant). In contrast, when this filter is applied to a range gate within a flow region, the filter output becomes non-zero because of inter-pulse RBC scatterer displacement that in turn results in phase changes in the pulsed Doppler ensemble (see Figure 4.4). As such, in a B-flow image frame (without the overlay of B-mode background), dark pixels correspond to tissue range gates that remain stationary between frames, while bright pixels correspond to range gates within flow regions, as shown in Figure 4.10.

4.4.2. *Flow vector estimation*

In practical Doppler applications, the detected Doppler frequencies are usually converted into flow velocity values by applying the Doppler equation shown in [4.7] and [4.11] for the CW and pulsed modes, respectively. For this mapping between Doppler frequency and flow velocity to be accurate, one prerequisite that needs to be satisfied is that the other parameters in the Doppler equation (c_o, f_o, ϑ, φ) must be known quantities. Otherwise, the frequency-to-velocity conversion task becomes algebraically ambiguous in that there is more than one unknown for a single equation. In arterial flow measurement scenarios, c_o tends to remain relatively constant (i.e. ultrasound wave speed does not vary significantly within soft tissues), while f_o (i.e. ultrasound frequency) is a fixed parameter specified by the sonographer. However, arteries may exhibit tortuous geometries so that ϑ and φ (i.e. beam-flow angle) may be very different from one region to another. As such, assuming the beam-flow angle to be of a constant value (e.g. 60°), as is typically done in clinical Doppler measurements (Lui et al. 2005), may not be appropriate. There is a need to redesign the Doppler measurement approach to accommodate applications with multi-directional flow patterns.

Over the past decade, there has been an innovative thrust towards the design of ultrasound techniques that can estimate flow vectors that describe both the flow speed and the flow direction (Jensen et al. 2016). These techniques intend to avoid the angle uncertainty inherent in the Doppler equation when mapping between Doppler frequency and flow velocity. Flow vector estimation can be performed using several approaches. One of them, known as vector Doppler, seeks to perform Doppler sensing from more than one beam-flow angle to obtain multiple Doppler frequency measurands. By doing this, the flow vector can be estimated by setting up multiple instances of the Doppler equation and solving for both the velocity and angle within a multiple-equation, two-unknown mathematical framework (Yiu and Yu 2016). Alternatively, it is possible to intentionally create transverse oscillations in the field profile during beamforming to facilitate flow estimation in the lateral direction in addition to axial flow estimation (Udesen and Jensen 2006). Other non-Doppler methods such as speckle tracking (Bohs et al. 2000) and directional cross-correlation (Jensen 2003) have been developed to estimate flow vectors. Regardless of which flow vector computation method is used, they can all be used to generate vector flow maps that are useful for assessing complicated flow patterns, such as the flow disturbance at the carotid bifurcation. Some clinical scanners have already implemented vector flow imaging as a new modality, as demonstrated in recent clinical studies (Hansen et al. 2015).

4.4.3. *High-frame-rate flow imaging*

Although conventional Doppler ultrasound techniques (CW Doppler, pulsed Doppler and CFI) have enabled non-invasive flow measurement applications, they have fallen short of achieving time-resolved tracking of spatio-temporal flow dynamics over the entire field of view. In particular, the spectrograms acquired from CW Doppler and pulsed Doppler only show time-varying flow dynamics at a single range gate (or sample volume) in the field of view, and, fundamentally, they do not provide flow information at multiple spatial locations. On the other hand, CFI shows flow information over the entire field of view. However, its video-range frame rate (let us say 20 fps at best) does not yield adequate time resolution (at best 50 ms) to coherently track fast-changing flow dynamics occurring during different phases of the cardiac cycle.

In general, data acquisition time is the key factor that governs the CFI frame rate f_{CFI}. As shown in [4.16], f_{CFI} is directly proportional to the pulse repetition frequency f_{PRF} and inversely proportional to the number of firings N per line and the number of scanlines L. Thus, two apparent strategies to improve the frame rate are to decrease L and/or N. However, the first option narrows the width of the field of view and the second leads to a coarser Doppler resolution according to [4.13]. It could also be tempting to simply increase f_{PRF}, but doing so reduces the maximum imaging depth because the pulse repetition frequency is ultimately limited by the time of flight of pulse echoes, which is directly related to the maximum axial depth to be probed (Yu 2018).

To increase the CFI frame rate without concomitantly reducing the imaged view, it is critical to redefine the entire imaging paradigm by using alternative data acquisition strategies. One such approach is to merge all the transmit scanlines together by firing broad, unfocused beams on transmission using the plane-wave excitation principle and then simultaneously forming all the beamlines on receipt (Tanter and Fink 2014). Similarly, it is possible to adopt a zonal firing strategy on transmission and then perform parallel beamforming within each zone on receipt (Mo et al. 2003). Another way to perform fast data acquisition makes use of the synthetic transmit aperture technique. This method works by sequentially performing spherical firings from a set of point sources (Jensen and Nikolov 2004) so that CFI data can be acquired recursively, and the frame rate can theoretically approach the pulse repetition frequency (Nikolov and Jensen 2003).

Using unfocused transmission schemes, CFI frame rates of well above 1,000 fps have been achieved (Bercoff et al. 2011). High-frame-rate CFI has also been integrated with B-flow imaging (section 4.4.1) to form a new technique called color-encoded speckle imaging that offers simultaneous visualization of mean flow velocity estimates and flow speckle at over 1,000 fps (Yiu and Yu 2013). A sample frame of this new imaging technique is shown in Figure 4.11(a). Unfocused transmission schemes have been further harnessed to facilitate vector flow estimation and mapping (section 4.4.2) at high frame rates (Jensen and Oddershede 2006; Yiu et al. 2014). These new techniques have greatly enhanced the visualization of complex cardiovascular (Goddi et al. 2017; Au et al. 2020) and urinary tract (Ishii et al. 2017) flow fields. Figure 4.11(b) shows an example of a vector flow image of the femoral bifurcation obtained using high-frame-rate, unfocused imaging.

4.4.4. *Flow mapping in 3D*

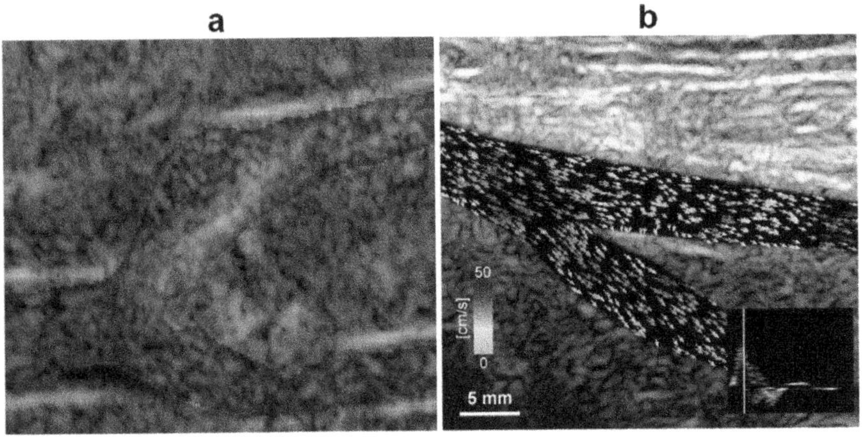

Figure 4.11. *Two high-frame-rate ultrasound flow imaging techniques: (a) color-encoded flow speckle imaging; (b) vector flow imaging*

From an imaging standpoint, CW Doppler and pulsed Doppler can be considered as single-point flow measurement modes in that they can acquire flow information at one spatial location in the field of view. The implementation of pulsed Doppler can potentially be modified to provide flow information over multiple range gates along the same scanline (Evans and McDicken 2000). Nonetheless, multi-gate pulsed Doppler is still merely a 1D flow mapping modality. On the other hand, the advent of CFI has effectively demonstrated the ability to use ultrasound to derive 2D maps of flow velocities. An important limitation remains, because these 2D flow maps only provide a single-plane snapshot of the more complex, three-dimensional flow patterns occurring within the arteries or veins. Out-of-plane flow that may be present over the image plane inherently cannot be tracked with 2D CFI.

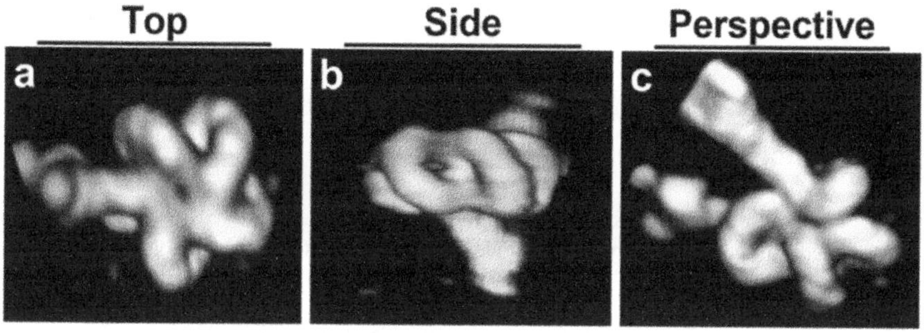

Figure 4.12. *3D color flow imaging of a helical toroid phantom from different graphical projections: (a) top, (b) side and (c) perspective*

It is possible to extend the formulation of CFI to the third dimension to generate 3D flow volumes (Fenster et al. 2001). In early studies, special transducer setups involving motorized sweeping of a 1D array transducer were devised to facilitate the acquisition of multiple slices of mono-planar CFI for 3D flow volume generation (Picot et al. 1993). Figure 4.12 shows an example of a 3D CFI volume obtained from a helical toroid flow phantom (Chee et al. 2021). The volume rate of this 3D flow imaging approach tends to be limited because of the need to mechanically sweep the array transducer. To overcome this issue, 2D array transducers have been developed to acquire data from volumetric flow using electronic beam steering (Christensen et al. 2015; Ramalli et al. 2015). Such an approach can readily provide real-time volumetric imaging rates. Indeed, the next generation of 3D ultrasound flow imaging technology focuses on incorporating high-frame-rate imaging principles (section 4.4.3) into the operation of 2D array transducers to obtain 3D flow volumes at a very rapid rate of over 1,000 volumes per second (Correia et al. 2016). There is also strong interest in deriving flow vectors (section 4.4.2) in a 3D space (Holbek et al. 2016).

4.5. Summary

Since its initial conceptualization, Doppler ultrasound has been widely used in clinical diagnosis. CW Doppler has found widespread use in fetal heart monitoring. Pulsed Doppler has been extensively adopted in many clinical ultrasound scanners to facilitate the detection of cardiovascular anomalies. CFI has established itself as a real-time, non-invasive diagnostic tool for high-level visualization and detection of blood flow within a field of view. Innovations in this field are highly active, and new developments are emerging regularly. These novel innovations are poised to expand Doppler ultrasound's clinical diagnostic value. It is expected that the new capacities they offer will benefit the clinical management of major cardiovascular diseases such as atherosclerosis and will improve patient outcome.

4.6. References

Arbeille, P., Desombre, C., Aesh, B., Philippot, M., Lapierre, F. (1995). Quantification and assessment of carotid artery lesions: Degree of stenosis and plaque volume. *J. Clin. Ultrasound*, 23, 113–124.

Au, J.S., Yiu, B.Y.S., So, H., Chee, A.J.Y., Greaves, D.K., Hughson, R.L., Yu, A.C.H. (2020). Ultrasound vector projectile imaging for detection of altered carotid bifurcation hemodynamics during reductions in cardiac output. *Med. Phys.*, 47, 431–441.

Bercoff, J., Montaldo, G., Loupas, T., Savery, D., Meziere, F., Fink, M., Tanter, M. (2011). Ultrafast compound Doppler imaging: Providing full blood flow characterization. *IEEE Trans. Ultrason. Ferroelectr. Freq. Contr.*, 58, 134–147.

Bohs, L.H., Geiman, B.J., Anderson, M.E., Gebhart, S.C., Trahey, G.E. (2000). Speckle tracking for multi-dimensional flow estimation. *Ultrasonics*, 38, 369–375.

Burton, R.F. (2000). *Physiology by Numbers: An Encouragement to Quantitative Thinking*, 2nd edition. Cambridge University Press, Cambridge.

Chee, A.J.Y., Ishii, T., Yiu, B.Y.S., Yu, A.C.H. (2021). Helical toroid phantom for 3-D flow imaging investigations. *Phys. Med. Biol.*, 66, 045029.

Chiao, R.Y., Mo, L.Y., Hall, A.L., Miller, S.C., Thomenius, K.E. (2000). B-mode blood flow (B-flow) imaging. *Proc IEEE Ultrason. Symp.*, 1469–1472.

Christiansen, T.L., Rasmussen, M.F., Bagge, J.P., Moesner, L.N., Jensen, J.A., Thomsen, E.V. (2015). 3D imaging using row–column-addressed arrays with integrated apodization II: Transducer fabrication and experimental results. *IEEE Trans. Ultrason. Ferroelectr. Freq. Contr.*, 62, 959–971.

Cobbold, R.S.C. (2007). *Foundations of Biomedical Ultrasound*. Oxford University Press, Oxford.

Correia, M., Provost, J., Tanter, M., Pernot, M. (2016). 4D ultrafast ultrasound flow imaging: In vivo quantification of arterial volumetric flow rate in a single heartbeat. *Phys. Med. Biol.*, 61, L48–L61.

Evans, D.H. and McDicken, W.N. (2000). *Doppler Ultrasound: Physics, Instrumentation and Signal Processing*, 2nd edition. Wiley, New York.

Fenster, A., Downey, D.B., Cardinal H.N. (2001). Three-dimensional ultrasound imaging. *Phys. Med. Biol.*, 46, R66–R99.

Ferrara, K. and DeAngelis, G. (1997). Color flow mapping. *Ultrasound Med. Biol.*, 23, 321–345.

Foster, F.S., Pavlin, C.J., Harasiewicz, K.A., Christopher, D.A., Turnbull, D.H. (2000). Advances in ultrasound biomicroscopy. *Ultrasound Med. Biol.*, 26, 1–27.

Goddi, A., Bortolotto, C., Fiorina, I., Raciti, M.V., Fanizza, M., Turpini, E., Boffelli, G., Calliada, F. (2017). High-frame rate vector flow imaging of the carotid bifurcation. *Insights Imag.*, 8, 319–328.

Hansen, K.L., Moller-Sorensen, H., Pedersen, M.M., Hansen, P.M., Kjaergaard, J., Lund, J.T., Nilsson, J.C., Jensen, J.A., Nielsen, M.B. (2015). First report on intraoperative vector flow imaging of the heart among patients with healthy and diseased aortic valves. *Ultrasonics*, 56, 243–250.

Holbek, S., Ewertsen, C., Bouzari, H., Pihl, M.J., Hansen, K.L., Stuart, M.B., Thomsen, C., Nielsen, M.B., Jensen, J.A. (2016). Ultrasonic 3-D vector flow method for quantitative in vivo peak velocity and flow rate estimation. *IEEE Trans. Ultrason. Ferroelec. Freq. Contr.*, 64, 544–554.

Ishii, T., Yiu, B.Y.S., Yu, A.C.H. (2017). Vector flow visualization of urinary flow dynamics in a bladder outlet obstruction model. *Ultrasound Med. Biol.*, 43, 2601–2610.

Jensen, J.A. (2003). Directional velocity estimation using focusing along the flow direction I: Theory and simulation. *IEEE Trans. Ultrason. Ferroelec. Freq. Contr.*, 50, 857–872.

Jensen, J.A. (2007). Medical ultrasound imaging. *Prog. Biophys. Mol. Biol.*, 93, 153–165.

Jensen, J.A. and Nikolov, S.I. (2004) Directional synthetic aperture flow imaging. *IEEE Trans. Ultrason. Ferroelec. Freq. Contr.*, 51, 1107–1118.

Jensen, J.A. and Oddershede, N. (2006). Estimation of velocity vectors in synthetic aperture ultrasound imaging. *IEEE Trans. Med. Imag.*, 25, 1637–1644.

Jensen, J.A., Nikolov, S.I., Yu, A.C.H., Garcia, D. (2016). Ultrasound vector flow imaging: Part I. Sequential systems. *IEEE Trans. Ultrason. Ferroelec. Freq. Contr.*, 63, 1704–1721.

Johnston, K.W., Haynes, R.B., Douville, Y., Lally, M.E., Brown, P.M., Cobbold, R.S.C. (1985). Accuracy of carotid Doppler peak frequency analysis: Results determined by receiver operating characteristic curves and likelihood ratios. *J. Vasc. Surg.*, 2, 515–523.

Kaneko, Z. (1986). First steps in the development of the Doppler flowmeter. *Ultrasound Med. Biol.*, 12, 187–195.

Kasai, C., Namekawa, K., Koyano, A., Omoto, R. (1985). Real-time two-dimensional blood flow imaging using an autocorrelation technique. *IEEE Trans. Sonics Ultrason.*, 32, 458–464.

Lovstakken, L., Bjaerum, S., Martens, D., Torp, H. (2006). Blood flow imaging – A new real-time, 2-D flow imaging technique. *IEEE Trans. Ultrason. Ferroelec. Freq. Contr.*, 53, 289–299.

Lui, E.Y., Steinman, A.H., Cobbold, R.S.C., Johnston, K.W. (2005) Human factors as a source of error in peak Doppler velocity measurement. *J. Vasc. Surg.*, 42, 972–979.

Mo, L.Y.L., Ji, T.L., Chou, C.H., Napolitano, D., McLaughlin, G.W., DeBusschere, D. (2003). Zone-based color flow imaging. *Proc. IEEE Ultrason. Symp.*, 29–32.

Moon, T.K. and Stirling, W.C. (2000). *Mathematical Methods and Algorithms for Signal Processing*. Prentice-Hall Inc., Upper Saddle River, NJ.

Nikolov, S.I. and Jensen, J.A. (2003). In-vivo synthetic aperture flow imaging in medical ultrasound. *IEEE Trans. Ultrason. Ferroelec. Freq. Contr.*, 50, 848–856.

Picot, P.A., Rickey, D.W., Mitchell, R., Rankin, R.N., Fenster, A. (1993). Three-dimensional colour Doppler imaging. *Ultrasound Med. Biol.*, 19, 95–104.

Ramalli, A., Boni, E., Savoia, A.S., Tortoli, P. (2015). Density-tapered spiral arrays for ultrasound 3D imaging. *IEEE Trans. Ultrason. Ferroelectr. Freq. Contr.*, 62, 1580–1588.

Tanter, M. and Fink, M. (2014). Ultrafast imaging in biomedical ultrasound. *IEEE Trans. Ultrason. Ferroelec. Freq. Contr.*, 61, 102–119.

Udesen, J. and Jensen, J.A. (2006). Investigation of transverse oscillation method. *IEEE Trans. Ultrason. Ferroelec. Freq. Contr.*, 53, 959–971.

White, D.N. (1982). Johann Christian Doppler and his effect, a brief history. *Ultrasound Med. Biol.*, 8, 583–591.

Whittingham, T.A. (2007). Medical diagnostic applications and sources. *Prog. Biophys. Mol. Biol.*, 93, 84–110.

Yiu, B.Y.S. and Yu, A.C.H. (2013). High-frame-rate ultrasound color-encoded speckle imaging of complex flow dynamics. *Ultrasound Med. Biol.*, 39, 1015–1025.

Yiu, B.Y.S. and Yu, A.C.H. (2016). Least-squares multi-angle Doppler estimators for plane wave vector flow imaging. *IEEE Trans. Ultrason. Ferroelec. Freq. Contr.*, 63, 1733–1744.

Yiu, B.Y.S., Lai, S.S.M., Yu, A.C.H. (2014). Vector projectile imaging: Time-resolved dynamic visualization of complex flow patterns. *Ultrasound Med. Biol.*, 40, 2295–2309.

Yu, A.C.H. (2018). A brief review of ultrasound imaging and video. In *Handbook of Speckle Filtering and Tracking in Cardiovascular Ultrasound Imaging and Video*, Loizou, C., Pattichis, C., D'hooge, J. (eds). IET Press, London.

Yu, A.C.H., Johnston, K.W., Cobbold, R.S.C. (2007). Frequency-based signal processing in ultrasound color flow imaging. *Can. Acoust.*, 35(2), 11–23.

5

Cardiac Ultrasound Imaging

Konstantina PAPANGELOPOULOU, Marta ORLOWSKA, Sjoerd NOOIJENS and Jan D'HOOGE
Katholieke Universiteit Leuven, Belgium

5.1. Introduction to cardiac ultrasound

Cardiac ultrasound, i.e. echocardiography, provides real-time images with a relatively high temporal resolution. Not surprisingly, it is thus the most widely used tool for the diagnosis, management and follow-up of different cardiac pathologies in current clinical practice. Over the past 60 years, the application of ultrasound as a means to image the heart has greatly evolved and nowadays includes the use of M-mode, 2D imaging, Doppler, as well as more novel techniques such as 3D and contrast echocardiography.

Transthoracic echocardiography (TTE) is a noninvasive, safe, low-cost and readily available technique. This makes it an ideal adjunct to standard clinical examination. Furthermore, modalities such as transesophageal (TEE or TOE), intracardiac echocardiography (ICE) and intravascular ultrasound (IVUS) have also been integrated into clinical practice, not only for diagnostic purposes, but also to guide invasive interventions to treat valvular heart disease, coronary disease and several cardiac defects. For example, transcatheter atrial septal defect closure is performed with TEE for echocardiographic guidance.

For a color version of all the figures in this chapter, see www.iste.co.uk/bridal/innovative.zip.

Innovative Ultrasound Imaging Techniques,
coordinated by S. Lori BRIDAL. © ISTE Ltd 2024.

5.1.1. *Heart disease, anatomy and function*

Cardiovascular diseases (CVD) remain the leading cause of death in Europe, as well as worldwide, even though, at least for high-income countries, the absolute numbers seem to be declining (Townsend et al. 2022; WHO 2021). According to the World Health Organization, in 2019, about 32% of total deaths around the globe were attributed to CVD. The main cause of CVD is ischemic heart disease (WHO 2021). CVD's heavy toll in terms of worldwide mortality is higher for men (1,325/100,000) than for women (1,029/100,000), according to estimates reported in 2017 (Townsend et al. 2022). Since acquired CVD is generally treatable, and most importantly preventable, timely and accurate diagnosis is crucial. Therefore, incorporating imaging of the heart into everyday clinical practice is vital.

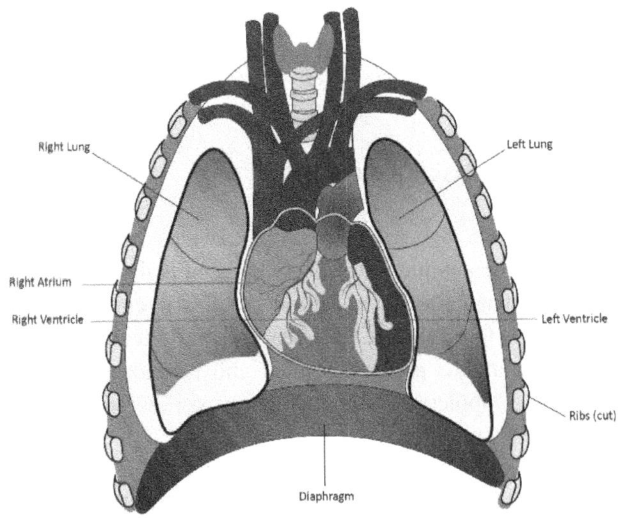

Figure 5.1. *The heart is surrounded by the lungs and the rib cage and is located just above the diaphragm in the mediastinum of the thoracic cavity*

The heart is located in the mediastinum of the thoracic cavity and is surrounded by the lungs and the rib cage (see Figure 5.1). It has a conical shape with its base at the level of the third costal cartilage and its apex pointing downwards, on the left of the sternum. About two-thirds of the heart are most commonly situated on the left of the midline. It "sits" on the diaphragm with its right side facing anteriorly and its left side facing posteriorly. The heart is enclosed in a double layered sac, the so-called pericardium. Between its two layers, there is a small amount of serous fluid that protects the heart and also allows it to move with each heartbeat. The heart itself has three distinct layers. The first is the endocardium: a thin, inner layer that serves as a barrier between the blood and the cardiac muscle. This cardiac muscle makes up the middle cardiac layer and is called the myocardium. Finally, the outer layer is called the epicardium and is comprised of elastic connective tissue and fat that further protects the heart.

There are four cardiac chambers: two atria and two ventricles (see Figure 5.2). The right atrium receives deoxygenated blood from the body through the inferior and superior vena cava and the coronary sinus. The deoxygenated blood then flows to the right ventricle and, through the pulmonary artery, reaches the lungs where gas exchange takes place. The left atrium, in turn, receives the newly oxygenated blood from the lungs, through the pulmonary veins. Subsequently, the blood moves into the left ventricle. Finally, via the aorta and the arterial system, the oxygenated blood reaches the different organs and tissues of the body. The atria are connected with the ventricles through the atrioventricular valves (the mitral valve on the left and the tricuspid valve on the right side), whereas the ventricles are connected with their corresponding vessels via the semilunar valves (aortic valve on the left and pulmonic valve on the right side). Thus, the heart, blood vessels and blood make up the cardiovascular system, whose role is to provide the body with the necessary nutrients and to remove waste for disposal.

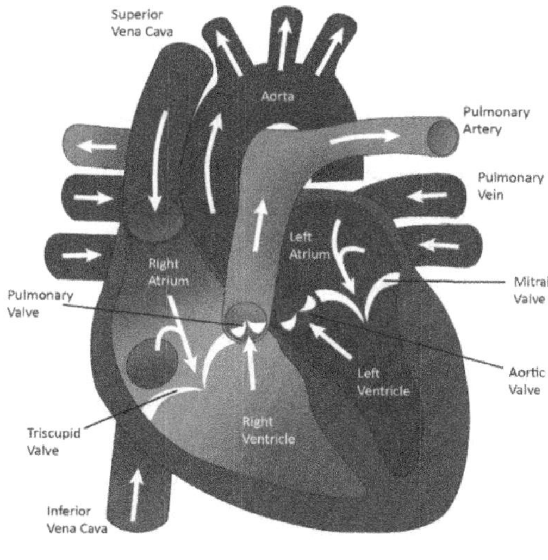

Figure 5.2. *Diagram showing the four cardiac chambers, their valves connecting them and the blood circulation with deoxygenated blood flowing through the right cardiac chambers to the pulmonary artery and the return of oxygenated blood to the left cardiac chambers for ejection to the body via the aorta*

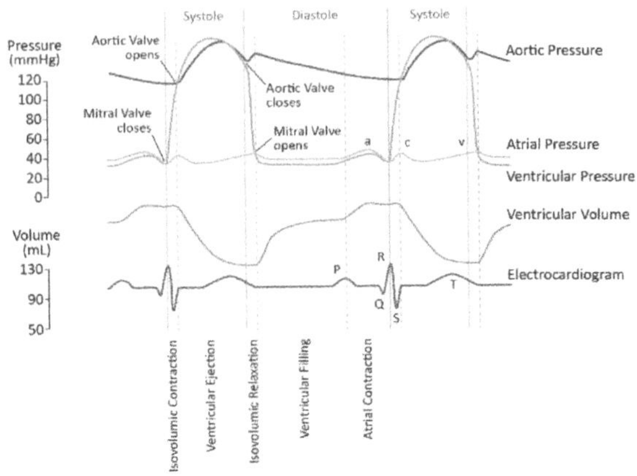

Figure 5.3. *Wigger's diagram of the cardiac cycle, showing pressure curves of the cardiac chambers and ventricular volume, with a simultaneous electrocardiogram recording. Each complete cardiac cycle is associated with electrical activity (detected on the electrocardiogram) that gives rise to myocardial contractions of the atria (during atrial contraction) and the ventricles (beginning during the phase of isovolumic contraction). The valves open and close as relative pressure values change. The ventricles are systematically filled and emptied of blood as shown by the modifications of the ventricular volume*

The flow of blood described above occurs during a series of alternating contractions and relaxations of the four cardiac chambers. Each cardiac cycle is made up of a complete sequence of these coordinated movements (see Figure 5.3):

1) **Atrial contraction (100–120 ms).** This is the first phase of the cardiac cycle, initiated by the electrical depolarization of the atria (i.e. the "P" wave on the electrocardiogram (ECG)). It leads to the contraction of the atrial cardiac muscle. The intra-atrial pressure thus rises, which leads to the rapid flow of blood in the ventricles.

2) **Isovolumic contraction (30 ms).** This phase begins with the ventricular electrical depolarization (i.e. the onset of the QRS complex on the ECG). As a result, the ventricular muscle starts to contract and the intraventricular pressure begins to rise, which causes the atrioventricular valves to close. At this stage, the semilunar valves are not open yet and thus there is no blood flow in or out of the ventricles, and no change in the ventricular volume is observed. As such, contraction is referred to as isovolumic or isovolumetric.

3) **Ventricular ejection (270 ms).** As the ventricular pressure rises further, the semilunar valves open and blood begins to flow into the great vessels (the

pulmonary artery on the right side and the aorta on the left side). This phase ends with the ventricular depolarization (i.e. the "T" wave on the ECG).

4) **Isovolumic relaxation (70–100 ms).** As the ventricular muscle begins to relax, the intraventricular pressure declines and the semilunar valves close, while the atrioventricular valves are also still closed. As a result, no volume changes are observed during this phase.

5) **Ventricular filling (430 ms).** Following atrial contraction and ejection from the ventricles, blood again gradually accumulates into the atria from the veins and the intra-atrial pressure begins to rise while the intraventricular pressure continues to fall. As a result, the atrioventricular valves open and blood flows from the atria to the ventricles.

5.1.2. *Typical clinical measurements*

The most common method to display cardiac ultrasound images is 2D echocardiography (with frame rates from 40 to 80 fps). This is merely a gray-scale display representing echoes returned from the visualized cardiac region, i.e. the field of view. The shade of gray of each pixel depends on the amplitude of the returning echo signal. This is the basis of cardiac imaging, since it is not only the main modality used to estimate cardiac morphology and function, but it is also used as a guide for the application of other ultrasound modalities, such as Doppler echocardiography.

In order to acquire good quality and clinically meaningful images, we need to avoid tissues that are strong reflectors or absorbers of ultrasound energy, such as the bones and the lungs. The ultrasound probe thus needs to be positioned at the intercostal spaces, at specific anatomic locations on the subject's thorax, the so-called acoustic windows. This helps to bypass the bones, as well as to bring the ultrasound probe closer to the heart. Both the American Society of Echocardiography (ASE) as well as the European Association of Cardiovascular Imaging (EACVI) have published guidelines on how to perform a complete echocardiographic examination and offer a thorough description of the echocardiographic views that should be acquired, along with the required cardiac measurements (Galderisi et al. 2017; Mitchell et al. 2019).

Very briefly, during scanning, the patient lies on the examination table, on the left lateral decubitus position with their left arm under their head. This way the heart is closer to the chest wall, and the intercostal spaces widen. The ultrasound transducer is then placed on one of several predefined positions on the thorax corresponding to one of the standard echocardiographic windows. The four main positions allow the acquisition of the standard echocardiographic views: parasternal, apical, sub-costal and suprasternal (see Figure 5.4).

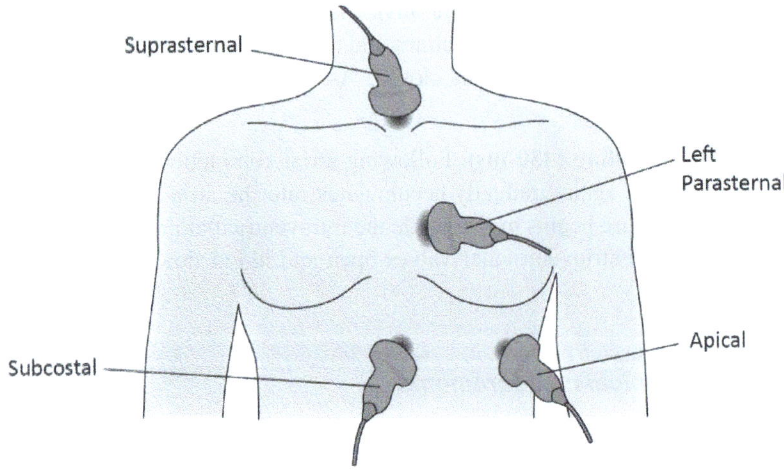

Figure 5.4. *Illustration of four standard positions used to obtain complementary views of the heart in echocardiography*

From the parasternal window, we can obtain a long axis view of the heart (see Figure 5.5(a)), as well as a series of short axis views at different levels, starting from the base and moving towards the apex of the heart (see Figure 5.5(b)). The parasternal long axis view provides valuable information about the cardiac morphology. It is used for the measurement of the thickness of the myocardial walls, the internal dimensions of the heart, the left atrium and the aortic annulus at different instances during the cardiac cycle (Lang et al. 2006). These values provide a first estimate of the cardiac structures, their anatomy and their function. Through the apical window, and with small manipulations of the ultrasound probe, a series of images of the heart can be acquired, with the left ventricular apex being the closest structure to the transducer (see Figure 5.5(c)). The minimal number of views that should be acquired through this window are the so-called apical four-, apical two-, apical three-, apical five-chamber and the right ventricle (RV)-focused view (Mitchell et al. 2019). These views offer qualitative as well as quantitative information related to the function of the ventricles and also provide insight regarding the structure and competency of three of the cardiac valves. For example, the apical four- and apical two-chamber views are used to estimate cardiac volumes, mainly left ventricular and atrial volumes. Finally, the sub-costal view is primarily used to assess the diameter and respiratory variation of the inferior vena cava (an indirect estimate of the right atrial pressure), whereas the suprasternal view gives an overview of part of the aorta and the aortic arch, along with the proximal part of the cervical arteries.

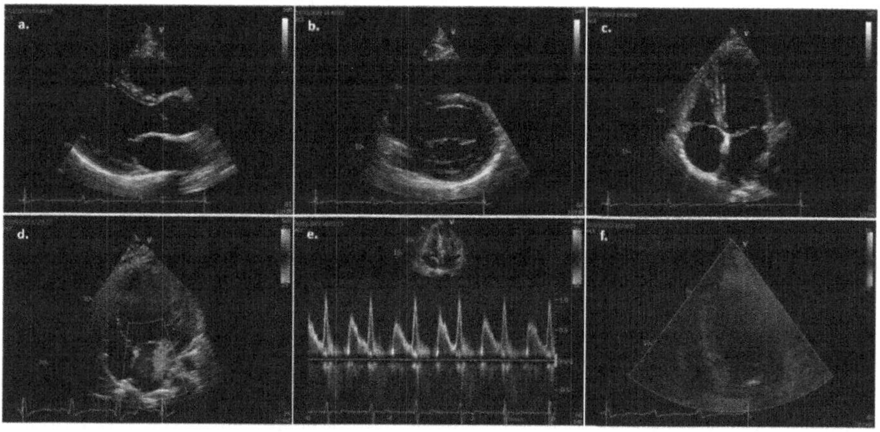

Figure 5.5. *Illustration of views that can be acquired through the acoustic windows shown in Figure 5.4: parasternal long axis (PLAX) (a) and short axis (PSAX) view (b) obtained through the left parasternal window. (c) The apical four-chamber view (AP4) acquired through the apical window. Illustration of color flow Doppler (d), transmitral flow assessed with pulsed wave (PW) Doppler (e) and Tissue Doppler Imaging (TDI)(f)*

Doppler echocardiography makes up an integral part of most echocardiographic examinations. It offers information on blood flow and can thus indicate abnormal blood flow patterns within and/or through the heart due, for example, to valvular stenosis or insufficiency or due to a shunt (i.e. an abnormal communication between two cardiac structures caused by a genetic or acquired defect). An easy way to visualize the blood flow within the heart is with color flow Doppler imaging, which is an extension of single-gate pulsed Doppler. First, a desired region of interest (i.e. the "color box") is selected within the 2D gray-scale image. Within this box, the velocity estimated for each pixel is represented by a specific color superimposed on the background gray-scale image so that the operator can relate the anatomy to the flow (see Figure 5.5(d)). Color flow Doppler can be applied in all imaging views. By convention, laminar flow is represented by a series of different shades of red and blue, where red and blue depict flow in the direction towards and away from the transducer, respectively, and where higher velocities are represented by brighter hues. Turbulent flow can be a sign of pathology. It is represented by a mosaic of colors, green or yellow, depending on the specific ultrasound imaging system.

In addition to visual assessment of blood flow with color flow Doppler, accurate measurement of the blood velocity at specific locations within the heart is an indispensable part of a complete echocardiographic examination. This is accomplished with a Doppler spectrogram, where the spectral velocity of flow at a specific location over time is represented graphically. Values above baseline represent the movement towards the transducer, whereas values below baseline represent the movement away from the transducer. Spectral Doppler techniques include Continuous Wave (CW) Doppler, Pulsed Wave (PW) Doppler (or pulsed Doppler) and high pulse repetition frequency (PRF) Doppler. Briefly, with PW Doppler, ultrasound pulses are transmitted at a given pulse repetition frequency and the probe detects the returning signals during the intervals in between. As described in section 4.2, this technique can be used to estimate flow velocities at a specific location as a function of time. However, in cardiac imaging, it can typically only be used to measure velocities up to about 1.5 m/s before aliasing occurs. Since CW Doppler (described in section 4.1) transmits and receives ultrasound signals continuously, it can detect higher velocities without aliasing. However, CW Doppler has a limited ability to localize flow as it can only describe the flow along the transmit direction of the ultrasound pulse but not the depth at which it occurs. In practice, this information needs to come from knowledge of normal physiologic velocity distributions with the heart. High PRF Doppler is a form of PW Doppler with the distinction that multiple sample volumes are used, each one at a depth that is a multiple integer of the depth of the initial sample volume. If the initial sample volume is placed at one half of the distance of the actual region of interest, and given the fact that depth is inversely correlated with PRF, then higher PRF can be achieved, leading to the detection of higher velocities. This modality can thus overcome the limitation of conventional PW Doppler regarding aliasing, at the expense of a relatively small range ambiguity.

In the clinical setting, the velocities that are of interest are mainly those of blood flow between two separate chambers (e.g. flow from the atria to the ventricles and from the ventricles to the great vessels). Most normal cardiac velocities are below 1.5 m/s, and thus, PW Doppler can be used in most cases. For example, transmitral flow is routinely assessed since it is an indicator of left ventricular diastolic function (i.e. filling properties) (see Figure 5.5(e)) (Nagueh et al. 2016). Furthermore, echocardiography can be used to make hemodynamic measurements that have historically been obtained invasively. For example, velocity measured at the left ventricular outflow track (and, more specifically, the velocity time integral) can be used for the noninvasive measurement of left ventricular cardiac output, an index of systolic function and cardiac competence. CW Doppler, as already mentioned, is used for the assessment of higher velocities. In the case of cardiac pathology, these velocities usually represent abnormal turbulent flow due to a stenotic orifice (e.g. blood flow from the left ventricle to the aorta in case of aortic stenosis) or due to regurgitation (e.g. abnormal backflow of blood from the left ventricle to the left atrium through an incompetent mitral valve).

Tissue Doppler imaging (TDI) also makes use of movement-based signal analysis. By appropriately adjusting the gain and velocity filtering settings, this modality can be used to estimate higher-amplitude, lower-velocity signals than those associated with echoes from moving blood that arise from the movement of the myocardial walls during the cardiac cycle. TDI estimations can be displayed and stored in the form of color Doppler TDI or in the form of PW-TDI. In current clinical practice, TDI is used for the velocity assessment of the mitral and tricuspid annulus as they move throughout the cardiac cycle (see Figure 5.5(f)). The early diastolic velocity of the mitral annulus is part of the current diastolic function assessment algorithm (Nagueh et al. 2016), whereas the systolic component of the tricuspid annulus should be used for the systolic function assessment of the right ventricle (Lang et al. 2006).

Although 2D echocardiography, supplemented with color and spectral Doppler, offers unique insight into cardiac anatomy and function, and provides valuable information that can be used in everyday clinical practice to diagnose, treat and follow-up many cardiac pathologies, it suffers from the fact that it remains a 2D representation of a complex 3D structure. This means that the operator must mentally project the acquired image into a 3D space, making several assumptions about the anatomical relationship between the different cardiac structures. In addition, given the fact that the available echocardiographic windows are, to a large extent, predefined and limited due to the surrounding anatomy (i.e. the lungs and the bones), the cardiac structures of interest can only be investigated based on specific anatomical planes. All the different aspects of the 3D structure cannot be visualized. For example, with 2D echocardiography, it is never possible to image the tricuspid valve in a transverse plane. It can, therefore, be challenging to detect pathologies, and this is particularly true for congenital heart disease where chamber morphology and function can be very distinct.

An important innovation towards overcoming this limitation is the development of 3D echocardiography. Currently, three different methods of acquiring 3D datasets can be used. With multi-plane imaging, multiple 2D views of the same structure, acquired from different planes can be displayed side by side simultaneously. By using the so-called live 3D imaging, data can be acquired in real time; usually a pyramidal volume of 30° x 60° is acquired. Such a narrow sector is used to preserve a sufficient temporal and spatial resolution. It is possible to obtain real-time, full-volume data, but only at the expense of temporal and spatial resolution. Finally, with multi-beat ECG-gated acquisition, the final image is created by stitching together several sub-sectors, usually two to six, acquired over sequential cardiac cycles. Gated acquisition can also be applied in conjunction with color flow Doppler. The multi-beat ECG-gated technique increases spatial and temporal resolution; however, this technique cannot be applied in patients with irregular rhythms, and cardiac shifting, caused by the patient's breathing or probe movement can cause stitching artifacts, i.e. misalignment of the acquired sub-volumes. Current guidelines recommend the incorporation of 3D imaging in everyday clinical practice, mainly for the more accurate measurement of cardiac volumes and the more detailed assessment of valvular pathology (Lang et al. 2012). More specifically, assessment of the left ventricular volume using 3D imaging has been shown to be more accurate and reproducible than 2D echocardiography, when using cardiovascular magnetic resonance (CMR) as the reference method (Mor-Avi et al. 2008). 3D measurements have been shown to be more accurate for the estimation of the severity of mitral stenosis, even when they are being compared with hemodynamic measurements which is the historical gold standard. (Pérez de Isla et al. 2007). It has been shown that 2D echocardiography consistently underestimates mitral regurgitation, when compared to 3D echocardiography (Marsan et al. 2009).

Transthoracic echocardiography (TTE) is a readily available and safe imaging modality, making it a highly cost-effective technique for cardiac anatomy and function assessment. One of its main limitations, however, is the fact that the heart lies inside the thoracic cavity, behind the ribs, the sternum and the lungs. Therefore, TTE efficacy can be restricted due to attenuation of the ultrasound beam. In some cases, attenuation effects can make ultrasonic imaging of the heart impossible, for example, in patients with lung disease. Since the heart is in close proximity to the esophagus, a transesophageal echocardiographic (TEE or TOE) imaging approach is ideal to image several cardiac structures, especially those located at the base of the heart, such as the left atrium and the pulmonary veins.

Currently, TEE examination is recommended whenever TTE images do not provide sufficient diagnostic information (Hahn et al. 2022), making it an indispensable alternative for cardiovascular imaging. The ultrasound probe used for TEE emits ultrasound waves with higher frequencies compared to the TTE probe (about 3–7 MHz for an adult TEE) as the required penetration depth is less. While the patient is in the left lateral decubitus position, the flexible probe is inserted in the patient's mouth and advanced to the patient's esophagus as the patient actively swallows to facilitate the process. The probe can be rotated up to 180°, flexed, advanced and withdrawn in order to facilitate the acquisition of the required views. All the imaging techniques that were described for TTE imaging (2D and 3D imaging, as well as Doppler echocardiography) can also be applied during a TEE examination. The American Society of Echocardiography, in collaboration with the Society of Cardiovascular Anesthesiologists, provides detailed recommendations for a complete and thorough TEE examination and offers additional protocol sequences when focused imaging of specific structures is preferred (Hahn et al. 2022). Since TEE is a semi-invasive imaging modality and may cause patient discomfort, it is most often adopted only in a clinical environment, and it is called upon to answer specific clinical questions. For example, TEE is essential for the detection of embolic sources and it should be performed whenever an embolic source of cardiac origin is suspected (Cohen et al. 2021). In addition, TEE should always be performed for the diagnosis of aortic pathologies, for example, dissection of the aorta, for the assessment of prosthetic valve function and the severity of mitral valve regurgitation, as well as whenever there is a clinical suspicion of infective endocarditis. Apart from its diagnostic role in the clinical routine, TEE is an essential tool in guiding therapeutic interventions, such as valvular replacement, both during cardiac surgery, as well as during transcatheter interventions in the cath-lab environment (Flachskampf et al. 2014).

Intracardiac echocardiography (ICE) is an important and relatively new modality among cardiac imaging technologies, in which a catheter with an ultrasound transducer at its tip can be inserted through the patient's vein and advanced towards the heart. It currently has a limited number of applications and is mainly used to guide electrophysiological procedures and percutaneous interventions (Bartel et al. 2014; Enriquez et al. 2018). A large number of pathologies can now be treated percutaneously, with the use of dedicated catheters and devices. Percutaneous procedures have proven to be more effective than pharmacologic treatments alone, as, for example, in the case of catheter ablation of cardiac arrhythmias (Asad et al. 2019). Furthermore, percutaneous treatment has been proven to be safer than open heart surgery, as, for example, in the case of atrial septal defect closure (Du et al. 2002). ICE offers real-time imaging of cardiac structures, enabling the localization of the targeted structure, while simultaneously enabling consideration of anatomical variability. It thus provides guidance during interventions and has been proven more helpful and effective than TEE (Bartel et al. 2014). Indeed, compared to TEE, it does not require general anesthesia, it does not obscure fluoroscopy, which is essential for percutaneous interventions, and it generates images with higher resolution. Volumetric ICE has been developed, and, although not yet widely used, holds promise for an even better and more representative visualization of cardiac structures. Despite these advantages of ICE, its applicability in the clinical setting is still limited, mainly due to the high cost of the equipment (Bartel et al. 2014; Enriquez et al. 2018).

5.1.3. *Unmet clinical needs*

Although echocardiography is an excellent tool for imaging of the cardiovascular system and provides invaluable information that can guide the diagnosis and treatment of patients, it still suffers from several shortcomings. The major shortcoming is its highly variable image quality, which is very patient specific and hard to predict, together with the occurrence of multiple artifacts such as shadowing and reverberations. These artifacts arise from incorrect assumptions related to wave propagation during image reconstruction but correcting for this type of artifact is far from trivial. In addition, the temporal resolution of a conventional echocardiographic examination is about 50–70 Hz enabled by reconstructing several (typically 2) image lines for every ultrasound pulse transmitted (i.e. Multi-Line Acquisition (MLA)). Even though this is much faster than, for example, cardiac magnetic resonance imaging (Lin and Alessio 2009), it is still not able to temporally resolve short-lived cardiac events, like those occurring during the isovolumic phases of the cardiac cycle (Jasaityte and D'hooge 2010).

Another common issue with echocardiography is the underestimation of cardiac volumes. Both 2D and 3D echocardiography have been proven to underestimate cardiac volumes, when compared with the gold standard, i.e. cardiac magnetic resonance imaging (Hoffmann et al. 2014). 3D echocardiographic measurements, although shown to correlate better with the corresponding ones derived from magnetic resonance imaging, still underestimate the "ground truth" values. This holds true both for left ventricular (Sugeng et al. 2010), as well as for the right ventricular volumes (Lang et al. 2015) and is a consequence of the limited spatial resolution.

Cardiac volumes and systolic function of the left ventricle should be performed using the modified Simpson's technique, which has been established as the most reliable method and is proposed in current guidelines (Mor-Avi et al. 2008). Briefly, the endocardial border of the left ventricle is delineated at end-diastole and end-systole, both in apical four and two chamber views, and then the cavity is divided into a series of ellipsoidal discs. The volume of each disc is calculated, and then all volumes are summed to derive the total ventricular volume. This technique, however, still has several pitfalls, since it requires accurate tracing of the endocardium, which cannot always be performed if image quality is poor. In addition, it uses two apical views of the left ventricle, which include most, but not all myocardial walls. As a result, it does not consider possible motion abnormalities of the myocardial walls that may not be visible within the two selected views. An additional pitfall of 2D echocardiography is the so-called foreshortening effect. The true apex of the heart is not visualized in the apical four chamber view. Instead the ultrasound beam travels through a plane superior to the level of the apex. This makes the left ventricle look more rounded and less bullet-shaped, as should be the case in a correctly acquired apical view.

The above-mentioned limitations underline the fact that, even though echocardiography is a vital tool for CVD diagnosis, treatment and follow-up, there still remains room for improvement and implementation of newer techniques that will be able to more accurately and reliably image the cardiac structures.

5.2. High-frame-rate imaging (in 2D)

High-frame-rate (HFR) imaging may allow for better assessment of cardiac function (Cikes et al. 2014). To keep the field of view and spatial resolution adequate while increasing the temporal resolution, two types of HFR approaches have been proposed. One is based on the simultaneous transmission of multiple focused beams (MLT, i.e. multi-line transmit) in different directions (Tong et al. 2013a; Tong et al. 2014; Ramalli et al. 2018). The other is based on defocused waves, i.e. diverging or plane waves (DW/PW) (Denarie et al. 2013; Papadacci et al. 2014; Porée et al. 2016) along with massive parallel beamforming (Shattuck et al. 1984) (see sections 2.1.2.2 and 2.1.2.3 for additional information). The choice to use one of these methods should be based on various factors, such as system requirements, computational load, energy transfer to the body, achievable frame rate, motion artifacts and image quality. Irrespective of which HFR approach is used, it is important to remember that higher temporal resolution comes at the cost of image quality. Indeed, the main drawback of HFR imaging is the reduced image quality and signal-to-noise ratio (SNR), which limit the potential of HFR for real-time display on the ultrasound system or for the quantification of cardiac function using traditional methods. More recently, new approaches towards improvement of the HFR images have been developed which are mentioned in the two sections below, followed by a description of the clinical potential of HFR imaging.

5.2.1. *Multi-line transmit*

Images obtained with the MLT approach suffer from reduced SNR and contrast due to potential artifacts arising from the interference between the main lobes and the side lobes of the transmitted and received beams that appear as ghost-like artifacts on the images. In the last two decades, multiple authors have presented mitigation schemes to overcome this issue. For example, Tong et al. (2014b) observed that the crosstalk intensity was suppressed by increasing the MLT beam opening angle, reducing the number of MLT beams or by using proper apodization on transmit and receive. Nevertheless, finding the best apodization for an ultrasound imaging system is not trivial since the apodization is known to influence the ultrasound beam formation in many different ways and the best choice depends on the specific application. In their study, a 4MLT-2MLA imaging approach using a Tukey apodization scheme was proposed for a typical cardiac transducer. This imaging system could generate a 90° sector image without significant loss in the image quality at approximately 306 Hz. It was further experimentally tested in vitro and in vivo in Tong et al. (2014b) that MLT can be very competitive as compared to conventional imaging while improving the frame rate by a factor of 4. It was also shown that MLT can be combined with MLA to provide images with a 12- to 16-fold increase in frame rate (about 340–450 Hz) without significantly compromising spatial resolution and SNR. Although the application of MLA can cause discontinuities between neighboring lines in the image, this can be alleviated by implementing so-called synthetic transmit beams (STBs) (Hergum et al. 2007). Finally, Zurakhov et al. (2018) recently showed that even better artifact rejection can be obtained along with increased spatial resolution by applying a predefined receive apodization after assessment of the interference magnitude.

To increase the frame rate even more (i.e. to have more MLT beams), it may be possible to suppress the crosstalk further by using coded excitation, as has been proposed for synthetic aperture imaging in Misaridis and Jensen (2005). Coded excitation based on two or more orthogonal transmit pulses whose mutual cross-correlation is very small has been used to suppress crosstalk in many applications. When simultaneously transmitting two or more mutually orthogonal codes, the received signals contain information from all codes. This information can then be separated through a decoding process. This approach was explored for echocardiographic applications in Tong et al. (2019). It was demonstrated that coded excitation could be used to suppress MLT crosstalk, although apodization is still needed when the number of MLT beams is larger than the number of orthogonal codes. Nevertheless, this approach can be beneficial in terms of SNR and penetration depth. Moreover, Demi et al. (2012, 2015) implemented orthogonal frequency-division multiplexing to create distinctive parallel beams in transmission. With the proposed method, multiple distinguishable narrow beams with different center frequencies were transmitted in parallel resulting in a reduction of the unwanted side lobes and an increase in the amplitude of the main beam compared with standard parallel beamforming but with possible amplitude variations due to distinct attenuation properties at different frequencies.

Another approach for reducing crosstalk between simultaneously transmitted beams is based on advanced beamforming schemes. Rabinovich et al. (2015) demonstrated that minimum variance beamforming can reduce transmit crosstalk better than simple delay-and-sum (DAS) beamforming. Furthermore, in Matrone et al. (2019), different coherence-based beamformers, which exploit the spatial coherence of backscattered signals across an array transducer, were investigated. The analysis performed on an experimental phantom and in vivo cardiac acquisitions, showed that advanced beamforming techniques can provide better image quality than DAS, by lowering crosstalk artifacts in reception and increasing image resolution and contrast at the same time. However, such improvements depend on the design parameters of the algorithms, which must be properly tuned.

Finally, it is worth mentioning that harmonic imaging remains an option for MLT (Prieur et al. 2013; Demi et al. 2015), although the high-energy content in transmission must be divided between simultaneous transmissions due to mechanical and thermal index considerations that limits the power output.

5.2.2. *Plane waves and diverging waves*

Another approach for obtaining HFR is based on defocused waves. These sequences insonify a wider region of interest simultaneously and, thus, can provide a higher frame rate than the MLT approach by doing all image reconstruction on receive. The behavior and implementation of plane wave and diverging wave imaging are similar, however, for cardiac applications, DW is preferred since the field of view for a single plane wave is limited by the transducer aperture and thus the acoustic window. Nevertheless, the use of a single defocused wave to reconstruct an image significantly affects the image quality, i.e. the contrast, SNR and the lateral resolution. Compounding of images reconstructed from single defocused wave transmits has been introduced to overcome this issue. Coherent compounding can be applied in a relatively straightforward manner by coherently summing images reconstructed from consecutive DWs to obtain high-quality images of the entire heart at an HFR over a full field of view (Montaldo et al. 2009; Papadacci et al. 2014). This provides a strong improvement of the imaging quality, even with a small number of transmit events, and it still strongly increases temporal resolution (by around a factor of 10) compared to standard imaging sequences (see Figure 5.6). On the contrary, to reduce the speckle noise in receive compounding, a Thomson's multi-taper approach has been proposed (Jensen et al. 2012). This approach aims to smooth the speckle by incoherently combining the acquired B-mode images after applying different apodization windows on the same original data. Although it has been shown that the multi-taper approach can be used for speckle reduction, it decreases the spatial resolution at the same time. Therefore, Toulemonde et al. (2015) proposed combining the coherent compounding technique with Thomson's multi-taper method to take advantage of coherent and incoherent approaches. That way, the coherent part of the method improves the resolution and contrast, whereas the incoherent part reduces the speckle noise.

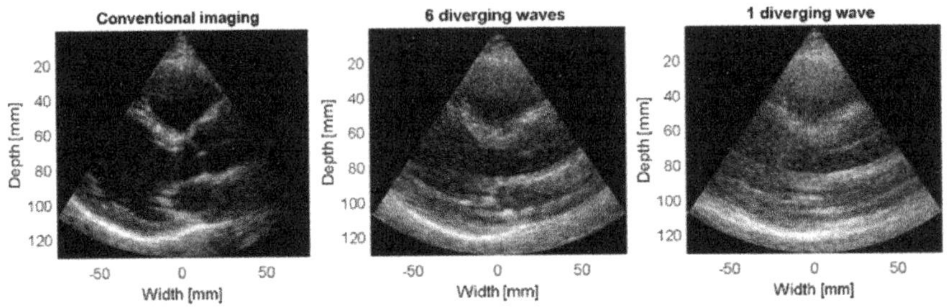

Figure 5.6. *Cardiac B-mode images obtained using conventional imaging sequence, six diverging waves and one diverging wave*

It is important to recall that compounding many images can introduce motion artifacts. Especially in cardiac imaging, compounding data acquired based on many transmits can introduce noticeable image degradations (e.g. lower SNR, lateral shifting, grating-lobe formation). Hence, it is advisable to integrate motion compensation into coherent compounding processes (Denarie et al. 2013; Gammelmark and Jensen 2014). The motion compensation method can be based on auto- or cross-correlation, which is calculated between images from successive transmits. After obtaining the information about displacement between transmits, the movement on the images is compensated and then coherent compounding is performed. Finally, to modify the impact of motion on compounding, a different order of the transmits from the same emission sequence can be implemented. Specifically, Porée et al. (2016) recommended the use of a triangular transmit sequence to avoid bias in Doppler motion estimates.

All methods mentioned above present the main drawback: how they decrease the effective frame rate. To increase SNR and contrast of the images and keep the high frame rate, Hadamard (Gong et al. 2017) or cascade imaging (Zhao and Luo 2018; Zhang et al. 2019) can be implemented. For example, Zhao and Luo (2018) proposed the use of orthogonal Golay pair-coded DW sequence. Specifically, two DWs at different steering angles coded by an orthogonal Golay pair are transmitted simultaneously, thus compensating for the frame rate reduction caused by the transmission of complementary codes. Moreover, Zhang et al. (2019) suggested to use sub-apertures which transmit a train of DWs that are weighted in both spatial and temporal directions with a coding matrix containing polarity coefficients. His results showed that decoded signals, which were beamformed and coherently compounded, significantly improved image quality in comparison to standard HFR recording at the same frame rate. However, thermal effects of such long pulse trains could be a limitation.

5.2.3. *Clinical potential*

First, high-frame-rate imaging enables the detection of brief events during the cardiac cycle such as isovolumic contraction and relaxation periods. Analysis of these cardiac mechanical phases at high temporal resolution could potentially provide important diagnostic or prognostic information. Moreover, the HFR approach can allow for the implementation of several measurement algorithms on the same set of images, hence within the same heartbeat, instead of requiring operators to sequentially activate numerous different acquisition modes, each adapted to a specific type of measurement. For example, speckle-tracking echocardiography (STE) is a clinical tool that is widely used to non-invasively assess regional myocardial function through the quantification of regional motion and deformation. However, in current clinical practice, STE is based on conventional B-mode imaging at a modest frame rate (typically lower than 80 Hz). This frame rate only visualizes the cardiac motion in a rough way, and it is, therefore, recommended to use this type of data for strain measurements only. To estimate time-dependent parameters, such as tissue velocity, acceleration or strain rate, finer time resolution is required. This can currently be obtained by recording a new set of images using a tissue Doppler imaging mode (TDI). Recently, novel STE, specifically developed for HFR recordings, has been tested (Grondin et al. 2017; Joos et al. 2018; Porée et al. 2018; Orlowska et al. 2020). It was shown that estimated strain measurements based on HFR STE are comparable to those measured with clinical STE, while the clinical markers of velocity, acceleration and strain rate obtained with HFR STE were in the same range as those computed from TDI. Furthermore, since the acquisition for B-mode and Doppler imaging is identical for HFR approach, blood flow can be estimated simultaneously at each pixel in a wide 2D region of interest (Berkoff et al. 2011). Ramalli et al. (2020) showed that HFR can achieve sufficiently high frame rates to provide quantitative use of Color Doppler imaging (CDI). Specifically, peak diastolic intraventricular pressure gradients, which have been described to be a marker for the diagnosis of diastolic function, were obtained with HFR CDI and were not statistically different from those calculated from standard color M-mode (the gold standard reference). Finally, mechanical activation imaging could also benefit from higher temporal resolution since the mechanical activation is followed by brief myocardial motion with a duration on the order of a few milliseconds. Recently, Kvåle et al. (2019) investigated the feasibility of mechanical activation imaging of the left ventricular myocardium using HFR imaging for the purpose of detecting conduction abnormalities. This study indicated that HFR together with novel signal processing methods has the potential to be a valuable tool for mechanical activation detection.

Furthermore, HFR imaging could provide insight into the intrinsic myocardial mechanical properties, such as stiffness or viscosity, by assessing the characteristics of the propagation of shear waves through the myocardium. Shear wave imaging (SWI) requires a source to create a shear wave (see section 3.4) that can be external/active (e.g. acoustic radiation force (Bouchard et al. 2009)) or internal/natural (e.g. closure of the valves (Vos et al. 2017)). Currently, there are a number of studies which investigate SWI using both types of sources. Using an external shear wave source, Villemain et al. (2019) found myocardial stiffness significantly higher in hypertrophic cardiomyopathic patients than in healthy volunteers. Furthermore, a pilot study in pediatric cancer patients was carried out and demonstrated the feasibility of using cardiac shear waves generated by an external source (Song et al. 2016). Although active-source SWI requires special transducers/excitations to create the shear waves, it can be used to measure myocardial stiffness in real time throughout the cardiac cycle, which allows, for example, the quantification of stiffness variations between systole and diastole (Pernot et al. 2011). Unfortunately, it has been shown that the feasibility of active-source SWI is lower than natural-source SWI (Keijzer et al. 2020). Natural SWI in the human heart allows detection of shear waves in the intraventricular septum created by the closure of the cardiac valves in 92% of cases (Santos et al. 2019). Natural SWI has the potential to become a valuable noninvasive method for the assessment of diastolic myocardial properties in heart transplant recipients (Petrescu et al. 2020) as well as patients with hypertensive heart disease (Cvijic et al. 2020). Nevertheless, the results obtained by Keijzer et al. (2019) suggest that measurement precision should be improved by averaging over multiple heartbeats due to the variability between measurements.

5.3. Volumetric imaging

Volumetric cardiac ultrasound imaging (3DUS) enables the use of ultrasound to investigate the heart in 3D rather than only imaging a single plane as is the case for traditional "2D" imaging (2DUS). The following sections will review why one would move to volumetric ultrasound imaging of the heart and what the ultrasound imaging pipeline would look like in theory, i.e. if all practical limits could be ignored. Then, we will discuss the limitations that are encountered in practice and several strategies that have been adopted to work around or deal with these limitations. Finally, we will briefly look forward toward the changes and improvements that are needed before volumetric ultrasound imaging can be used routinely by cardiologists. For more background on the topic, we refer to the following review papers: Karadayi et al. (2009); Prager et al. (2010); Roh (2014); Huang and Zeng (2017); Osipov et al. (2018, 2020).

5.3.1. *Why 3DUS of the heart*

The first and most obvious improvement in moving to 3D cardiac ultrasound is that the volumetric information will provide a clinician with the 3D anatomical context. In other words, volumetric imaging can reveal how cross-sections and slices of the heart relate to the organ as a whole. This 3D anatomical context allows the clinician to verify that a certain imaging plane is in the optimal position. To put this into perspective, for 2DUS, a clinician needs to keep track of the structures of the heart by mentally reconstructing the volume while moving the imaging plane. This takes extensive training to master and contributes to the operator dependency found in 2DUS (Fenster and Downey 2000). Choosing "perfect" anatomical views and imaging planes helps to identify the true dimensions of the organ and prevents foreshortening as the imaging plane is (verifiably) not skewed with respect to the heart (Fenster and Downey 1996). Furthermore, problems caused by out-of-plane motion can be avoided with 3DUS as information that is not viewed a specific plane will still be present in the volume.

Since 3DUS obtains information from the entire heart, it is possible to estimate volumes without any assumptions. This is not the case for 2DUS where, for example, the left ventricular cavity is often assumed to be ellipsoidal and the estimation of the radius is based on a single plane. Therefore, 3DUS provides a better estimation of the cavity volume, which tracked over time gives the stroke volume, a clinically relevant measure for cardiac performance.

Furthermore, during routine echocardiographic tests, 3DUS can simultaneously investigate and display multiple anatomical views taken from the same acoustic window (parasternal long/short axis views or apical 3/4/5 chamber views). This means that no time is wasted finding the next anatomical view.

Finally, mechanical manipulation of the probe during transesophageal echocardiography (TEE) is difficult as the small probe is mounted on a catheter in the esophagus. If such a probe has volumetric capabilities based on electronic repositioning (i.e. steering) in both the azimuth and elevation direction, the probe can be held in place while still allowing clinicians to alter the imaging plane.

Thus, in short, volumetric cardiac ultrasound imaging allows for the detection of verifiably optimal anatomical views and better assessment of the dimensions of the heart, thereby reducing operator dependency. Furthermore, clinical efficiency is improved because multiple anatomical views can be investigated simultaneously. Finally, 3DUS allows easier (electronic) probe manipulation for TEE.

5.3.2. *Ideal configuration for 3DUS of the heart*

For both 2DUS and 3DUS of the heart, the probe needs to be positioned in the intercostal space and, from there, the ultrasound beam can be directed to obtain a field of view including the whole heart. To control the ultrasound beam (i.e. steering and focusing), the array elements must be small and close to one another ($<\lambda/2$) in order to avoid grating lobes (and therefore artifacts) to appear during beam steering. For 3DUS, this implies going from a 1D array probe to a 2D matrix probe. Ideally, each array element is individually connected to an independent controllable electronic channel of the ultrasound system. The acquired data is beamformed and mapped on a regular Cartesian grid during scan conversion. Although this is essentially the same as what is done in 2D, the computational load is significantly higher in 3D. Finally, whereas traditional 2DUS data can easily be displayed on a 2D screen, 3DUS data may render the problem of representing the volumetric information on the 2D display much more technically complex.

In practice, the hardware specifications cited above are not feasible/economically justified. The number of elements scales quadratically with the aperture size, thereby demanding an ultrasound system that can control thousands of elements simultaneously. Furthermore, to keep the modality operating in real time, more image lines need to be reconstructed in the same amount of time. In this section, we will discuss these practical limitations and possible solutions for them, starting with those based on hardware, then beamforming and finally those relying on improvements in software and data management.

5.3.3. *Hardware challenges*

As mentioned above, the ideal probe for echocardiography has an aperture filled with elements that are small along the direction in which the beam needs to be controlled. For 2DUS, this is not a problem as 64 rectangular elements (0.3 mm by 10 mm) would result in a 2 cm by 1 cm aperture. However, a matrix array with an aperture of just 1 by 1 cm^2 would need 1,024 (32 by 32 grid, each 0.3 by 0.3 mm^2) elements! This type of matrix probe is hard to manufacture and the small elements have a higher electrical impedance than large, rectangular ones, making it hard to match the impedance with that of the ultrasound system driving it (Turnbull and Foster 1991). This problem remains important for non-PZT elements (i.e. pMUT/cMUT). A cable the size of a garden hose would be needed to individually connect these 1,024 elements to an ultrasound system. Therefore, as the element count increases, the cable size could become a limiting factor. Furthermore, current clinical ultrasound systems are often limited to 256 independent electronic channels, so higher channel counts would require specialized hardware (Prager et al. 2010). In short, it is not yet feasible to manufacture or connect a fully- wired dense matrix array on clinical systems. Possible solutions are to lower the channel count by either connecting more elements to each channel or by reducing the number of elements altogether.

5.3.4. *Hardware – multiplexing*

A possible way to lower the channel count is by connecting more elements to each channel by building a probe that is "row/column" addressed (Morton and Lockwood 2003; Seo and Yen 2009). For such a probe, instead of connecting each element individually, one channel will be connected to an entire row or an entire column of the matrix array. Obviously, this reduces the number of channels needed to connect an N x N matrix array from N^2 to 2N, resulting in a linear increase of the channel count for an increasing aperture size. As a result, all elements along a row (or column) will get the same delay and apodization value during transmit; similarly, all data received will be an integration of all elements on the row/column.

During transmit with the row/column array, either the rows alone or the columns alone are used, which means the probe is only capable of controlling the beam in one direction (azimuth or elevation). In the perpendicular direction, the elements will essentially function as a large rectangular element, resulting in an unfocused beam in this direction; the specific nature of the unfocused beam results from the aperture size and optional curvature of the probe surface (Démoré et al. 2009) or an acoustic lens (Bouzari et al. 2017). In receive, the perpendicular set of channels is used, allowing beam control in the perpendicular direction. Therefore, instead of controlling the beam in all directions during both transmit and receive, the row/column array separates the beam control in two subsequent orthogonal in-plane controls (i.e. during transmit and receive). In short, the row/column array can control the beam in 3D, but not as effective as a fully wired matrix array could. Indeed, as the transmit and receive beams need to overlap, this subsequent approach implies that focusing outside of the transducer's aperture is not possible, thereby limiting the field of view of the row/column addressed array to its aperture size. Moreover, by only focusing "once" in each direction, the row/column array uses its aperture half as effectively. This could theoretically be overcome by doubling the number of elements in each direction as the channel count scales linearly. However, in echocardiography, the room for expanding the aperture will be limited by the limited size of the intercostal acoustic window.

Several probes have been proposed where a switch is added to each channel connecting them to a set of elements so that only one of the channels can be used at a given time (multiplexing) (Provost et al. 2014). Repeating a sequence for each of the multiplexed sets and subsequently combining the results (assuming linearity) can approximate the functionality of a fully-wired array at the cost of a reduced frame rate. An example of this is phased sub-array imaging (PSA) (Johnson et al. 2005a, 2005b), where small subsets of the probe are used during transmit and receive and then coherently weighted and summed to result in the final image.

Finally, the most advanced way to reduce the channel count is to move part of the post-processing into the probe itself (Larson 1993; Savord and Solomon 2003; Blaak et al. 2009). This two-stage beamforming strategy relies on sub-aperture processing (SAP), where a group of elements are pre-beamformed by set delays at the probe, essentially resulting in a larger, steered "element". After the pre-beamforming, the data is transferred from the probe to the system with only one cable per sub-aperture, drastically reducing the cable count. At the system level, the second stage of beamforming is done, followed by post-processing and subsequent display. If the beamforming can be perfectly split in two stages, then the performance of SAP is equal to that of a fully wired array. However, hardware constraints limit the processing possibilities in the first stage (i.e. in the probe), so simplifications need to be made. For example, only linear steering capability and a constant apodization inside the sub-aperture may be enabled (Zhao et al. 2015). Furthermore, the increased amount of electrical circuits in the probe could give rise to heating problems, power consumption concerns and a bulky probe that is not ergonomic.

5.3.5. *Hardware – sparse arrays*

Sparse arrays provide a more obvious way to reduce the channel count, because their aperture is only sparsely populated (i.e. not completely filled). Thereby, they use fewer elements for a fixed aperture size and require fewer channels. The reduced channel count comes at a cost in performance, mainly in terms of image contrast, caused by increased grating lobes as a result of the increased average pitch (i.e. distance between elements). The resolution is usually less affected, because this correlates with the size of the overall aperture, which is not changed. Several groups have investigated the design process for sparse arrays, i.e. decide where the active elements will be located. Some made use of optimization algorithms (genetic algorithms, simulated annealing) to iteratively change and assess the element distribution (Haupt 1994; Roux et al. 2016a, 2016b, 2017). These algorithms are computationally expensive, especially when more degrees of freedom (non-gridded element positions) and more steering angles are used during optimization. Other groups based their element positions on the favorable properties of Fermat's spiral, which results in a distribution with a uniform but nonperiodic element density, i.e. the pitch is not constant (Vígano et al. 2009; Martínez-Graullera et al. 2010; Ramalli et al. 2015; Nooijens et al. 2020). The pitch dictates the position of the grating lobes, which will therefore also not be constant. This means that the grating lobes are spread out in space to form a "grating plateau" rather than accumulating to a high intensity grating lobe.

5.3.6. *Hardware – motorized probes and motion tracking*

Normally, ultrasound images do not have an absolute coordinate system, instead the lateral and depth positions are relative to the center of the aperture, the absolute position of which is unknown. However, if the position and rotation of a 2DUS probe are known and tracked while it is used to scan the entire heart, it becomes possible to digitally combine all the acquired slices into a 3D volume. There are two main ways of defining the probe's position: by using motors to move the probe in a precise way (mechanical solutions) or by accurately tracking the probe while it is moved "freely" by the clinician (tracking solutions). Both solutions make use of 2DUS hardware that is readily available in clinics, making them a relatively cheap option for volumetric imaging since there is little need for hardware changes. The motors or trackers can be mounted on the existing systems (Fenster et al. 2011; Roh 2014).

Theoretically, a robotic arm can be used to precisely control the position and rotation of a 2DUS probe to allow repeated scanning of some predefined volume. However, although this has been developed, this solution is too bulky to integrate in a clinical workflow. More often, small motors that can be integrated into the probe while maintaining its ease of handling are used. For example, a "wobbler" probe based on a 2DUS aperture mechanically tilted in elevation, while electronic steering is performed in azimuthal axis is frequently used in, for example, obstetrics. However, this is not a suitable option for cardiac imaging because of the relatively small acoustic window. As such, for cardiac applications, a probe rotating around its center axis normal to the aperture has been proposed (e.g. Nguyen-Dinh et al. 2001; Blancher et al. 2004; Voormolen et al. 2006). The advantage of these mechanical probes is that there is no need for calibration (in contrast to the tracking solutions described below); however, the moving parts can degrade over time due to heat accumulation or abrasion, which can decrease the long-term reliability.

Attaching a tracking mechanism to a 2DUS probe enables the tracking of the position and pose (e.g. rotation and tilting) of the probe while allowing the clinician to freely move the probe to cover the organ. Tracking of the probe can be done by either adding a sensor to the probe or by attaching it to an articulated arm, a jointed instrument that measures the angle of each joint to track the position of a clamp. There are several types of sensors that can be used, for example, acoustic, magnetic or optical, but they all follow the same principle: several transducers or receivers are positioned in the room to track the target or emitter attached to the probe. The tracking system must be calibrated and may need to be recalibrated periodically to avoid calibration drift. The need for calibration takes time, and also allows an assessment of the performance of the tracking system, which is harder to assess for the integrated motor parts of the mechanical solutions. Because the probe is tracked rather than repeatedly covering a predefined volume, the tracking solution is better adapted to expand the field of view of a static (or slow moving) object, than it is to investigate one volume over time. This means that in the echocardiographic context, mechanical solutions might be more suitable than tracking solutions. However, when probe tracking is combined with ECG gating, it is possible to combine multiple anatomical views to construct a static volume of the heart.

5.3.7. *Beamforming – challenges and solutions*

To expand 2DUS to 3DUS beamforming, we "just" have to add the elevational direction. Although there are many similarities between 2D and 3D modes, it is not that straightforward to change from one to the other in practice. To investigate a volume rather than a sector, we need to image lines in both the azimuth and elevation directions. In other words, if we needed 60 lines for a 2DUS sector, we would need 3,600 lines for an equivalent 3DUS volume. Using a focused beam for each image line (i.e. SLT imaging) would result in a frame rate of ~128 Hz for 2DUS but just over 1 Hz for 3DUS, which is too low for evaluation of an organ contracting with a period of ~1s or less (i.e. a normal heart rate of 60–80 beats per minute).

As in the 2DUS case, the most straightforward way to increase the frame rate is to either use fewer scan lines in the same volume (decreasing line density) or to decrease the size of the volume. These choices will sacrifice the resolution or the field of view, respectively. For 3DUS there is also the option of bi- or tri-plane imaging, where two or three planes are imaged instead of an entire volume (Sugeng et al. 2003; Franke 2007). An added advantage is that they can be displayed without any rendering techniques, as they are essentially two or three simultaneously recorded B-mode images that can be shown on the display side-by-side.

Other strategies rely on the assumption that the cardiac cycle is periodic. Acquisitions from several heartbeats are combined to create a new dataset with a higher, "virtual" frame rate. Using the data from an ECG lead can help to determine at what point in the cardiac cycle each image was acquired or trigger data acquisition for distinct sub-volumes. However, gating only works when the heart rhythm is constant, and it is not a real-time technique and can therefore not be used for image guidance during interventions, for example.

More advanced techniques to increase the frame rate follow the same strategies as for 2DUS (discussed in section 5.2); however, there are some additional considerations in the 3DUS case. In echocardiography, apertures are small and a relatively large volume must be covered. For 3D diverging wave imaging (Provost et al. 2014), this implies that the energy of the wave will be spread over an increasing "area" rather than "a line". In other words, the energy will decrease quadratically with increasing depth, which can limit the maximum penetration depth and SNR at larger depths. Furthermore, the higher number of parallel reconstruction lines required per diverging wave transmit leads to a high computational load. To prevent this from becoming a bottleneck for the frame rate, in practice, GPU-based beamformers are used.

Using multi-line transmission (MLT) can, just like for the 2DUS case, increase the frame rate while preserving resolution and penetration depth. However, cross-talk artifacts can reduce the image quality (Tong et al. 2014b; Ortega et al. 2016). As mentioned in the previous section (see section 5.2.1), this artifact can be reduced by using window functions for the apodization (Tong et al. 2014b). The number of simultaneously transmitted lines in 3DUS MLT is higher, which means that the energy output of the probe increases. This may give rise to safety concerns in terms of an increased Thermal Index (TI) and an increased probe surface temperature, although countermeasures have been explored for the 2D case (Santos et al. 2015).

One technique that is unique to 3DUS is multi-plane transmission (Chen et al. 2017, 2019) which is a combination of an unfocused wave in one direction (azimuthal or elevational), and MLT in the perpendicular direction. This technique is called multi-plane transmit (MPT) and can be seen as the middle ground alternative to DWI and MLT. As the waves are partially focused (MLT direction), MPT maintains resolution and penetration depth better than DWI does, and increases the temporal resolution more than would be possible with MLT alone.

5.3.8. *Software challenges*

When moving from 2DUS to 3DUS, most steps of the post-processing and data management remain very similar, although the scale on which they happen increases drastically. The quantity of data that passes each of the stages of beamforming scales quadratically. This can become a bottleneck for real-time volumetric imaging. For example, saving volumes rather than frames may increase data sizes from several megabytes to tens of GB, so regular storage options may no longer be sufficient and data transfer speed may begin to impact processing. These problems can (partially) be addressed by increasing the hardware capabilities and GPU-based software acceleration.

A more fundamental problem is that displaying a 3D (or 4D) dataset on a 2D screen is not trivial. By displaying several slices of the dataset (usually perpendicular or parallel to each other), we can work around this problem. This would nevertheless require a clinician to move the positions of the slices and mentally reconstruct the volume, or accept that a large part of the dataset is simply not displayed. For a fast-moving structure like the heart, scrolling through the slice positions would probably require the display to be paused. Other techniques rely on either automated segmentation or a combination of segmentation and rendering techniques, both of which are complete research fields in themselves and therefore mostly outside the scope of this chapter and the reader is referred to the following reviews: Kaufman and Mueller (2005); Osipov et al. (2018).

5.4. References

Asad, Z.U.A., Yousif, A., Khan, M.S., Al-Khatib, S.M., Stavrakis, S. (2019). Catheter ablation versus medical therapy for atrial fibrillation: A systematic review and meta-analysis of randomized controlled trials. *Circulation: Arrhythmia and Electrophysiology*, 12(9), e007414.

Bartel, T., Müller, S., Biviano, A., Hahn, R.T. (2014). Why is intracardiac echocardiography helpful? Benefits, costs, and how to learn. *European Heart Journal*, 35(2), 69–76.

Bercoff, J., Montaldo, G., Loupas, T., Savery, D., Mézière, F., Fink, M., Tanter, M. (2011). Ultrafast compound Doppler imaging: Providing full blood flow characterization. *IEEE Transactions on Ultrasonics, Ferroelectrics, and Frequency Control*, 58(1), 134–147.

Blaak, S., Yu, Z., Meijer, G.C.M., Prins, C., Lancee, C.T., Bosch, J.G., de Jong, N. (2009). Design of a micro-beamformer for a 2D piezoelectric ultrasound transducer. In *2009 IEEE International Ultrasonics Symposium*, October 2009, Rome, 1338–1341.

Blancher, J., Léger, C., Nguyen, L.D. (2004). Time-varying, 3-D echocardiography using a fast-rotating probe. *IEEE Transactions on Ultrasonics, Ferroelectrics, and Frequency Control*, 51(5), 634–639.

Bouchard, R.R., Hsu, S.J., Wolf, P.D., Trahey, G.E. (2009). In vivo cardiac, acoustic-radiation-force-driven, shear wave velocimetry. *Ultrasonic Imaging*, 31(3), 201–213.

Bouzari, H., Engholm, M., Beers, C., Stuart, M.B., Nikolov, S.I., Thomsen, E.V., Jensen, J.A. (2017). Curvilinear 3-D imaging using row-column-addressed 2-D arrays with a diverging lens: Feasibility study. *IEEE Transactions on Ultrasonics, Ferroelectrics, and Frequency Control*, 64(6), 978–988.

Chen, Y., Tong, L., Ortega, A., Luo, J., D'hooge, J. (2017). Feasibility of multiplane-transmit beamforming for real-time volumetric cardiac imaging: A simulation study. *IEEE Transactions on Ultrasonics, Ferroelectrics, and Frequency Control*, 64(4), 648–659.

Chen, Y., Pernot, M., Papadacci, C., D'hooge, J., Luo, J. (2019). Multi-plane-transmit (MPT) volumetric imaging based on a matrix array: Experimental validation. In *2019 IEEE International Ultrasonics Symposium (IUS)*, October 2019, Glasgow, 1890–1893.

Cikes, M., Tong, L., Sutherland, G.R., D'hooge, J. (2014). Ultrafast cardiac ultrasound imaging: Technical principles, applications, and clinical benefits. *JACC: Cardiovascular Imaging*, 7(8), 812–823.

Cohen, A., Donal, E., Delgado, V., Pepi, M., Tsang, T., Gerber, B., Soulat-Dufour, L., Habib, G., Lancellotti, P., Evangelista, A. et al. (2021). EACVI recommendations on cardiovascular imaging for the detection of embolic sources: Endorsed by the Canadian Society of Echocardiography. *European Heart Journal – Cardiovascular Imaging*, 22(6), e24–e57.

Cvijic, M., Bézy, S., Petrescu, A., Santos, P., Orlowska, M., Chakraborty, B., Duchenne, J., Pedrosa, J., Vanassche, T., D'hooge, J. et al. (2020). Interplay of cardiac remodelling and myocardial stiffness in hypertensive heart disease: A shear wave imaging study using high-frame rate echocardiography. *European Heart Journal – Cardiovascular Imaging*, 21(6), 664–672.

Daae, A.S., Wigen, M.S., Fadnes, S., Løvstakken, L., Støylen, A. (2021). Intraventricular vector flow imaging with blood speckle tracking in adults: Feasibility, normal physiology and mechanisms in healthy volunteers. *Ultrasound in Medicine & Biology*, 47(12), 3501–3513.

Demi, L., Verweij, M.D., Van Dongen, K.W. (2012). Parallel transmit beamforming using orthogonal frequency division multiplexing applied to harmonic imaging – A feasibility study. *IEEE Transactions on Ultrasonics, Ferroelectrics, and Frequency Control*, 59(11), 2439–2447.

Demi, L., Ramalli, A., Giannini, G., Mischi, M. (2015). In vitro and in vivo tissue harmonic images obtained with parallel transmit beamforming by means of orthogonal frequency division multiplexing. *IEEE Transactions on Ultrasonics, Ferroelectrics, and Frequency Control*, 62(1), 230–235.

Demore, C.E., Joyce, A.W., Wall, K., Lockwood, G.R. (2009). Real-time volume imaging using a crossed electrode array. *IEEE Transactions on Ultrasonics, Ferroelectrics, and Frequency Control*, 56(6), 1252–1261.

Denarie, B., Tangen, T.A., Ekroll, I.K., Rolim, N., Torp, H., Bjåstad, T., Lovstakken, L. (2013). Coherent plane wave compounding for very high frame rate ultrasonography of rapidly moving targets. *IEEE Transactions on Medical Imaging*, 32(7), 1265–1276.

Du, Z.D., Hijazi, Z.M., Kleinman, C.S., Silverman, N.H., Larntz, K., Amplatzer Investigators (2002). Comparison between transcatheter and surgical closure of secundum atrial septal defect in children and adults: Results of a multicenter nonrandomized trial. *Journal of the American College of Cardiology*, 39(11), 1836–1844.

Enriquez, A., Saenz, L.C., Rosso, R., Silvestry, F.E., Callans, D., Marchlinski, F.E., Garcia, F. (2018). Use of intracardiac echocardiography in interventional cardiology: Working with the anatomy rather than fighting it. *Circulation*, 137(21), 2278–2294.

Fenster, A. and Downey, D.B. (1996). 3-D ultrasound imaging: A review. *IEEE Engineering in Medicine and Biology Magazine*, 15(6), 41–51.

Fenster, A. and Downey, D.B. (2000). Three-dimensional ultrasound imaging. *Annual Review of Biomedical Engineering*, 2(1), 457–475.

Fenster, A., Parraga, G., Bax, J. (2011). Three-dimensional ultrasound scanning. *Interface Focus*, 1(4), 503–519.

Flachskampf, F.A., Wouters, P.F., Edvardsen, T., Evangelista, A., Habib, G., Hoffman, P., Hoffmann, R., Lancellotti, P., Pepi, M. (2014). Recommendations for transoesophageal echocardiography: EACVI update 2014. *European Heart Journal – Cardiovascular Imaging*, 15(4), 353–365.

Franke, A. (2007). Real-time three-dimensional echocardiography in stress testing: Bi- and triplane imaging for enhanced image acquisition. *Cardiology Clinics*, 25(2), 261–265.

Galderisi, M., Cosyns, B., Edvardsen, T., Cardim, N., Delgado, V., Di Salvo, G., Donal, E., Sade, L.E., Ernande, L., Garbi, M. et al. (2017). Standardization of adult transthoracic echocardiography reporting in agreement with recent chamber quantification, diastolic function, and heart valve disease recommendations: An expert consensus document of the European Association of Cardiovascular Imaging. *European Heart Journal – Cardiovascular Imaging*, 18(12), 1301–1310.

Gammelmark, K.L. and Jensen, J. (2014). 2-D tissue motion compensation of synthetic transmit aperture images. *IEEE Transactions on Ultrasonics, Ferroelectrics, and Frequency Control*, 61(4), 594–610.

Gong, P., Song, P., Chen, S. (2017). Ultrafast synthetic transmit aperture imaging using Hadamard-encoded virtual sources with overlapping sub-apertures. *IEEE Transactions on Medical Imaging*, 36(6), 1372–1381.

Grondin, J., Sayseng, V., Konofagou, E.E. (2017). Cardiac strain imaging with coherent compounding of diverging waves. *IEEE Transactions on Ultrasonics, Ferroelectrics, and Frequency Control*, 64(8), 1212–1222.

Hahn, R.T., Saric, M., Faletra, F.F., Garg, R., Gillam, L.D., Horton, K., Khalique, O.K., Little, S.H., Mackensen, G.B., Oh, J. et al. (2022). Recommended standards for the performance of transesophageal echocardiographic screening for structural heart intervention: From the American Society of Echocardiography. *Journal of the American Society of Echocardiography*, 35(1), 1–76.

Haupt, R.L. (1994). Thinned arrays using genetic algorithms. *IEEE Transactions on Antennas and Propagation*, 42(7), 993–999.

Hergum, T., Bjastad, T., Kristoffersen, K., Torp, H. (2007). Parallel beamforming using synthetic transmit beams. *IEEE Transactions on Ultrasonics, Ferroelectrics, and Frequency Control*, 54(2), 271–280.

Hoffmann, R., Barletta, G., Von Bardeleben, S., Vanoverschelde, J.L., Kasprzak, J., Greis, C., Becher, H. (2014). Analysis of left ventricular volumes and function: A multicenter comparison of cardiac magnetic resonance imaging, cine ventriculography, and unenhanced and contrast-enhanced two-dimensional and three-dimensional echocardiography. *Journal of the American Society of Echocardiography*, 27(3), 292–301.

Huang, Q. and Zeng, Z. (2017). A review on real-time 3D ultrasound imaging technology. *BioMed Research International*, 6027029, 20. https://doi.org/10.1155/2017/6027029.

Jasaityte, R. and D'hooge, J. (2010). Strain rate imaging: Fundamental principles and progress so far. *Imaging in Medicine*, 2(5), 547.

Jensen, A.C., Nasholm, S.P., Nilsen, C.I.C., Austeng, A., Holm, S. (2012). Applying Thomson's multitaper approach to reduce speckle in medical ultrasound imaging. *IEEE Transactions on Ultrasonics, Ferroelectrics, and Frequency Control*, 59(10), 2178–2185.

Johnson, J.A., Karaman, M., Khuri-Yakub, B.T. (2005a). Coherent-array imaging using phased subarrays. Part I: Basic principles. *IEEE Transactions on Ultrasonics, Ferroelectrics, and Frequency Control*, 52(1), 37–50.

Johnson, J.A., Oralkan, O., Ergun, S., Demirci, U., Karaman, M., Khuri-Yakub, B.T. (2005b). Coherent array imaging using phased subarrays. Part II: Simulations and experimental results. *IEEE Transactions on Ultrasonics, Ferroelectrics, and Frequency Control*, 52(1), 51–64.

Joos, P., Porée, J., Liebgott, H., Vray, D., Baudet, M., Faurie, J., Tournoux, F., Cloutier, G., Nicolas, B., Garcia, D. (2018). High-frame-rate speckle-tracking echocardiography. *IEEE Transactions on Ultrasonics, Ferroelectrics, and Frequency Control*, 65(5), 720–728.

Karadayi, K., Managuli, R., Kim, Y. (2009). Three-dimensional ultrasound: From acquisition to visualization and from algorithms to systems. *IEEE Reviews in Biomedical Engineering*, 2, 23–39.

Kaufman, A.E. and Mueller, K. (2005). Overview of volume rendering. *The Visualization Handbook*, 7, 127–174.

Keijzer, L.B., Strachinaru, M., Bowen, D.J., Geleijnse, M.L., van der Steen, A.F., Bosch, J.G., de Jong, N., Vos, H.J. (2019). Reproducibility of natural shear wave elastography measurements. *Ultrasound in Medicine & Biology*, 45(12), 3172–3185.

Keijzer, L.B., Caenen, A., Voorneveld, J., Strachinaru, M., Bowen, D.J., van de Wouw, J., Sorop, O., Merkus, D., Duncker, D.J., van der Steen, A.F. et al. (2020). A direct comparison of natural and acoustic-radiation-force-induced cardiac mechanical waves. *Scientific Reports*, 10(1), 18431.

Kvåle, K.F., Bersvendsen, J., Remme, E.W., Salles, S., Aalen, J.M., Brekke, P.H., Edvardsen, T., Samset, E. (2019). Detection of regional mechanical activation of the left ventricular myocardium using high frame rate ultrasound imaging. *IEEE Transactions on Medical Imaging*, 38(11), 2665–2675.

Lang, R.M., Bierig, M., Devereux, R.B., Flachskampf, F.A., Foster, E., Pellikka, P.A., Picard, M.H., Roman, M.J., Seward, J., Shanewise, J. et al. (2006). Recommendations for chamber quantification. *European Journal of Echocardiography*, 7(2), 79–108.

Lang, R.M., Badano, L.P., Tsang, W., Adams, D.H., Agricola, E., Buck, T., Faletra, F.F., Franke, A., Hung, J., de Isla, L.P. et al. (2012). EAE/ASE recommendations for image acquisition and display using three-dimensional echocardiography. *European Heart Journal – Cardiovascular Imaging*, 13(1), 1–46.

Lang, R.M., Badano, L.P., Mor-Avi, V., Afilalo, J., Armstrong, A., Ernande, L., Flachskampf, F.A., Foster, E., Goldstein, S.A., Kuznetsova, T. et al. (2015). Recommendations for cardiac chamber quantification by echocardiography in adults: An update from the American Society of Echocardiography and the European Association of Cardiovascular Imaging. *European Heart Journal – Cardiovascular Imaging*, 16(3), 233–271.

Larson III, J.D. and Hewlett Packard Co (1993). 2-D phased array ultrasound imaging system with distributed phasing. U.S. Patent 5(229), 933.

Lin, E. and Alessio, A. (2009). What are the basic concepts of temporal, contrast, and spatial resolution in cardiac CT? *Journal of Cardiovascular Computed Tomography*, 3(6), 403–408.

Marsan, N.A., Westenberg, J.J., Ypenburg, C., Delgado, V., van Bommel, R.J., Roes, S.D., Nucifora, G., van der Geest, R.J., de Roos, A., Reiber, J.C. et al. (2009). Quantification of functional mitral regurgitation by real-time 3D echocardiography: Comparison with 3D velocity-encoded cardiac magnetic resonance. *JACC: Cardiovascular Imaging*, 2(11), 1245–1252.

Martínez-Graullera, O., Martín, C.J., Godoy, G., Ullate, L.G. (2010). 2D array design based on Fermat spiral for ultrasound imaging. *Ultrasonics*, 50(2), 280–289.

Matrone, G., Ramalli, A., D'hooge, J., Tortoli, P., Magenes, G. (2019). A comparison of coherence-based beamforming techniques in high-frame-rate ultrasound imaging with multi-line transmission. *IEEE Transactions on Ultrasonics, Ferroelectrics, and Frequency Control*, 67(2), 329–340.

Misaridis, T. and Jensen, J.A. (2005). Use of modulated excitation signals in medical ultrasound. Part III: High frame rate imaging. *IEEE Transactions on Ultrasonics, Ferroelectrics, and Frequency Control*, 52(2), 208–219.

Mitchell, C., Rahko, P.S., Blauwet, L.A., Canaday, B., Finstuen, J.A., Foster, M.C., Horton, K., Ogunyankin, K.O., Palma, R.A., Velazquez, E.J. (2019). Guidelines for performing a comprehensive transthoracic echocardiographic examination in adults: Recommendations from the American Society of Echocardiography. *Journal of the American Society of Echocardiography*, 32(1), 1–64.

Montaldo, G., Tanter, M., Bercoff, J., Benech, N., Fink, M. (2009). Coherent plane-wave compounding for very high frame rate ultrasonography and transient elastography. *IEEE Transactions on Ultrasonics, Ferroelectrics, and Frequency Control*, 56(3), 489–506.

Mor-Avi, V., Jenkins, C., Kühl, H.P., Nesser, H.J., Marwick, T., Franke, A., Ebner, C., Freed, B.H., Steringer-Mascherbauer, R., Pollard, H. et al. (2008). Real-time 3-dimensional echocardiographic quantification of left ventricular volumes: Multicenter study for validation with magnetic resonance imaging and investigation of sources of error. *JACC: Cardiovascular Imaging*, 1(4), 413–423.

Morton, C.E. and Lockwood, G.R. (2003). Theoretical assessment of a crossed electrode 2-D array for 3-D imaging. In *IEEE Symposium on Ultrasonics*, October, 1, 968–971.

Nagueh, S.F., Smiseth, O.A., Appleton, C.P., Byrd, B.F., Dokainish, H., Edvardsen, T., Flachskampf, F.A., Gillebert, T.C., Klein, A.L., Lancellotti, P. et al. (2016). Recommendations for the evaluation of left ventricular diastolic function by echocardiography: An update from the American Society of Echocardiography and the European Association of Cardiovascular Imaging. *European Journal of Echocardiography*, 17(12), 1321–1360.

Nguyen-Dinh, A., Mauchamp, P., Felix, N., Dufait, R., Auclair, P., Flesch, A. (2001). Integrated mechanism based multiplane/3D ultrasonic imaging probes. In *IEEE Ultrasonics Symposium. Proceedings. An International Symposium (Cat. No. 01CH37263)*, October, 2, 1147–1150.

Nooijens, S., Ramalli, A., Ingram, M., Fournelle, M., Bertrand, A., D'hooge, J. (2020). Design of a sparse ellipsoidal array for volumetric ultrasound imaging of the prostate. *IEEE International Ultrasonics Symposium (IUS)*, September, 1–3.

Orlowska, M., Ramalli, A., Petrescu, A., Cvijic, M., Bezy, S., Santos, P., Pedrosa, J., Voigt, J.U., D'hooge, J. (2020). A novel 2-D speckle tracking method for high-frame-rate echocardiography. *IEEE Transactions on Ultrasonics, Ferroelectrics, and Frequency Control*, 67(9), 1764–1775.

Ortega, A., Provost, J., Tong, L., Santos, P., Heyde, B., Pernot, M., D'hooge, J. (2016). A comparison of the performance of different multiline transmit setups for fast volumetric cardiac ultrasound. *IEEE Transactions on Ultrasonics, Ferroelectrics, and Frequency Control*, 63(12), 2082–2091.

Osipov, L.V., Kulberg, N.S., Leonov, D.V., Morozov, S.P. (2018). 3D ultrasound: Current state, emerging trends and technologies. *Biomedical Engineering*, 52, 199–203. https://doi.org/10.1007/s10527-018-9813-0.

Osipov, L.V., Kulberg, N.S., Leonov, D.V., Morozov, S.P. (2020). 3D ultrasound: Visualization of volumetric data. *Biomedical Engineering*, 54(2), 149–154.

Papadacci, C., Pernot, M., Couade, M., Fink, M., Tanter, M. (2014). High-contrast ultrafast imaging of the heart. *IEEE Transactions on Ultrasonics, Ferroelectrics, and Frequency Control*, 61(2), 288–301.

Pérez de Isla, L., Casanova, C., Almería, C., Rodrigo, J.L., Cordeiro, P., Mataix, L., Aubele, A.L., Lang, R., Zamorano, J.L. (2007). Which method should be the reference method to evaluate the severity of rheumatic mitral stenosis? Gorlin's method versus 3D-echo. *European Journal of Echocardiography*, 8(6), 470–473.

Pernot, M., Couade, M., Mateo, P., Crozatier, B., Fischmeister, R., Tanter, M. (2011). Real-time assessment of myocardial contractility using shear wave imaging. *Journal of the American College of Cardiology*, 58(1), 65–72.

Petrescu, A., Bézy, S., Cvijic, M., Santos, P., Orlowska, M., Duchenne, J., Pedrosa, J., Van Keer, J.M., Verbeken, E., von Bardeleben, S. et al. (2020). Shear wave elastography using high-frame-rate imaging in the follow-up of heart transplantation recipients. *Cardiovascular Imaging*, 13(11), 2304–2313.

Porée, J., Posada, D., Hodzic, A., Tournoux, F., Cloutier, G., Garcia, D. (2016). High-frame-rate echocardiography using coherent compounding with Doppler-based motion-compensation. *IEEE Transactions on Medical Imaging*, 35(7), 1647–1657.

Porée, J., Baudet, M., Tournoux, F., Cloutier, G., Garcia, D. (2018). A dual tissue-Doppler optical-flow method for speckle tracking echocardiography at high frame rate. *IEEE Transactions on Medical Imaging*, 37(9), 2022–2032.

Prager, R.W., Ijaz, U.Z., Gee, A.H., Treece, G.M. (2010). Three-dimensional ultrasound imaging. *Proceedings of the Institution of Mechanical Engineers, Part H: Journal of Engineering in Medicine*, 224(2), 193–223.

Prieur, F., Dénarié, B., Austeng, A., Torp, H. (2013). Correspondence-multi-line transmission in medical imaging using the second-harmonic signal. *IEEE Transactions on Ultrasonics, Ferroelectrics, and Frequency Control*, 60(12), 2682–2692.

Provost, J., Papadacci, C., Arango, J.E., Imbault, M., Fink, M., Gennisson, J.L., Tanter, M., Pernot, M. (2014). 3D ultrafast ultrasound imaging in vivo. *Physics in Medicine & Biology*, 59(19), L1.

Rabinovich, A., Feuer, A., Friedman, Z. (2015). Multi-line transmission combined with minimum variance beamforming in medical ultrasound imaging. *IEEE Transactions on Ultrasonics, Ferroelectrics, and Frequency Control*, 62(5), 814–827.

Ramalli, A., Boni, E., Savoia, A.S., Tortoli, P. (2015). Density-tapered spiral arrays for ultrasound 3-D imaging. *IEEE Transactions on Ultrasonics, Ferroelectrics, and Frequency Control*, 62(8), 1580–1588.

Ramalli, A., Dallai, A., Guidi, F., Bassi, L., Boni, E., Tong, L., Fradella, G., D'hooge, J., Tortoli, P. (2018). Real-time high-frame-rate cardiac B-mode and tissue Doppler imaging based on multiline transmission and multiline acquisition. *IEEE Transactions on Ultrasonics, Ferroelectrics, and Frequency Control*, 65(11), 2030–2041.

Ramalli, A., Bézy, S., Orlowska, M., Boni, E., Voigt, J.-U., D'hooge, J. (2020). High frame rate color Doppler to measure intraventricular pressure gradients. *2020 IEEE International Ultrasonics Symposium (IUS)*, Las Vegas, 1–4. https://doi.org/10.1109/IUS46767.2020.9251332 10.1109/IUS46767.2020.9251332.

Roh, Y. (2014). Ultrasonic transducers for medical volumetric imaging. *Japanese Journal of Applied Physics*, 53(7S), 07KA01.

Roux, E., Ramalli, A., Liebgott, H., Cachard, C., Robini, M.C., Tortoli, P. (2016a). Wideband 2-D array design optimization with fabrication constraints for 3-D US imaging. *IEEE Transactions on Ultrasonics, Ferroelectrics, and Frequency Control*, 64(1), 108–125.

Roux, E., Ramalli, A., Tortoli, P., Cachard, C., Robini, M.C., Liebgott, H. (2016b). 2-D ultrasound sparse arrays multidepth radiation optimization using simulated annealing and spiral-array inspired energy functions. *IEEE Transactions on Ultrasonics, Ferroelectrics, and Frequency Control*, 63(12), 2138–2149.

Santos, P., Tong, L., Ortega, A., Løvstakken, L., Samset, E., D'hooge, J. (2015). Acoustic output of multi-line transmit beamforming for fast cardiac imaging: A simulation study. *IEEE Transactions on Ultrasonics, Ferroelectrics, and Frequency Control*, 62(7), 1320–1330.

Santos, P., Petrescu, A.M., Pedrosa, J., Orlowska, M., Komini, V., Voigt, J.U., D'hooge, J. (2019). Natural shear wave imaging in the human heart: Normal values, feasibility, and reproducibility. *IEEE Transactions on Ultrasonics, Ferroelectrics, and Frequency Control*, 66(3), 442–452.

Savord, B. and Solomon, R. (2003). Fully sampled matrix transducer for real time 3D ultrasonic imaging. In *IEEE Symposium on Ultrasonics*, October, 1, 945–953.

Seo, C.H. and Yen, J.T. (2009). A 256 x 256 2-D array transducer with row-column addressing for 3-D rectilinear imaging. *IEEE Transactions on Ultrasonics, Ferroelectrics, and Frequency Control*, 56(4), 837–847.

Shattuck, D.P., Weinshenker, M.D., Smith, S.W., von Ramm, O.T. (1984). Explososcan: A parallel processing technique for high speed ultrasound imaging with linear phased arrays. *The Journal of the Acoustical Society of America*, 75(4), 1273–1282.

Siddiqui, W.T., Usman, T., Atiq, M., Amanullah, M.M. (2014). Transcatheter versus surgical closure of atrial septum defect: A debate from a developing country. *Journal of Cardiovascular and Thoracic Research*, 6(4), 205.

Song, P., Bi, X., Mellema, D.C., Manduca, A., Urban, M.W., Pellikka, P.A., Chen, S., Greenleaf, J.F. (2016). Pediatric cardiac shear wave elastography for quantitative assessment of myocardial stiffness: A pilot study in healthy controls. *Ultrasound in Medicine & Biology*, 42(8), 1719–1729.

Sugeng, L., Kirkpatrick, J., Lang, R.M., Bednarz, J.E., DeCara, J.M., Lammertin, G., Spencer, K.T. (2003). Biplane stress echocardiography using a prototype matrix-array transducer. *Journal of the American Society of Echocardiography*, 16(9), 937–941.

Sugeng, L., Mor-Avi, V., Weinert, L., Niel, J., Ebner, C., Steringer-Mascherbauer, R., Bartolles, R., Baumann, R., Schummers, G., Lang, R.M. et al. (2010). Multimodality comparison of quantitative volumetric analysis of the right ventricle. *JACC: Cardiovascular Imaging*, 3(1), 10–18.

Tong, L., Gao, H., D'hooge, J. (2013a). Multi-transmit beam forming for fast cardiac imaging – A simulation study. *IEEE Transactions on Ultrasonics, Ferroelectrics, and Frequency Control*, 60(8), 1719–1731.

Tong, L., Ortega, A., Gao, H., D'hooge, J. (2013b). Fast three-dimensional ultrasound cardiac imaging using multi-transmit beam forming: A simulation study. In *IEEE International Ultrasonics Symposium (IUS)*, July, 1456–1459.

Tong, L., Ramalli, A., Jasaityte, R., Tortoli, P., D'hooge, J. (2014). Multi-transmit beam forming for fast cardiac imaging – Experimental validation and in vivo application. *IEEE Transactions on Medical Imaging*, 33(6), 1205–1219.

Tong, L., He, Q., Ortega, A., Ramalli, A., Tortoli, P., Luo, J., D'hooge, J. (2019). Coded excitation for crosstalk suppression in multi-line transmit beamforming: Simulation study and experimental validation. *Applied Sciences*, 9(3), 486.

Toulemonde, M., Basset, O., Tortoli, P., Cachard, C. (2015). Thomson's multitaper approach combined with coherent plane-wave compounding to reduce speckle in ultrasound imaging. *Ultrasonics*, 56, 390–398.

Townsend, N., Kazakiewicz, D., Lucy Wright, F., Timmis, A., Huculeci, R., Torbica, A., Gale, C.P., Achenbach, S., Weidinger, F., Vardas, P. (2022). Epidemiology of cardiovascular disease in Europe. *Nature Reviews Cardiology*, 19(2), 133–143.

Turnbull, D.H. and Foster, F.S. (1991). Beam steering with pulsed two-dimensional transducer arrays. *IEEE Transactions on Ultrasonics, Ferroelectrics, and Frequency Control*, 38(4), 320–333.

Viganó, M.C., Toso, G., Caille, G., Mangenot, C., Lager, I.E. (2009). Sunflower array antenna with adjustable density taper. *International Journal of Antennas and Propagation*, 624035, 10. https://doi.org/10.1155/2009/624035.

Villemain, O., Correia, M., Mousseaux, E., Baranger, J., Zarka, S., Podetti, I., Soulat, G., Damy, T., Hagège, A., Tanter, M. et al. (2019). Myocardial stiffness evaluation using noninvasive shear wave imaging in healthy and hypertrophic cardiomyopathic adults. *JACC: Cardiovascular Imaging*, 12(7 Part 1), 1135–1145.

Voormolen, M.M., Krenning, B.J., Lancee, C.T., Ten Cate, F.J., Roelandt, J.R., van der Steen, A.F. (2006). Harmonic 3-D echocardiography with a fast-rotating ultrasound transducer. *IEEE Transactions on Ultrasonics, Ferroelectrics, and Frequency Control*, 53(10), 1739–1748.

Vos, H.J., van Dalen, B.M., Heinonen, I., Bosch, J.G., Sorop, O., Duncker, D.J., van der Steen, A.F., de Jong, N. (2017). Cardiac shear wave velocity detection in the porcine heart. *Ultrasound in Medicine & Biology*, 43(4), 753–764.

WHO (2021). Cardiovascular diseases (CVDs) [Online]. Available at: https://www.who.int/news-room/fact-sheets/detail/cardiovascular-diseases-(cvds) [Assessed 5 January 2022].

Zhang, Y., Li, H., Lee, W.N. (2019). Imaging heart dynamics with ultrafast cascaded-wave ultrasound. *IEEE Transactions on Ultrasonics, Ferroelectrics, and Frequency Control*, 66(9), 1465–1479.

Zhao, F. and Luo, J. (2018). Diverging wave compounding with spatio-temporal encoding using orthogonal Golay pairs for high frame rate imaging. *Ultrasonics*, 89, 155–165.

Zhao, K.Q., Bjastad, T.G., Kristoffersen, K. (2015). Error analysis of subaperture processing in 1-D ultrasound arrays. *IEEE Transactions on Ultrasonics, Ferroelectrics, and Frequency Control*, 62(4), 663–672.

Zurakhov, G., Tong, L., Ramalli, A., Tortoli, P., D'hooge, J., Friedman, Z., Adam, D. (2018). Multiline transmit beamforming combined with adaptive apodization. *IEEE Transactions on Ultrasonics, Ferroelectrics, and Frequency Control*, 65(4), 535–545.

6

Ultrasound Contrast Agents: Microvascular Characterization

Simona TURCO[1], Peiran CHEN[1], Andrej LYSHCHIK[2], Ahmed EL KAFFAS[3] and Massimo MISCHI[1]

[1] *Eindhoven University of Technology, The Netherlands*

[2] *Thomas Jefferson University Hospital, Philadelphia, USA*

[3] *Stanford Medicine, California, USA*

6.1. Introduction

Dynamic contrast-enhanced ultrasound (DCE-US) is a powerful imaging tool that provides diagnostic information by combining standard anatomical imaging with vascular assessment through interpretation of the transport kinetics of ultrasound contrast agents (UCAs). These consist of solutions of gas-filled microbubbles encapsulated in a biocompatible shell with a diameter distribution ranging from 1 μm to 10 μm (Feinstein 2004; Faez et al. 2013). Their size is similar to that of red blood cells (6–8 μm), but larger than the gaps in the endothelial layers making up the vessel walls (a few hundred nanometers). As such, UCAs can pass through the circulatory system down to the capillary level, while remaining intravascular. This makes them especially suited for assessment of the microcirculation.

When UCAs are insonified by ultrasound waves near their resonance frequency, they can generate strong nonlinear echoes (Correas et al. 2001; Sboros 2008; Mischi

---

For a color version of all the figures in this chapter, see www.iste.co.uk/bridal/innovative.zip.

Innovative Ultrasound Imaging Techniques,
coordinated by S. Lori BRIDAL.

et al. 2018). In DCE-US, the passage of intravenously injected UCAs through an organ is recorded by an ultrasound imaging system through contrast-specific imaging sequences, which enhance the nonlinear echoes from UCAs while suppressing the linear echo signals from surrounding tissues (Frinking et al. 2000). DCE-US may thus provide real-time assessment of blood flow, enabling physiological quantification for many established clinical applications.

Physiological quantification is typically performed by analyzing the temporal evolution of the UCA concentration in the organ or tissue of interest. By looking at the changes in the acoustic intensity over time, time–intensity curves (TICs) can be extracted to describe UCA temporal kinetics (see Figure 6.1). These can be analyzed using principles of indicator dilution theory. Although its use in the context of DCE-US started only a few decades ago, indicator dilution theory has a very long history. Initially focused on the cardiovascular domain, first reports of indicator dilution methods date back to 1761, when Haller compared pulmonary circulation times through inflated and collapsed lungs by injecting a colored liquid into the vena cava (large vein returning blood from the body to the heart) of an animal to provide an indicator of the blood's circulation (Fox 1962; Jhanji et al. 2008). Other important milestones include the measurement of blood volume and flow in 1827 by Hering (Tigerstedt 1921), and its extension by Stewart to measure cardiac output in 1897 (Stewart 1921). The cardiac output (blood volume per unit time) can be estimated based on the rate of change in the concentration of the indicator. Thus, given a measurement of the indicator's concentration over time, t, the cardiac output equals the injected dose of the indicator divided by the area under the concentration-time curve (concentration $(t)\cdot t$). This principle is formulated by the well-known Stewart–Hamilton equation for calculation of the cardiac output. This technique was then further reviewed by Hamilton to take indicator recirculation (during the second and later passages of the indicator bolus) into account through exponential fitting of the early downslope of the dilution curve.

While traditional indicator dilution methods require invasive sampling of the indicator concentration in the tissue of interest, the advent of contrast-enhanced imaging techniques such as DCE-US has enabled minimally invasive measurement of the indicator concentration (or a surrogate thereof) with unprecedented temporal resolution. Moreover, while only macro-scale, tissue- or organ-level analysis was once feasible, contrast-enhanced imaging has enabled the addition of the spatial dimension, permitting hemodynamic assessment down to the micro-scale, image-pixel level resolution. In parallel, temporal, spatial and spatio-temporal analysis methods have been developed to provide a more comprehensive interpretation of the UCA dynamics in both time and space. This can provide real-time assessment of the vascular function and architecture on both the macro- and micro-scale. As a result,

DCE-US has proven useful for many established and emerging clinical applications, especially in cardiology and oncology.

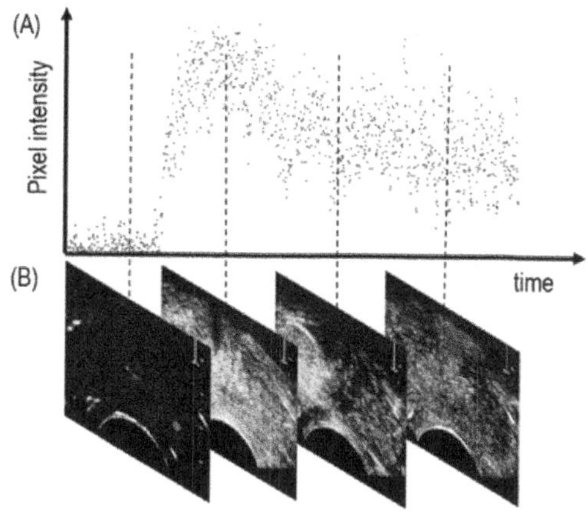

Figure 6.1. *(A) Example of a time–intensity curve (TIC) obtained by recording changes in video intensity at one imaging pixel (blue dot in (B)). (B) Selected frames of the DCE-US video from which the TIC in (A) has been extracted*

Contrast echocardiography, i.e. the use of DCE-US for cardiac assessment, has been used for over 40 years. Applications range from assessment of myocardial perfusion and viability to the evaluation of coronary artery disease. Moreover, because the formation of new vessels, a process known as angiogenesis (Folkman 1984), plays a fundamental role in many physiological and pathological processes, UCAs have been employed to assess angiogenic vasculature in many pathologies such as cancer, atherosclerosis, diabetes, placental insufficiency, hyperlipidemia and arthritis. DCE-US has thus emerged as a useful imaging modality for a range of clinical domains beyond cardiology, including radiology, gastrointestinal imaging and perinatology (Kono et al. 2017; Bertolotto et al. 2018; Mischi et al. 2018; Sidhu et al. 2018; Erlichman et al. 2020; Hwang et al. 2020; Villemain et al. 2020).

In this chapter, we review the methods that have been developed and used for assessment of the microvasculature by DCE-US. Starting from fundamental concepts describing the physics of the UCA acoustic response behind contrast-specific imaging sequences, we discuss the conversion from acoustic intensity to UCA concentration, a fundamental step for quantification known as calibration. Then, we describe the methods that have been proposed for temporal, spatial and spatio-temporal analysis of UCA kinetics, with emphasis on physics- and physiology-driven approaches. Finally, we provide an overview of the clinical utility of UCAs, including established applications and emerging trends. The chapter is concluded by a discussion of current challenges and future perspectives.

6.2. Ultrasound contrast agents and their acoustic response

Historically, UCAs have evolved through three distinct generations (Calliada et al. 1998; Appis et al. 2015; Paefgen et al. 2015). The first generation consisted of air bubbles without a stabilizing shell, such as Echovist® (Schering, Berlin, Germany). These UCAs were used in clinical practice in the early 90s. Echovist was made by mixing a solution with galactose microcrystals, but the resulting UCA was not sufficiently stable in blood flow and failed to cross the transpulmonary circulation (Calliada et al. 1998; Correas et al. 2001). The second generation of UCAs were composed of air bubbles encapsulated by a stabilizing shell, such as albumin (Albunex®, Molecular Biosystems, San Diego, CA, USA) or galactose and palmitic acid (Levovist®, Schering) (Calliada et al. 1998; Cosgrove 2006; Sboros 2008). The third generation is more advanced. The microbubbles are filled with air or perfluorocarbon gases encapsulated by a shell of albumin, phospholipids or polymers. This generation is widely employed in current clinical routine (Piscaglia et al. 2012; Faez et al. 2013; Paefgen et al. 2015; Appis et al. 2015).

When insonified by an acoustic field, UCA microbubbles can produce a strong echo signal due to the large difference in acoustic impedance at the interface between blood and the microbubble's gas core. Given that the diameter of microbubbles is much smaller than the ultrasound wavelength, at low UCA concentration, the backscattered acoustic intensity can, to a first approximation, be characterized as a Rayleigh scattering process (Calliada et al. 1998). However, UCAs also demonstrate resonant behavior. Gas-filled microbubbles are much more compressible than the surrounding tissue and blood. When insonified by ultrasound waves, the wall of the microbubble oscillates with particular efficiency at the resonant frequency of the microbubble. This frequency depends on the microbubble diameter, and for the typical range of diameters present in UCAs (1–10 μm), it coincidentally falls within the acoustic frequency ranges available on most clinical systems for diagnostic ultrasound imaging (2–10 MHz). This oscillation can become very nonlinear and the oscillation dynamics for a single non-coated microbubble can be described by the Rayleigh–Plesset equation as:

$$\rho r\frac{\partial^2 r}{\partial t^2}+\frac{3\rho}{2}\left(\frac{\partial r}{\partial t}\right)^2=\left(\frac{2\sigma}{r_0}+P_0-P_v\right)\cdot\left[\left(\frac{r_0}{r}\right)^{3k}-1\right]-p(t). \quad [6.1]$$

This equation describes the changes in bubble radius r from the resting or equilibrium position r_0 that occur when a microbubble is insonified by a time-varying acoustic pressure field $p(t)$, and where the bubble is in a surrounding fluid with density ρ. Other variables are σ, the surface tension, κ, the polytropic gas exponent of the gas encapsulated in the bubble, P_v, the vapor pressure exerted by the gas in the bubble on the surrounding liquid, and P_0, the hydrostatic pressure. A later formulation known as the RPNNP equation (Rayleigh, Plesset, Noltingk, Neppiras, Poritsky) takes into account shell elasticity and damping effects. Both equations show that bubble oscillations can become nonlinear to produce an asymmetric expansion and compression wavefront. As a result, when the driving pressure amplitude exceeds the range for which the microbubble behaves as a linear harmonic oscillator, higher frequency components at multiples of the fundamental frequency (i.e. the frequency of the incident ultrasound wave, f_0) are formed. Moreover, some microbubbles present compression-only behavior at low acoustic power (e.g. bubbles with phospholipid shells that can buckle as they are compressed). This behavior can be associated with the appearance of frequency components at half the fundamental frequency (sub-harmonic). An evolution of the RPNNP model proposed by Marmottant et al. (2005) shows how coated microbubbles enable additional oscillation modes, such as buckling behavior, when the microbubble surface becomes smaller than the elastic shell. This effect occurs at a low pressure threshold for lipid-coated microbubbles, thanks to the reduced surface tension provided by the lipid monolayer as it buckles (Marmottant et al. 2005; Dollet et al. 2008). Note that alternative descriptions of microbubble oscillations based on liquid enthalpy balance were proposed by Herring (1941) and Gilmore (1952), relaxing some of the assumptions of the RPNNP equations and admitting fluid compressibility. Furthermore, increasing the acoustic pressure will ultimately lead to acoustic bubble destruction. The mechanical index (MI) can be used to gauge the mechanical interaction between the acoustic field and UCAs as:

$$MI = \frac{P_{neg}[MPa]}{\sqrt{f[MHz]}}, \qquad [6.2]$$

with f being the ultrasound frequency and P_{neg} being the peak negative acoustic pressure. In clinical imaging, an MI lower than 0.3 is typically used to limit microbubble destruction during imaging.

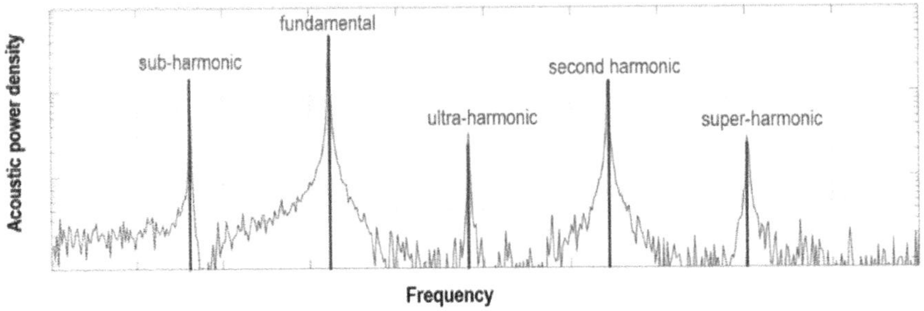

Figure 6.2. *Schematic representation of the distribution of acoustic power backscattered from a single UCA microbubble (frequency response). At certain driving pressure thresholds, several components can emerge at frequencies smaller and higher than the fundamental frequency, which can be selectively imaged by using contrast-specific scanning sequences*

6.2.1. *Contrast-specific imaging*

As shown in Figure 6.2, the frequencies exploited for contrast-specific imaging can be sub-harmonic (about half of the fundamental frequency), ultra-harmonic (between the fundamental and second harmonic frequencies), second and higher harmonics (multiples of the fundamental, second harmonic and above – $2f_0$, $3f_0$, etc.), and super-harmonics (between the higher harmonics). In conventional brightness mode (B-mode) ultrasound imaging, the scanner transmits and receives at the same frequency (fundamental frequency). To exploit the characteristic nonlinear acoustic response of UCA microbubbles, several contrast-specific ultrasound imaging sequences have been developed to selectively receive at frequencies other than the fundamental frequency, thereby enhancing the intensity of signals from UCA microbubbles relative to that from surrounding tissue (Correas et al. 2001; de Jong et al. 2000; Cosgrove 2006; Quaia 2007).

Contrast-specific imaging can be achieved by harmonic imaging, which combines the use of expensive broadband transducers with frequency selective filters, or by power modulation imaging and phase modulation imaging, whereby the transmitted pulses are modulated in phase and/or amplitude, and a smart linear combination of the received pulses is used to suppress the linear signal from the surrounding structures while enhancing the nonlinear signals from UCAs. For example, the Cadence Contrast Pulse Sequencing method combines amplitude and phase modulation by transmitting three consecutive pulses with different amplitudes and phases (e.g. $1/2p_{t1}(t)$, $-p_{t2}(t)$ and $1/2p_{t3}(t)$), and then applying a suitable linear combination of the received echoes (e.g. $2\cdot[p_{r1}(t) + p_{r2}(t) + p_{r3}(t)]$) (de Jong et al.

2000; Correas et al. 2001; Cosgrove 2006; Quaia 2007). This way the linear echoes are cancelled out, while the nonlinear echoes are enhanced.

6.2.2. *Calibration to assess UCA concentration*

Quantitative analysis of the UCA temporal kinetics by, for example, indicator dilution methods, requires estimation of the UCA concentration as a function of time, $C(t)$. Thus, a direct relationship between the received echo signal power and the UCA concentration needs to be established. This process is referred to as calibration. The acoustic response of UCA microbubbles to a pressure field depends on the backscatter coefficient, which is the scattering cross-section per unit volume, and the attenuation coefficient. Assuming low MI (so that bubble destruction can be neglected), low contrast concentration (to neglect interaction forces between microbubbles) and isotropic scattering, the frequency-dependent backscatter coefficient $\beta(f)$ and the UCA concentration are linearly related as:

$$\beta(f) = \frac{\rho_n \Sigma_{tot}(f)}{4\pi}, \qquad [6.3]$$

where $\Sigma_{tot}(f)$ is the normalized frequency-dependent total scattering cross-section (i.e. the normalized scattering cross-section of the microbubbles' size distribution) and ρ_n is the number of microbubbles per unit volume. This can then be related to the backscattered acoustic intensity $I(f)$ as a function of the transmitted acoustic intensity I_0 as:

$$I(f) = \frac{dV}{z^2}\frac{\rho_n \Sigma_{tot}(f)}{4\pi} I_0 = \frac{dV}{z^2}\beta(f) I_0. \qquad [6.4]$$

In [6.4], dV is the volume of insonified contrast particles and z is the distance between dV and the transducer. In addition, the contrast particles cause attenuation of the backscattered acoustic intensity due to several effects, including acoustic wave damping due to viscous and thermal friction, diffusion or scattering of the acoustic energy in different directions and microbubble destruction. These effects, however, are negligible for low UCA concentrations and low MI.

In practice, the size distribution of microbubbles is unknown. This hampers the estimation of the backscatter coefficient. Moreover, accurate calibration is further complicated by the multiple transformations that the signal undergoes during the acquisition process as it is converted from acoustic intensity to electrical voltage, and finally to quantized video intensity (with 2^8=256 gray levels when 8 bits are used for quantization). If all the steps in the acquisition chain are carefully accounted for, a signal that is linearly proportional to the UCA concentration can still be obtained so that relative quantification can be achieved. Briefly, quantification requires accounting for each conversion in the data acquisition process. The first step is the electromechanical conversion from acoustic intensity to voltage performed by the US transducer and providing a "raw" radiofrequency signal (RF). This is followed by demodulation and conversion into a quantized signal by a log-like compression (LC), which typically also includes a gamma transformation to compensate the nonlinear relationship between video intensity, input voltage and the time-gain compensation applied to account for the increasing attenuation with depth (Wiencek et al. 1993; Rognin et al. 2008; Mischi et al. 2003).

The squared amplitude of the raw RF signal is directly proportional to the UCA concentration; thus, linearization could simply be achieved by squaring the raw signal (Rognin et al. 2008; Payen et al. 2013). However, the raw RF signal is rarely made available by the US scanner manufacturers. Thus, signal linearization requires reversal of all the transformations applied to establish a relative acoustic intensity, which reflects local UCA concentration. Accounting for all the acquisition steps, the video intensity (quantized gray-level, QL) can be related back to the RF signal (V) as (Rognin et al. 2008):

$$QL(V) = \text{unit8}\left[(2^8 - 1)\frac{20dB}{LC_{DR}}\left(\frac{V}{V_{max}}10^{\frac{LC_{DR}}{20dB}}\right)\right] \qquad [6.5]$$

where LC_{DR} is the dynamic range of the log compression (expressed in dB), $V_{\max}$ is the maximum amplitude of the received RF signal, and unit8 is the unsigned integer quantization operator. Since the UCA concentration is linearly related to the square of the amplitude of the RF signal (V^2), signal linearization can be achieved by inversion of [6.5].

Appropriate application of signal linearization allows for data comparison between different acquisitions, studies and centers using different US scanner and/or scanner settings, facilitating the establishment of standardized acquisition and analysis protocols. As shown by Rognin et al. (2008) and Gauthier et al. (2011), quantification can be performed as accurately with linearized video signals as with raw RF signals if the gain has been appropriately chosen so as to avoid signal saturation or truncation, and if the dynamic range is sufficiently high. In this case, the measured TIC can be related to the UCA concentration $C(t)$ as:

$$I(t) = aC(t) + b, \qquad [6.6]$$

where a is a proportionality constant related to the UCA total scattering cross-section, and b is the baseline signal intensity.

6.3. Analysis of UCA kinetics

During a DCE-US imaging examination, UCA can be administered following two different protocols, namely bolus injection and constant infusion, and the changes in the acoustic intensity over time are measured in a region of interest (ROI). As shown schematically in Figure 6.3, the bolus administration protocol aims for fast injection of the contrast agent, to mimic a Dirac pulse, which is required for the accurate application of most kinetic models. The dilution of the contrast agent, showing typical wash-in and wash-out phases, is then recorded downstream in the organ or tissue of interest. In the constant infusion protocol, a high-intensity pulse can first be applied to destroy all microbubbles in the ROI, after which the replenishment of inflowing microbubbles is sampled until a steady intensity plateau is established. The replenishment kinetics and the amplitude of the plateau are related to blood flow and volume.

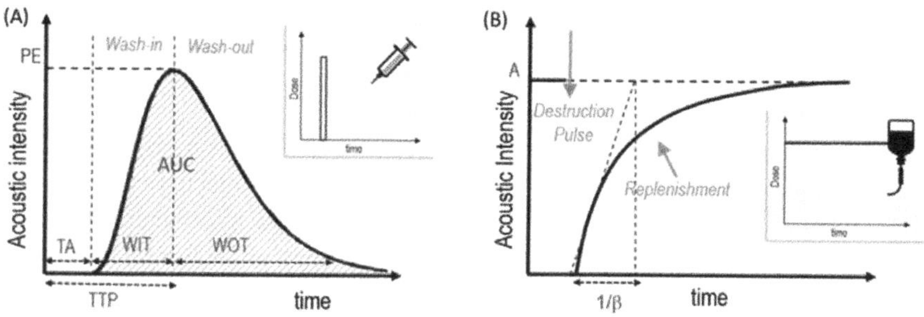

Figure 6.3. *Schematic comparison of the bolus injection and constant infusion protocols. (A) In the bolus injection protocol, a dose of UCA is administered intravenously to approximate a Dirac distribution. The dilution of the contrast agent in the downstream ROI shows a contrast wash-in phase, during which the acoustic intensity rises from background level to a peak value, followed by a wash-out phase. (B) In the constant infusion protocol, after application of a destructive pulse, the acoustic intensity rises steadily until it reaches a plateau. The symbols are further described in Table 6.1*

Analysis of the TIC obtained from either the bolus injection or the constant infusion protocols allows the estimation of parameters that are related to the physiology of the investigated organ or tissue. Importantly, these parameters may be altered by the development of pathological conditions, thus providing a means for vascular assessment that aids the detection, diagnosis and monitoring of many conditions. Given its wider application in clinical practice, the focus of the following section is mostly on quantitative methods developed for the bolus injection protocol.

However, a brief overview of methods used to extract the perfusion parameter from TICs obtained by the constant infusion protocol is also provided.

6.3.1. *Analysis with a bolus injection*

After a bolus injection of a dose of UCA, microbubbles are first filtered through the pulmonary circulation, and then travel through the circulatory system to reach the ROI at different times. Recording the changes in the video intensity over time at the detection site, TICs can be obtained at each imaging pixel (see Figure 6.1). These TICs are related to the changes in UCA concentration, $C(t)$, provided that appropriate, calibrated linearization has been performed, i.e. the relationship between the gray level and bubble concentration has been established (see equation [6.5]). When appropriately normalized, $C(t)$ can thus be interpreted as the probability distribution of the particle transit time through the circulation. In other words, at each time point t, the normalized $C(t)$ can be interpreted as the probability that the UCA particles need a time t to transit from the injection to the detection site, where the TIC is measured (organ or tissue of interest).

Empirical analysis of time and amplitude features of the linearized TIC allows the calculation of a set of parameters that are related to the injected contrast dose and to the perfusion conditions in the ROI. Since these parameters are only indirectly related to blood flow and volume, and the units of measurement depend on the way the TIC amplitude is calibrated, these parameters are often referred to as semi-quantitative. An overview of semi-quantitative parameters commonly used in clinical practice is provided in Table 6.1. These parameters have proven useful for many clinical applications, including cancer diagnostics and treatment monitoring. In a study on prostate cancer patients, perfusion parameters were able to discriminate prostate cancer aggressiveness, with AT and TTP showing the best performance (Maxeiner et al. 2019). Larger AT and TTP, as well as higher WIR and PE, were also observed in breast tumor tissue, compared with the surrounding normal tissue (Cao et al. 2014). Moreover, the ratio between perfusion parameters in the tumor core relative to its periphery was highly correlated with the microvascular density, center/periphery ratio, measured by histological analysis of ex vivo tumor tissue, suggesting that CEUS perfusion parameters are able to reflect the microvascular distribution in breast tumors (Li et al. 2018). Semi-quantitative CEUS parameters have also shown utility for monitoring cancer treatments that affect tumor vasculature. A large study involving patients with gastrointestinal stromal tumors, renal cell carcinomas and hepatocellular carcinomas showed that the changes in AUC (area under the curve) from baseline to day 30 after anti-angiogenic treatment were predictive of treatment success (Lassau et al. 2014). However, semi-quantitative assessment may suffer from intra- and inter-patient variability, thus limiting the reproducibility and repeatability of the obtained parameters (Lassau et al. 2017), especially when linearization is not performed appropriately (Averkiou et al. 2020).

Alternatively, the temporal evolution of the UCA concentration can be interpreted using indicator dilution theory. This enables the estimation of quantitative parameters that are directly related to the underlying physiology. An indicator is any substance that exhibits the same flow dynamics as a substance of interest (e.g. blood) without perturbing the system, and that can be selectively measured. In an indicator dilution method, a known amount of indicator particles (e.g. UCAs) are injected upstream in the circulation and measured downstream over time. If the dose of the indicator, m, is known, and $C(t)$ is measured at the detection site, the Stewart–Hamilton equation permits calculation of the blood flow F and volume V as (Stewart 1921; Hamilton et al. 1928):

$$F = \frac{m}{\int_0^{\infty} C(t)dt} = \frac{m}{\text{AUC}} \quad [6.7]$$

$$V = F\frac{\int_0^{\infty} tC(t)dt}{\int_0^{\infty} C(t)dt} = F \cdot \text{MTT} \quad [6.8]$$

where AUC is the area under the indicator dilution curve, $C(t)$, and MTT is the mean transit time, i.e. the mean time needed for the indicator particles to pass through the circulatory system once.

In DCE-US, the portion of the injected UCA that reaches the ROI is not known. Moreover, only a function that is linearly related to $C(t)$ is normally available. As a result, equations [6.7] and [6.8] are only valid in a relative sense, provided that the other basic assumptions of the indicator dilution theory are respected. For a single-input single-output flow system, these assumptions are as follows:

– Volume and flow are constant during the measurement. This is respected as long as the time of the measurement is kept short enough.

– The system is stationary, thus the distribution of transit times does not vary over time. This assumption holds as long as the transit time fluctuations occur on a time scale that is much longer than the duration of the TIC.

– The indicator is injected instantaneously. This can be considered valid as long as the injection time is much shorter than the MTT, and as long as its presence does not perturb the flow, which is verified for the small amount of contrast agent used in practice.

– The flow of indicator particles is the same as for fluid particles. This is respected if there is complete mixing between the contrast and the fluid.

– Recirculation of the indicator is not present.

Semi-quantitative parameter	Description	Protocol	Units	Related to
Peak enhancement (PE)	Maximum TIC intensity	Bolus injection	Amplitude	Blood volume, contrast dose
Time to peak (TTP)	Time to maximum TIC intensity	Bolus injection	Time	Blood flow
Time of appearance (AT)	Time at which the TIC amplitude rises above baseline level	Bolus injection	Time	Blood flow
Wash-in time (WIT)	Difference between AT and TTP	Bolus injection	Time	Blood flow
Wash-out time (WOT)	Time interval between TIC maximum and TIC descent to baseline value	Bolus injection	Time	Blood flow
Wash-in rate (WIR)	Wash-in gradient	Bolus injection	Amplitude/time	Blood flow
Wash-out rate (WOR)	Wash-out gradient	Bolus injection	Amplitude/time	Blood flow
Area under the curve (AUC)	Integral of the TIC	Bolus injection	Amplitude/time	Blood flow, contrast dose
Replenishment plateau (A)	TIC intensity at plateau	Constant infusion	Amplitude	Blood volume
Replenishment rate (β)	Replenishment gradient	Constant infusion	Amplitude/time	Blood flow

Table 6.1. *Overview of semi-quantitative parameters typically extracted from contrast ultrasound TICs*

The last assumption is not valid in DCE-US, because the second and later passes of UCA particles add to the TIC and hide the wash-out phase (see Figure 6.4). Moreover, TIC measured by DCE-US may be corrupted by speckle noise, shadowing, acoustic reverberation and poor contrast mixing (Tang et al. 2011; Turco et al. 2016; Mischi et al. 2018). All these effects pose limitations for the calculation of quantitative and semi-quantitative parameters directly from the measured TICs. To obtain more reliable estimates of the MTT and AUC, TICs are typically time-filtered and then fit with a suitable mathematical model to cancel out the effects of noise and isolate the first-pass of the UCA bolus (see Figure 6.4). An overview of commonly used models is provided in Table 6.2 (Harabis et al. 2013; Turco et al. 2016, 2020; Mischi et al. 2018).

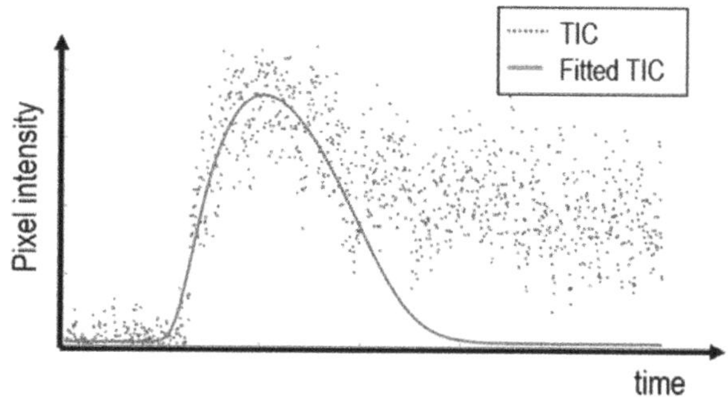

Figure 6.4. *Example of a TIC measured by DCE-US (blue dots), together with the fit obtained by a suitable mathematical model (orange line), which filters out the effects of noise and isolates the first pass of the indicator*

Several models for fitting indicator dilution curves are based on compartmental modeling. By this modeling technique, the indicator volume is divided into a number of exchanging compartments (see Figure 6.5). These are mathematical objects which permit lumping a certain amount of material into discrete objects for which the indicator concentration is well mixed and exhibits the same kinetic behavior (Cobelli et al. 2007). A compartment is typically characterized by a distribution volume, in which the indicator is uniformly distributed, and rate constants (in units of 1/time) that describe the fractional transfer in and out of the compartment. From a system-modeling perspective, a normalized indicator dilution curve from a bolus injection administration can also be interpreted as the impulse response of the dilution system. Assuming linearity and time-variance, the model parameters can be obtained by input–output analysis, aimed at extracting the impulse response from the known input and output (deconvolution). This approach offers an alternative to (nonlinear) model fitting of the indicator dilution curve (output) and is especially suited for analysis of DCE-US images, as the input-output analysis is independent of the actual injection site. It thus enables local characterization of the dilution system. From the impulse response, the MTT can be easily calculated as:

$$\text{MTT} = \int_0^\infty th(t)dt, \qquad [6.9]$$

where t is the time, and $h(t)$ is the impulse response of the system. The first model used to fit an indicator dilution curve was a mono-compartmental model, which was proposed by Hamilton et al. (1928) to fit the wash-out phase of the curve. He noted that the typical dilution curve exhibits an initial rise followed by a decrease that resembles a mono-exponential decay. Assuming a model with a single compartment, the decay is characterized by the time constant τ, which corresponds to the MTT.

Model	Equation	MTT estimator
Mono-compartment (Hamilton et al. 1928)	$C(t) = \text{AUC}\,\frac{1}{\tau}e^{-\frac{t}{\tau}}$	$\text{MTT} = \tau$
Erlang (n compartments) (Krejcie et al. 1996)	$C(t) = \text{AUC}\,\frac{e^{-\frac{t}{\tau}}\left(\frac{t}{\tau}\right)^{n-1}}{\tau(n-1)!}$	$\text{MTT} = n\tau;$ $n \in Z^+$
Gamma variate (Davenport 1983; Mischi et al. 2008)	$C(t) = \text{AUC}\,\frac{e^{-\frac{t}{\tau}}\left(\frac{t}{\tau}\right)^{n-1}}{\tau\Gamma(n)}$	$\text{MTT} = n\tau,$ $n \in R^+$
Lagged normal (order n) (Bassingthwaighte et al. 1966; Davis Jr and Kutner 1976)	$C(t) = \frac{\text{AUC}}{\sqrt{2\pi\sigma^2}}e^{\frac{-(t-\mu)^2}{2\sigma^2}} * \frac{1}{\tau_1}e^{-\frac{1}{\tau_1}t} * \ldots * \frac{1}{\tau_n}e^{-\frac{1}{\tau_n}t}$	$\text{MTT} = \mu + \tau_1 + \cdots + \tau_n$
Lognormal (Qian and Bassingthwaighte 2000)	$C(t) = \frac{\text{AUC}}{\sqrt{2\pi}\sigma t}e^{\frac{(ln\,(t)-\mu)^2}{2\sigma^2}}$	$\text{MTT} = e^{\mu+\frac{\sigma^2}{2}}$
Local density random walk (LDRW) (Bogaard et al. 1986)	$(t) = \text{AUC}\frac{e^{\lambda}}{\mu}\sqrt{\frac{\lambda\mu}{2\pi t}}e^{-\frac{\lambda}{2}\left(\frac{t}{\mu}+\frac{\mu_t}{t}\right)}$	$\text{MTT} = \mu_t$
First-time passage (FTP) (Bogaard et al. 1986)	$C(t) = \text{AUC}\,e^{\lambda}\sqrt{\frac{\lambda\mu}{2\pi t^3}}e^{-\frac{\lambda}{2}\left(\frac{t}{\mu_t}+\frac{\mu_t}{t}\right)}$	$\text{MTT} = \mu_t$
Modified LDRW (Kuenen et al. 2011)	$C(t) = \text{AUC}\sqrt{\frac{\kappa}{2\pi t}}e^{-\frac{\kappa}{2t}(t-\mu_t)^2}$	$\text{MTT} = \mu_t$
AUC = area under the curve; τ = time constant of single compartment; μ = mean of Gaussian distribution; σ = standard deviation of Gaussian distribution; λ = skewness parameter; μ_t = mean transit time; κ = local dispersion parameter.		

Table 6.2. *Overview of mathematical models suitable for fitting TICs obtained by the bolus injection protocol*

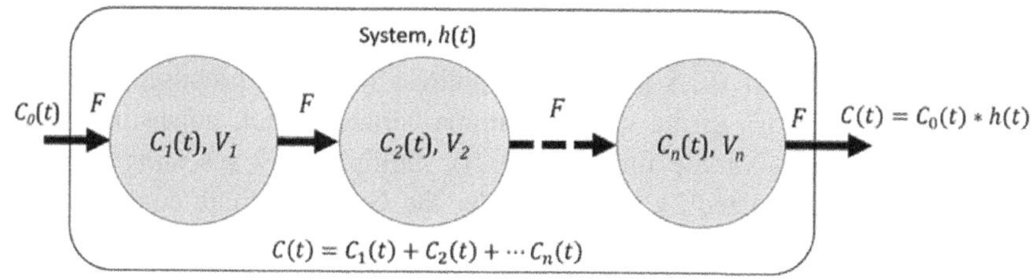

Figure 6.5. *Example of a compartmental model represented by the cascade of n compartments. Each compartment has a distribution volume V_i and concentration $C_i(t)$. The output of each compartment is the input to the next compartment. The total concentration measured at the detection site (e.g. ROI or single pixel) is the sum of the concentrations in each compartment. From a system analysis perspective, the measured concentration can also be seen as the convolution of the input concentration, $C_0(t)$, with the impulse response of the system, h(t)*

The Erlang model is the result of describing the dilution of the contrast agent as the transport through a cascade of n compartments. In the Erlang model, the input to each compartment is the output of the previous compartment (see Figure 6.5), and the compartments have the same volume V and rate constant $1/\tau$. With the initial conditions being that the concentration in the first compartment is a Dirac impulse of amplitude equal to the injected dose divided by V, i.e. $C_1(t{=}0) = \mathrm{m}/V$, while the concentration in all other compartments is zero, i.e. $C_i(t{=}0) = 0$, for $i \neq 1$, the solution to this compartmental model is an Erlang probability density function (PDF) multiplied by the AUC, as given in Table 6.2. Note that $C(t)$ is the output of the last compartment, given by the series of convolutions of the initial concentration with the impulse response of each compartment. Historically, the n-compartmental model is an extension of the simple mono-compartmental model, proposed by Hamilton et al. (1928) to fit the wash-out of indicator dilution curves, and of the two-compartmental model proposed by von Reth and Bogaard (1983) to describe the transport through the atrium and ventricle in the heart.

The Gamma-variate model is easily obtained from the Erlang model by allowing for a non-integer number of compartments. As a result, the Erlang PDF is generalized to a Gamma distribution by using the gamma operator $\Gamma(n)$, as shown in Table 6.2. When a TIC is fit by either the Erlang or Gamma-variate model, the MTT is easily obtained as $\mathrm{MTT} = n\tau$. As noted by Rizzo et al. (2017), however, the UCA kinetics can be very heterogeneous (especially in newly formed angiogenic vessels). Due to their tortuosity and small size, these vessels may exhibit a very slow wash-out, which, for analysis of a limited duration TIC, may resemble apparent microbubble trapping. As a result, the Gamma-variate model may not be able to appropriately describe all UCA kinetics. To address this, they proposed to add an "irreversible component" to the classic Gamma-variate model, consisting of the integral of the Gamma-variate function ($C_g(t)$), multiplied by a scaling factor a_1 ($0 < a_1 < 1$) and normalized by the area under the Gamma-variate curve (AUC_g). The irreversible component resembles a compartment where the contrast agent can flow in but do not flow out. When added to $C_g(t)$, this component enables better modeling of the slow wash-out, resulting in:

$$C(t) = C_g(t) + \frac{a_1}{AUC_g} \int_0^t C_g(\tau)\, d\tau \qquad [6.10]$$

Using a variational Bayesian method for pixel-wise parameter estimation, including an automatic relevance determination algorithm, the irreversible component can be excluded for TICs for which the classic Gamma-variate model is more appropriate (where no apparent trapping is present).

The lagged-normal model can also be interpreted as the result of the cascade of n compartments, but as opposed to the Erlang model, the input to the first compartment is a Gaussian PDF parametrized in μ and σ. The total concentration is then given by the convolution of this Gaussian input by the impulse response of each compartment. For the i-th compartment, this is given by $\frac{1}{\tau_i} e^{-\frac{1}{\tau_i} t}$, where $\frac{1}{\tau_i}$ is the rate constant for each compartment. The lagged-normal model was proposed to describe the transport of the indicator from a large artery to the microcirculation (Bassingthwaighte et al. 1966).

A non-compartmental model, which has been widely used for fitting TICs extracted from DCE-US loops, is the lognormal function. Mathematically, it represents the PDF of a random variable whose logarithm is normally distributed with mean μ and standard deviation σ. Although its application for TIC fitting has an empirical origin, the physiological relationship between the lognormal function and vascular hemodynamics can be found in the work of Qian and Bassingthwaighte (2000). They showed that in a network of bifurcating vessels, with asymmetric branching and random variations at each bifurcation, the flow distributes lognormally. In fact, an indicator dilution curve can be described equivalently as a probability distribution of particle flow or of particle transit times (Arditi et al. 2006).

In the context of physics-driven models, the local density random walk (LDRW) and the first-time passage (FTP) models are both solutions of the diffusion with drift equation (see Table 6.2). This very general equation has been used to describe UCA transport by modeling a vessel as a long tube of infinite length. Simplifying the transport process by considering only the spatial dimension z along the vessel, the diffusion with drift equation describes the changes of the indicator concentration in space and time as indicator particles are dragged by a carrier fluid (e.g. blood) with velocity v, as (Bogaard et al. 1984, 1986; Turco et al. 2016; Mischi et al. 2018):

$$\frac{\partial C(z,t)}{\partial t} = \frac{\partial}{\partial z}\left(D\frac{\partial C(z,t)}{\partial z}\right) - v\frac{\partial C(z,t)}{\partial z}, \qquad [6.11]$$

where D is the diffusion coefficient, which accounts for molecular diffusion and the flow profile projected along z. Equation [6.11] is also referred to as the convective dispersion equation because it can be interpreted as the superimposition of a convective term, which determines the linear drift and a diffusion term. While, normally, diffusion is due to Brownian motion, in the context of convection through a microvascular network, it is mainly determined by the multipath trajectories across the microcirculation. This has been described by Taylor (1953) as apparent dispersion.

The difference between the LDRW and the FTP models resides in the boundary conditions at the outlet. In the FTP model, a virtual absorbing barrier is present at the outlet so that only one passage of the contrast bolus is allowed. Conversely, the LDRW allows for multiple passages of the UCA particles at the same detection site (Sheppard 1962; von Reth and Bogaard 1983; Bogaard et al. 1986; Mischi et al. 2003, 2007). The parameters of the models are λ, a skewness parameter, and μ, the mean transit time (see Table 6.2). The former expresses the different contributions of convection and diffusion to particle transport along a certain distance L by its relationship with the Peclet number $\mathrm{Pe} = vL/D = 2\lambda$. The Peclet number is a standard parameter used to characterize fluid-dynamic systems.

A modified version of the LDRW model (mLDRW) was proposed by Kuenen et al. (2011) to put more emphasis on the dispersion features of the indicator transport across the microvascular bed. This model is obtained by locally solving equation [6.11] with the boundary condition that the contrast concentration follows a Gaussian distribution in space before entering the detection point. Using this new parametrization, the local contributions of dispersion and convection are no longer dependent on the travelled distance and can be described by the parameter $\kappa = \lambda/\mu = v_l^2/2D_l$, where v_l and D_l are the local velocity and local dispersion coefficient, respectively (see Table 6.2).

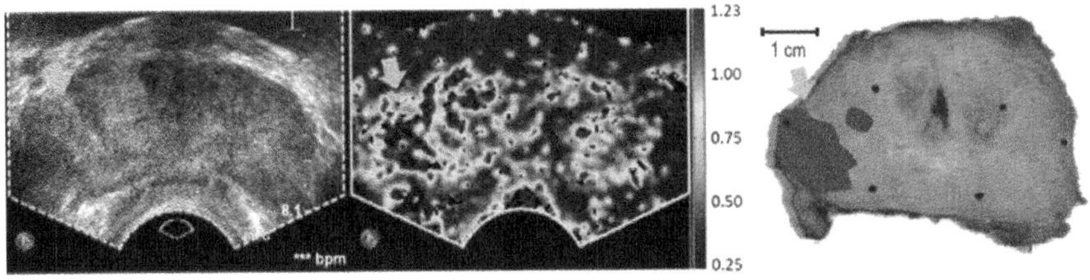

Figure 6.6. *Example of parametric analysis of DCE-US. On the left, the DCE-US recording shows the B-mode acquisition next to the contrast mode map of the parameter κ from the mLDRW model. On the right, the histological analysis of the prostate (performed after radical prostatectomy) shows the cancerous region marked in red. Data were recorded at the Amsterdam University Medical Center, Location AMC (The Netherlands). The area of high κ values shows a good match with the cancerous area in the pathology slice, as highlighted by the orange arrows. Reproduced and modified with permission from Turco et al. (2020)*

Parameter mapping

Parametric analysis of the TICs can provide important information on the microvascular perfusion by estimating semi-quantitative (Table 6.1) and quantitative parameters (Table 6.2). This can be performed by selecting an ROI (e.g. a suspicious nodule) and obtaining a mean TIC by averaging all the TICs in each pixel within the ROI or independently at each single pixel. The latter makes it possible to visualize the parameters in the whole area of interest as a color-coded map (see Figure 6.6). A clear advantage of a pixel-by-pixel analysis is the possibility of localizing suspicious areas that may not be so evident by looking at the raw data. Moreover, the spatial distribution of the parameters can also be very informative, especially for cancer diagnosis, where features such as high vascular heterogeneity and the presence of highly perfused tumor periphery compared to a poorly perfused, necrotic tumor center have been observed for many tumor types (Luo et al. 2009; Vilana et al. 2010; Fidler 2001; Sirsi et al. 2012; Liu et al. 2014). The main disadvantages of the pixel-by-pixel approach are the higher level of noise, requiring more attention in terms of denoising, and the long computation time needed to repeat nonlinear iterative curve fitting at each pixel. In current clinical imaging, the dimensions of a DCE-US frame can range from 500 up to 1,000 pixels in width and depth. Thus, the number of repetitions of the fitting procedure can easily reach 10^5–10^6. Due to the poor signal-to-noise ratio, classic nonlinear estimators such as least-squares approaches may lead to a high number of unreliable estimates when applied pixel-wise. Alternatively, more robust and efficient estimation procedures may be achieved by applying Maximum likelihood and Bayesian estimation frameworks (Kuenen et al. 2014; Rizzo et al. 2017). The latter also allows incorporation of prior knowledge about the UCA kinetics into the estimation process (Rizzo et al. 2017). A multi-model system identification approach able to select the best perfusion model according to the best fit can also mitigate the effects of frame rate, noise and wash-in time on the accuracy of the estimated parameters (Akhbardeh et al. 2019).

6.3.2. *Analysis with a constant infusion rate*

Besides the bolus injection protocol, estimation of perfusion parameters can also be performed with a constant infusion protocol by a destruction–replenishment method. Here, a perfusion pump is used to infuse the contrast agent until an estimated steady-state contrast signal is reached (post wash-in) within an imaging plane of interest. Perfusion parameters can then be estimated by transmitting a high-MI pulse to destroy all microbubbles in the field of view, and then recording the refill from inflowing microbubbles. This provides a general input function to the signal and a reference point, which enables more advanced and accurate quantification of blood flow and blood volume. In addition, this method allows evaluation of the reperfusion for several 2D imaging planes, as long as the steady-state is maintained (up 10–12 min) (Wei et al. 1998; Hudson et al. 2009). Different mathematical models have been derived to describe the replenishment kinetics. The simplest is the mono-exponential model developed by Wei et al. (1998) when the disruption-replenishment method was first introduced. It was proposed for use in the context of echocardiology where clear indications for clinical use are available. While it has not been established clinically for other indications, several studies in humans have shown the potential of the destruction–replenishment technique for diagnosis and longitudinal treatment monitoring applications (Williams et al. 2011; Hudson et al. 2014; el Kaffas et al. 2017). An overview of the main available models is provided in Table 6.3.

It is important to note that it is often difficult to establish a steady-state contrast signal (Dietrich et al. 2012). Moreover, imaging during the replenishment phase can influence the signal intensity because destruction of refilling microbubbles may occur for certain combinations of pressure and frame rate (Shi et al. 2001). These issues can be mitigated by implementing an intermittent imaging strategy (Porter et al. 1996). To apply this strategy, repeated destructive pulses are transmitted with sufficient delay to allow for full replenishment, each replenishment curve is then sampled only once, but with increasing delay relative to the corresponding destructive pulse. Therefore, the measured intensities on the replenishment curve are no longer affected by the scanning sequence.

By far the most commonly used in clinical and pre-clinical applications (Pollard et al. 2002; Krix et al. 2004; Huang-Wei et al. 2006; Zhou et al. 2018) for analysis of contrast replenishment after a destruction pulse, the model developed by Wei et al. (1998) describes the replenishment kinetics as the step response of a compartmental model with a single compartment. The replenishment plateau A (see Figure 6.3 and Table 6.3) reflects the fractional blood volume and is related to the input concentration to the compartment as $A=aC_0$, with a being a proportionality constant. The replenishment time constant τ, or equivalently, the replenishment rate $\beta=1/\tau$, is related to the blood flow. Relative perfusion can then be estimated by their product $A\beta = A/\tau$. An inherent assumption of this model is that a constant number of microbubbles enters the detection area. In other words, the model is valid only if microbubble destruction is negligible in feeding vessels traversed before entering the detection ROI. To relax this assumption, Wei's model was later extended to a multi-compartmental model, which can describe different replenishment kinetics in adjacent compartments (Lucidarme et al. 2003).

Model	Equation
Wei et al. (1998)	$C(t) = A\left(1 - e^{-\frac{t}{\tau}}\right)$
Krix et al. (2003)	$\{C(t) = M\sum_i g_i v_i t = Mv_{mean}t \quad t < t_{max} \; C(t) = \left[1 - \sum_i g_i \frac{d^2}{3} {v_i}^2 t^2\right] \quad t > t_{min}$
Arditi et al. (2006)	$C(t) = A\int_0^{\infty} P(\tau) perf\left[1.94\frac{Kd}{2\tau}(t-\tau)\right] d\tau$
Hudson et al. (2009)	$C(t) = \int_V B(x,y,z)F(x,y,z,t)dV$

Table 6.3. *Overview of models used to describe TICs obtained by a constant infusion protocol*

Because of its simplicity, Wei's model cannot account for more complex vasculature networks in which multiple vessels exhibit different refilling kinetics and are possibly oriented along different directions with respect to the imaging and destruction planes. To account for this scenario, Krix et al. (2003) proposed a piecewise description of the replenishment curve (Table 6.3). The model consists of a linear part up to time t_{max}, which considers the refilling of vessels perpendicular to the imaging plane, and a nonlinear part starting a time t_{min} for all the remaining vessels. In this model, the concentration is a function of the sum of the velocity in each vessel v_i, weighted by a factor g_i, and the thickness of the ROI d (effective width of the ultrasound beam).

The replenishment curve may also be influenced by the actual shape of the imaging and destruction volumes and by the point-spread function of the imaging system (Potdevin et al. 2004; Arditi et al. 2006). To include the effects of the imaging system, Arditi et al. (2006) described the replenishment curve as a perf function, defined as $\text{perf}(t) = 0.5(1+\text{erf}(t))$, averaged over of the probability distribution $P(\tau)$ of particle transit time (Table 6.3). The perf function is dependent on the parameters K, a transmit–receive diffraction parameter, d, the width of the destruction zone, and τ, the time needed for the microbubbles to refill half of the destruction zone. The authors indicate that any mathematical model describing the probability distribution of particle transit time for a bolus injection, such as the models summarized in Table 6.2, is a suitable option for $P(\tau)$.

Using a more general approach, Hudson et al. (2009) described the replenishment curve as the average over the investigated volume, V, of the product between a beam function, $B(x,y,z)$, and a time-dependent flow function, $F(x,y,x,t)$. The beam function was modeled as a truncated sinc function, which results from the diffraction pattern of ultrasound waves through a rectangular aperture (Cobbold 2006), while a lognormal model was adopted for the flow function.

6.3.3. *Spatial analysis*

In complex vascular networks, consisting of vessels of different sizes and branching that are oriented in different directions, UCA kinetics in the investigated ROI may be very heterogeneous. This is even more pronounced in pathological, angiogenic vasculature where the tortuosity and irregularity of newly formed vessels leads to complex hemodynamic patterns. Therefore, analysis of the spatial distribution of UCAs in the ROI may provide additional, important insights into vascular function and morphology. For example, a hallmark of many solid tumors is a well-perfused periphery accompanied by a poorly perfused, necrotic tumor core (Fidler 2001; Luo et al. 2009; Vilana et al. 2010; Liu et al. 2014).

Although it is still a relatively new field compared to temporal analysis, a few methods have been proposed for spatial analysis of DCE-US that show promise, especially for assessment of atherosclerotic plaque and cancer diagnostics (Molinari et al. 2010; Zhang et al. 2014; Saidov et al. 2016). The analysis can be performed directly on the linearized DCE-US data, by selecting a relevant frame of the DCE-US loop (e.g. frame at peak enhancement) or obtaining a single projection by applying an operation over the whole DCE-US loop or a part thereof. One common example is the maximum intensity projection (MIP), obtained by taking the maximum intensity value over time at each pixel. Alternatively, spatial analysis can be performed on parametric maps obtained by temporal analysis.

A method for 3D spatial analysis of DCE-US was developed to improve the characterization of thyroid nodules (Molinari et al. 2010). This method requires the acquisition of multiple 2D slices so as to obtain a 3D DCE-US volume. After a pre-processing step for image intensity compensation and normalization, a morphological operation is applied to detect microbubbles. This is followed by a histogram-based thresholding and reconstruction step to obtain a 3D skeleton of the vasculature. From this skeleton, a series of vascular trees (T_i) are obtained and mapped as m nodes (p_i) in the form $T_i=[p_1,p_2,.., p_m]$. This mapping permits the extraction of several parameters characterizing the vascular architecture, including the number of trees and branching nodes, the vascular density and the average vessel radius. Of particular interest for cancer diagnostics is the vascular tortuosity, which can be assessed by the distance metric (DM) and the sum-of-angle metric (SOAM) in 2D and 3D, respectively, as:

$$\mathrm{DM} = \frac{|p_m - p_i|}{\sum_{i=1}^{m-1} |p_i - p_{i+1}|}. \qquad [6.12]$$

$$\mathrm{SOAM} = \frac{\sum_{k=1}^{m-3} \sqrt{IP_k{}^2 + TP_k{}^2}}{\sum_{k=1}^{m-1} |p_k - p_{k+1}|}. \qquad [6.13]$$

In [6.13], IP is defined by the planar angle between two vectors connecting three nodes, and TP is obtained as the angle defining the torsion of the curve in a node. From the DM, the inflection count metric (ICM) can also be derived as the DM divided by the number of flexes in the path. The interested reader is referred to the original article from Molinari et al. (2010) for more information.

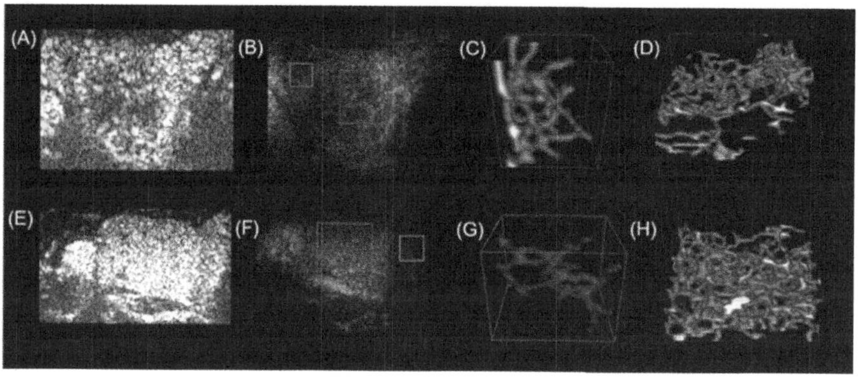

Figure 6.7. *(A, E) Single frames of the 3D DCE-US of benign and malignant thyroid nodules, respectively. (B, F) Maximum intensity projections of the vascular network; red rectangles indicate ROIs including the nodules, while green rectangles include a portion of the healthy thyroid parenchyma. (C, D) Three-dimensional skeleton of the vascular network in the healthy parenchyma and benign nodule, respectively. The vascular complexity measured by the DM showed DM = 58.2 in the nodule versus DM = 25.5 in the parenchyma. (G, H) Three-dimensional skeleton of the vascular network in the healthy parenchyma and malignant nodule, respectively. The vascular complexity measured by the DM showed larger differences (DM = 91.4 vs. DM = 17.6) compared to the benign case*

In a different approach proposed for carotid plaque characterization (Zhang et al. 2015), temporal averaging is first applied to obtain a multi-frame averaged image. This is followed by delineation of the plaque borders and segmentation of the intraplaque neovascularization (IPN). From the obtained segmented image, several quantitative spatial features are extracted, including the area ratio (AR), given by the ratio of the IPN area over the plaque area, the center deviation degree (CDD) and the radial deviation degree (RDD), calculated as the mean and standard deviation, respectively, of the normalized distance from the IPN to the plaque centroid. If n_p is the total number of pixels in the IPN, the CDD and RDD are calculated as:

$$\mathrm{CDD} = \frac{1}{n_p}\sum_{i=1}^{n_p}\left(\frac{d_i}{D_i}\right), \qquad [6.14]$$

$$\mathrm{RDD} = \sqrt{\frac{1}{n_p - 1}\sum_{i=1}^{n_p}\left(\frac{d_i}{D_i} - \mathrm{CDD}\right)^2}, \qquad [6.15]$$

where d_i is the distance between the i-th pixel in the IPN and the plaque center. To calculate D_i, the segment passing through the i-th pixel in the IPN, the plaque center and the plaque border is first drawn. D_i is then calculated as the distance between the plaque center and the intersection between the segment and the plaque border. The proposed features improved the distinction between low-grade and high-grade plaque compared to traditional features such as the area ratio.

According to the established concept that a vascular network can be well represented as a fractal bifurcating tree, a few studies have compared the fractal dimension of cancerous and normal vasculature (Baish and Jain 2000). Indeed, increased fractal dimension (FD) is typically found in chaotic vascular networks, such as those formed by tumor angiogenesis (Baish and Jain 2000). While fractal analysis of the vasculature is typically performed by microscopic analysis of tissue slices, which can only be acquired post-mortem or by invasive surgical procedures, DCE-US offers an opportunity for assessment of the vascular FD in vivo. In the method proposed by Saidov et al. (2016), the FD is calculated on perfusion maps obtained by temporal analysis of TICs (e.g. parametric map of wash-in rate). First, a sample size m of size L is defined and divided into sub-samples of smaller sizes ($m = L/4$, $m = L/16$, $m = L/64$, …); then, the mean and standard deviation of the selected perfusion parameter in each sample are calculated to obtain the relative dispersion (RD), i.e. the ratio between standard deviation and mean. The RD at different scales m follows a power law dependent on FD. The FD can be obtained by curve fitting with the following formula:

$$\frac{\mathrm{RD}(m)}{\mathrm{RD}(m_{ref})} = \left(\frac{m}{m_{ref}}\right)^{1-FD}, \qquad [6.16]$$

where m_{ref} represents an arbitrary sample size taken as reference. In a preclinical study, two prostate tumors with marked differences in microvascular density distribution were established in mice; the parameter FD was significantly different between the two different types of tumors and showed good agreement with the immunohistological analysis performed on ex vivo tumor tissue (Saidov et al. 2016).

In recent years, new revolutionary techniques have been proposed to overcome the diffraction limit of sound waves, providing ultrasound imaging with unparalleled spatial resolution (Errico et al. 2015; Bar-Zion et al. 2018; Couture et al. 2018; Solomon et al. 2018; Christensen-Jeffries et al. 2020). This family of techniques, collectively referred to as super-resolution ultrasound imaging, works by pinpointing the position of individual microbubbles across multiple DCE-US frames, enabling the reconstruction of super-resolved microvascular networks. Although super-resolution imaging is beyond the scope of this chapter, it is important to note that super-resolved images may provide an ideal starting point for a more accurate spatial analysis of the microvasculature in healthy and diseased tissue. This has already been shown in pre-clinical studies. Lin et al. (2017) assessed vessel tortuosity on super-resolved microvascular networks by the distance metric, demonstrating increased tortuosity in tumor-bearing compared to healthy rats. Spatial analysis of super-resolution microvascular images in renal tumor xenografts showed a significant correlation of features such as the inter-vessel distance and the distance metric, measured in vivo, with their histological counterparts, obtained ex vivo (Lowerison et al. 2020). Super-resolution imaging is covered in detail in Chapter 7.

6.3.4. *3D spatio-temporal analysis*

Although the temporal and spatial analysis of DCE-US has proven useful in the (semi)quantitative assessment of microvascular perfusion and architecture, UCA transport is intrinsically a three-dimensional spatio-temporal process. As such, methods that simultaneously take into account the spatio-temporal characteristics of UCA transport are necessary to fully exploit the wealth of information present in DCE-US sequences. This becomes even more important when 3D recordings are available.

A first approach for the spatio-temporal analysis of DCE-US sequences calculated the changes in spatial features over time to simultaneously assess vessel morphology and flow in ischemic tissue (Charalampidis et al. 2006). In particular, the FD over time, FD(t), is first calculated by using a modified version of a variational method; then a set of features, $F_{FD}^{(i)}$, are extracted by averaging FD(t) over a fixed period T as:

$$F_{FD}^{(i)} = \frac{1}{T} \sum_{t=t_i-T+1}^{t_i} \mathrm{FD}(t), \qquad [6.17]$$

where t_i is the last point in the interval for calculation of the i-th feature. The period T was chosen empirically by looking at the periodicity patterns in FD(t) to obtain a total set of four fractal features. In addition, the average image intensity at specific time points, $V(t)$, was used to derive a set of "volume" features as $F_V(i) = V(t_i)$, and a set of "volume-slope" features defined as $F_{VS}^{(i)} = [V(t_i + T_{VS}) - V(t_i)]/T_{VS}$, where T_{vs} is the interval between the two points at which the slope is taken; $F_V(i)$ and $F_{VS}(i)$ are related to arterial flow (Charalampidis et al. 2006). In general, combining full sets of features led to a reduced classification error for distinguishing ischemic vasculature, compared to using single features or subsets of features, suggesting that looking at the full time-evolution of spatial features may lead to more accurate assessment.

Under the hypothesis that the similarity between TICs in a spatial neighborhood reflects UCA dispersion through the multipath vascular trajectory, several spatial similarity measures were proposed for a local characterization of the microvascular architecture (Mischi et al. 2012; Kuenen et al. 2013; Schalk et al. 2015). Indeed, spatio-temporal modeling of UCA kinetics proved a monotonic relationship between the dispersion parameter κ from the mLDRW model (Table 6.2) and the degree of similarity between neighboring pixels. Similarity features can be obtained by comparing the TIC extracted at each pixel with the TICs in its surroundings. To make the estimation independent of the direction of blood flow, a ring-shaped kernel was adopted, with an inner diameter of 1 mm and an outer diameter 2.5 mm (Figure 6.8). The size of the ring was determined to account for the resolution of the imaging system and for the size threshold for which tumors require angiogenesis (2–3 mm in diameter) to grow further; this threshold is referred to as "angiogenic switch". This kernel is moved across the whole image to obtain spatial similarity maps.

Linear similarity can be estimated by calculating the spectral coherence, i.e. the correlation between two frequency spectra, as:

$$\rho(S_1(f), S_2(f)) = \frac{\int_{f_{min}}^{f_{max}} (S_1(f) - \underline{S_1})(S_2(f) - \underline{S_2}) df}{\sqrt{\int_{f_{min}}^{f_{max}} (S_1(f) - \underline{S_1})^2 df \int_{f_{min}}^{f_{max}} (S_2(f) - \underline{S_2})^2 df}} \quad [6.18]$$

where $S_1(f)$ and $S_2(f)$ are the frequency amplitude spectra of TICs $C_1(t)$ and $C_2(t)$, respectively, and $\underline{S}$ represents the mean value of $S(f)$ within the selected frequency bandwidth. For each pixel, the spectral coherence is calculated between the central TIC and all the TICs in the ring-shaped kernel and then averaged to obtain a single measure of coherence (Figure 6.8).

An alternative measure of linear similarity can be obtained in the time domain by looking at the temporal correlation between TICs as:

$$r(C_1(t), C_2(t)) = \frac{\int_0^{\infty} (C_1(t) - \underline{C_1})(C_2(t) - \underline{C_2}) dt}{\sqrt{\int_0^{\infty} (C_1(t) - \underline{C_1})^2 dt \int_0^{\infty} (C_2(t) - \underline{C_2})^2 dt}}. \quad [6.19]$$

However, while the spectral coherence is not influenced by phase shifts (delays) between TICs, for the temporal correlation, appropriate time windowing and TIC alignment need to be performed to remove any influence of the bolus arrival time on the obtained similarity measure.

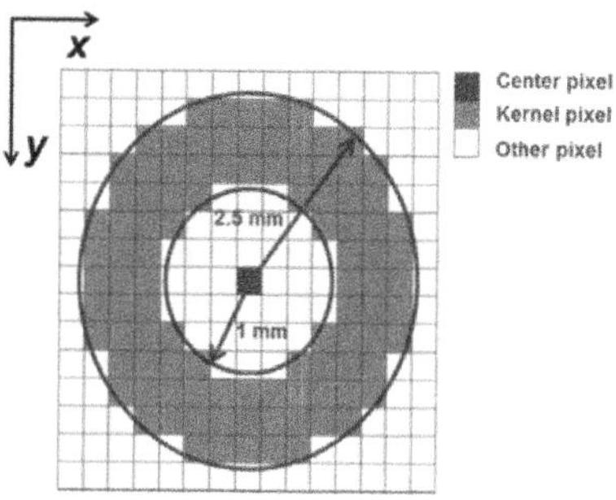

Figure 6.8. *Ring-shaped kernel adopted for spatio-temporal analysis of DCE-US loops. The TIC in the center pixel is compared with those within the ring; the ring size is chosen according to the imaging resolution and the scale at which early angiogenesis occurs*

Besides linear similarity measures, nonlinear similarity can be investigated by looking at the statistical dependency between TICs. If the intensity value at each pixel over time is modeled as a random variable, the discrete mutual information between the central TIC, C, and the random variable X, composed of all the TICs in the kernel except for the central one, is given by (Schalk et al. 2017):

$$I(X,C) = \sum_{x \in X} \sum_{c \in C} p_{X,C}(x,c) log_2 \left(\frac{p_{X,C}(x,c)}{p_X(x) p_C(c)} \right). \qquad [6.20]$$

Equation [6.20] depends on the joint probability mass function (PMF) between X and C, which is in practice quite complex to obtain. Assuming that the TICs in X are mutually independent, and dependent only on C, the joint PMF can be calculated in practice as $p_{X,C}(x,c) = \frac{N_C(x,c)}{N \cdot K}$, with $N_C(x,c)$ being the number of pixels for which X=x and C=c, N the number of pixels in the kernel excluding the central pixel, and K the total number of frames. Extension of these similarity measures in 3D is straightforward by extending the ring-kernel to a 3D spherical kernel (Schalk et al. 2015, 2018).

More comprehensive approaches for spatio-temporal analysis of DCE-US loops are based on modeling the UCA kinetics in time and space. In this context, van

Sloun et al. (2017a) proposed an approach based on local system-identification by which the impulse response in time and space (Green's function) of the convective dispersion equation (see [6.11]) is modeled as:

$$g(x,t|v,D) = \frac{1}{\sqrt{4\pi Dt}} exp\left(-\frac{(x-vt)^2}{4Dt}\right). \quad [6.21]$$

Also in this case, a ring-shaped kernel is used, whereby the central TIC is considered as the input to the system, while all other TICs in the kernel are possible outputs. From these, non-causal outputs, i.e. TICs whose arrival time is later than the central TIC, are first excluded. Since the distance between pixels is known, the convective velocity, v, and the dispersion coefficient, D, can be estimated separately by system input–output analysis, also allowing for the calculation of the Peclet number.

A blood velocity vector field can be obtained by analyzing the local propagation of microbubbles (van Sloun et al. 2018). Assuming UCA transport to be dominated by the convective component, the average velocity vector $\vec{v} = [v_{x,}v_y]$ within a circular kernel of radius R can be calculated as:

$$\vec{v}^T\vec{\tau} = \boldsymbol{L}, \quad [6.22]$$

where $\vec{\tau}$ is a vector constructed by looking at the time delays between each pair of TICs within the circular kernel, while $\boldsymbol{L}$ is a matrix constructed by looking at the pixel distance between each pixel in the kernel. To provide a measure of the complexity of the underlying vascular network, the Shannon entropy of the obtained velocity vector field, $H(V)$, was proposed, showing promise for differentiation of malignant and benign tissue in the prostate (van Sloun et al. 2018). The resulting velocity vector is actually a projection onto the 2D imaging plane of the 3D velocity vector field. Using a spherical kernel permits extension of [6.22] for analysis of 3D DCE-US loops (van Sloun et al. 2018), obtaining a 3D velocity vector $\vec{v} = [v_x, v_y, v_z]$. Importantly, this allows tracing the streamlines describing the trajectories of flow by a technique referred to as DCE-US tractography (van Sloun et al. 2018). Given a vector field $v[x(t)]$, this method is based on the resolution of the following ordinary differential equation:

$$\partial_t x(t) = v[x(t)], \quad [6.23]$$

which describes the trajectory of a microbubble starting at position x_0 at time t=0. From the obtained tractographic reconstruction, spatial analysis can be performed by extracting features such as the ICM, as a measure of vascular tortuosity, and the number of trajectories per unit volume as a measure of vascular density. These spatial features have been shown to enable tumor localization in prostate cancer, which was in agreement with the histopathological ground truth (van Sloun et al. 2018). This method can be extended to include dispersion by solving the convective dispersion equation in 3D, using a finite-element modeling approach (Wildeboer et al. 2018b). The obtained velocity and dispersion fields were used as mean and standard deviation, respectively, of a Gaussian process to compute the directional pathway by Monte Carlo sampling. This enabled a probabilistic tractography visualization of the dispersion and velocity fields in the prostate (Wildeboer et al. 2018b).

A fluid dynamic model to describe the velocity amplitude of the UCA bolus in time and space was proposed by de Senneville et al. (2018). Since the relationship between the video intensity and the local UCA concentration is rarely known in practice, the proposed model relates the microbubble transport ($\vec{v}$) directly to the changes in the video intensity in time and space, $I(\vec{r},t)$, as:

$$\partial_t I(\vec{r},t) + \vec{v}(\vec{r},t)\nabla I(\vec{r},t) = 0. \qquad [6.24]$$

The model consists of a transient term due to the temporal variations in video intensity ($\partial_t I$ term) and a transport term to take into account the intensity variations due to microbubble transport in space ($\vec{v}\nabla I$ term). An inherent assumption of this model is that UCA transport is dominated by the convective component. In fact, if a linear relationship between $I(t)$ and $C(t)$ exists, equation [6.24] can be obtained from a 2D convective dispersion equation in which the dispersion coefficient is zero. A quantitative evaluation of the overall microbubble transport in a selected ROI, Γ, is obtained by the parameter γ, referred to as the spatio-temporal averaged microbubble transport, as:

$$\gamma = \frac{\sum_{t=t_0}^{t_0+\Delta T} \sum_{\vec{r}\in\Gamma} I(\vec{r},t) \| V(\vec{r},t) \|_2}{\sum_{t=t_0}^{t_0+\Delta T} \sum_{\vec{r}\in\Gamma} I(\vec{r},t)}. \qquad [6.25]$$

This metric summarizes the UCA transport over a period ΔT, starting from the bolus arrival time, t_0, within an ROI, Γ. The symbol $\|\cdot\|_2$ represents the L2 norm. In equation [6.25], the amplitude of the velocity vector $\| V(\vec{r},t) \|_2$ is weighted by the intensity level. The intensity in the ROI is calculated as the sum of the intensities in each pixel over time. As a result, ROIs for which the microbubble transport (velocity in space and time) is similar, but the intensity in each pixel and/or the number of pixels in which UCA are passing varies, will have similar values of the parameter γ. In a study on pregnant rats, the proposed parameters γ outperformed other TIC-based parameters in the detection of placental insufficiency (Senneville et al. 2018).

In parallel, Wildeboer et al. (2018a) proposed a description of UCA transport as a three-dimensional convective dispersion process. Essentially, this method extends equation [6.9] to all spatial dimensions as:

$$\partial tC = \nabla \cdot (D\nabla C) - v\nabla C \quad [6.26]$$

where **D** is the dispersion tensor and **v** is the velocity vector. These are both locally constant and described as:

$$D = \left[D_{xx}\; D_{xy}\; D_{xz}\; D_{yx}\; D_{yy}\; D_{yz}\; D_{zx}\; D_{zy}\; D_{zz}\,\right]\; v = \left[v_x\; v_y\; v_z\,\right]. \quad [6.27]$$

Assuming $D_{xy} = D_{yx}$, $D_{yz} = D_{zy}$, and $D_{zx} = D_{xz}$, the number of unknowns reduces to six independent diffusion components and three independent velocity components. These are estimated by computing the concentration gradients by convolution of the DCE-US data with Gaussian spatial and temporal derivates. The resulting linear model is then solved by least squares minimization. Summary parameters characterizing the local dispersion and velocity of UCA transport were defined as:

$$D_{ADC} = \left|\frac{1}{3}(D_{xx} + D_{yy} + D_{zz})\right|, \quad v = \sqrt{v_x^2 + v_y^2 + v_z^2} \quad [6.28]$$

where D_{ADC} is the apparent dispersion coefficient, calculated as the magnitude of the trace of the dispersion tensor divided by three, and v is the local velocity magnitude. The parameter v showed promising performance in detecting clinically significant prostate cancer, achieving an accuracy of 80% (Wildeboer et al. 2019). When combined by machine learning with other parameters extracted from quantitative analysis methods such as mLDRW model fitting, spatio-temporal similarity analysis and system identification, and semi-quantitative parameters such as WIT, WIR, PE and AT (see Table 6.1), the diagnostic performance was further improved, achieving an accuracy of 81% (Wildeboer et al. 2019).

6.4. Current challenges and future perspectives

Analysis of the transport kinetics of UCA microbubbles combined with real-time DCE-US imaging has permitted minimally invasive quantification of hemodynamics parameters, aiding diagnosis and monitoring of different conditions in a broad range of clinical domains, including cardiology, oncology, radiology, urology, gastrointestinal imaging and perinatal care (Kono et al. 2017; Bertolotto et al. 2018; Mischi et al. 2018; Sidhu et al. 2018; Erlichman et al. 2020; Hwang et al. 2020; Villemain et al. 2020).

The wide implementation of quantitative DCE-US in clinical routine, however, is hindered by the limited availability of standardized acquisition protocols and calibration procedures. A few steps have been taken in this direction with the publication of different guidelines and recommendations for the clinical use of DCE-US (Claudon et al. 2013; Cantisani et al. 2015; Nolsøe and Lorentzen 2016; Sidhu et al. 2017; Dietrich et al. 2018) and quantification of tumor perfusion by DCE-US (Leen et al. 2012; Dietrich et al. 2012). Unfortunately, reproducibility is still hampered by the lack of a data standard that is compatible with quantification procedures. Ideally, with such a standard in place and all US scanner manufacturers complying with it, DCE-US could become a practical, functional and widely employed quantitative imaging modality.

In general, absolute calibration is not achievable and DCE-US quantification is typically performed on linearized data. Because of the unknown contrast dose input to the area of interest and the inability to retrieve the absolute contrast concentration, the Stewart–Hamilton equation cannot be applied in an absolute sense; thus, researchers have mostly focused on temporal features of UCA transport. Using system identification techniques (impulse response and Green's functions), as well as three-dimensional spatio-temporal modeling of UCA transport, vascular hemodynamics can be assessed locally, laying down the foundations for exciting developments in quantitative DCE-US.

Due to its simplicity, the bolus injection protocol is by far the most commonly used in both clinical and research settings. Several models have been developed to describe the UCA bolus kinetics in time and space. Generally, physics- and physiology-driven models provide interpretable parameters, and additionally offer the opportunity to gain knowledge and insights on the investigated processes; these should therefore be preferred over empirical, data-driven approaches. When conventional 2D DCE-US is employed, one of the main challenges of bolus injection methods is the search for the best suited imaging plane to observe UCA flow, since only one plane can be well imaged with a single UCA injection. Although, in comparison, the constant infusion protocol would allow for imaging multiple planes with a single contrast injection, its application is much more complex in practice. It requires the use of an injection pump, a dedicated image sequence including the application of high-pressure ultrasound bursts and the challenging attainment of a steady plateau (Dietrich et al. 2012). This has resulted in limited use and low compliance in clinical settings.

Another critical aspect of DCE-US quantification is concerned with data pre-processing to remove or reduce the corruption by noise and artifacts (Tang et al. 2011). Conventional methods are based on simple low-pass or band-pass filtering to reduce the effects of high-frequency noise and slow motion artifacts, while keeping the relevant frequency components capturing UCA kinetics. In addition, spatial smoothing can also be applied to increase the signal-to-noise ratio, especially in pixels with poor signal. More advanced spatio-temporal filtering techniques based on wavelets (Bar-Zion et al. 2015) and singular value decompositions (Wildeboer et al. 2020) have also been proposed, showing the ability to separate signal components coming from UCAs from those coming from clutter and noise. Since the resolution of the imaging system is typically anisotropic and dependent on the depth, dedicated solutions are needed for accurate spatial and spatio-temporal analysis. This can be achieved by spatial regularization filters (Schalk et al. 2018) or by employing adaptive kernel sizes (Wildeboer et al. 2019).

Since a DCE-US exam can require several minutes of data acquisition, motion artifacts are relatively common in DCE-US sequences. Motion can be due to intrinsic body movements, such as heart beats and breathing, or external causes, such as handheld probe tilting. Oftentimes motion compensation is required before the application of quantitative analysis techniques. When conventional 2D CEUS is employed, compensation of motion in the direction perpendicular to the imaging plane is very difficult to achieve. This happens when extrinsic or intrinsic motion causes the investigated ROI to go out of the imaging plane. Out-of-plane motion compensation currently mostly consists of identifying and removing the out-of-plane frames (Schäfer et al. 2015), possibly followed by interpolation strategies to retrieve the original temporal resolution. Conversely, techniques to compensate in-plane motion have been widely investigated. Most are based on image registration and motion tracking (e.g. speckle tracking) (Akkus et al. 2012; Bouhlel et al. 2014; Carvalho et al. 2014; Bakas et al. 2019). Singular value-decomposition filtering has also proven effective in reducing motion artifacts. Specific to DCE-US perfusion imaging, the use of the goodness-of-fit measures from TIC fitting can be used as a cost function for optimizing the registration procedure, resulting in improved image quality (Barrois et al. 2015).

Although currently limited to specialized centers, ultrasound systems allowing for 3D DCE-US are steadily becoming more available (Huang and Zeng 2017; Kaffas et al. 2020). Three-dimensional acquisitions present many advantages for quantitative DCE-US. Besides facilitating motion compensation in all directions, possibly avoiding the need for out-of-plane frame removal, 3D DCE-US permits recording the UCA transport process in the whole volume by a single bolus injection. Given that UCA dilution is intrinsically a three-dimensional spatio-temporal process, 3D acquisitions pave the way for applications of techniques that describe the UCA transport in all flow directions, accounting for full boundary conditions. This permits the relaxation of assumptions and approximations, and leads to the estimation of more accurate and comprehensive hemodynamic parameters. Although this comes at the cost of reduced spatio-temporal resolution, the recent introduction of ultrafast ultrasound imaging is enabling 3D DCE-US at increasingly higher temporal resolution (Montaldo et al. 2009; Couture et al. 2012; Viti et al. 2016). Combined with sparse sampling strategies, efficient implementation of ultrafast 3D DCE-US can be achieved, reducing the challenges in terms of hardware requirements (Roux et al. 2016).

Exciting developments are also taking place in the context of ultrasound molecular imaging, thanks to the introduction of targeted microbubbles (Lindner 2004; Deshpande et al. 2010; Pochon et al. 2010). Essentially, these are functionalized microbubbles, obtained by decorating the bubble shell with targeting ligands. When flowing in the microcirculation, targeted microbubbles can attach to specific molecules on the vessel wall, causing steady enhancement in areas where the target molecule is present. This is especially evident in the late phase of the DCE-US sequences, when all non-bound microbubbles have washed out. Although these bubbles are still not approved for clinical use, targeted microbubbles commercially known as BR55 (Pochon et al. 2010) (Bracco, Geneva, Switzerland) have proven safe and efficacious in clinical trials for detection of prostate, breast and ovarian cancer, raising promise for their clinical translation (Smeenge et al. 2017; Willmann et al. 2017). Quantification methods applied to targeted DCE-US have shown their ability to provide assessment of the relative binding degree (related to the concentration of the target molecule), while reducing acquisition time and simplifying the acquisition protocol (Chen et al. 2012; Sirsi et al. 2012; Turco et al. 2017, 2018).

More recently, nanobubbles with diameters of the order of 100 nm are being developed and optimized. Thanks to their size, they can pass through the gaps in the endothelial layers, enabling additional assessment of vessel permeability, one of the hallmarks of cancer angiogenic vasculature (Folkman 1984). This also widens the range of targeting options, because molecules beyond the vessel walls can be reached (Cai et al. 2015; Perera et al. 2015; Chen et al. 2017; Zhou et al. 2018). In the future, the combination of double injection (both microbubbles and nanobubbles) protocols with dedicated imaging sequences, as well as suitable modeling and quantification techniques, may pave the way for simultaneous assessment of perfusion, extravasation and molecular targets within a single DCE-US examination (Carr et al. 2011; Herbst et al. 2017).

Although the increasing number of extracted parameters poses important challenges in terms of the combination and interpretation of the wealth of available information, it also brings about exciting possibilities for multiparametric and multimodal approaches (El Kaffas et al. 2020). In this context, artificial intelligence (AI) can be employed to optimally harness the complementary information provided by different quantitative parameters and ultrasound imaging modality, including, for example, B-mode imaging and ultrasound elastography (Mannaerts et al. 2018; Akkus et al. 2019). Classic machine learning classifiers can exploit complex nonlinear relationships between features at a pixel or ROI level, possibly boosting the diagnostic accuracy (Căleanu et al. 2014; Kondo et al. 2017; Mannaerts et al. 2018). Although generally more data-hungry, deep learning strategies are alleviating the need for explicit development, validation and selection of hand-engineered features, allowing for end-to-end approaches with promising classification performance (Wu et al. 2014). To further take advantage of the morphological structures and spatial patterns in the images, convolutional neural networks (CNNs) can be used to learn and exploit the spatial relationships between pixels. By the recent extension to 3D, CNNs can also learn local temporal patterns, boosting their utility for data-driven analysis of UCA kinetics. However, deep learning has raised concern about the reliability and interpretability of the obtained predictions, especially in sensitive fields such as diagnostic imaging (Reyes et al. 2020). In response, methods to visualize, understand and possibly steer the decision processes of AI algorithms are being investigated (Wang et al. 2019; Zhang et al. 2020).

6.5. References

Akhbardeh, A., Sagreiya, H., El Kaffas, A., Willmann, J.K., Rubin, D.L. (2019). A multi-model framework to estimate perfusion parameters using contrast-enhanced ultrasound imaging. *Medical Physics*, 46, 590–600.

Akkus, Z., Hoogi, A., Renaud, G., Gerrit, L., van den Oord, S.C.H., Schinkel, A.F.L., de Jong, N., van der Steen, A.F.W., Bosch, J.G. (2012). Motion compensation method using dynamic programming for quantification of neovascularization in carotid atherosclerotic plaques with contrast enhanced ultrasound (CEUS). *Medical Imaging 2012: Ultrasonic Imaging, Tomography, and Therapy*. International Society for Optics and Photonics, 83200C.

Akkus, Z., Cai, J., Boonrod, A., Zeinoddini, A., Weston, A.D., Philbrick, K.A., Erickson, B.J. (2019). A survey of deep-learning applications in ultrasound: Artificial intelligence-powered ultrasound for improving clinical workflow. *Journal of the American College of Radiology*, 16, 1318–1328.

Appis, A.W., Tracy, M.J., Feinstein, S.B. (2015). Update on the safety and efficacy of commercial ultrasound contrast agents in cardiac applications. *Echo Research and Practice*, 2, R55–R62.

Arditi, M., Frinking, P.J.A., Xiang, Z., Rognin, N.G. (2006). A new formalism for the quantification of tissue perfusion by the destruction-replenishment method in contrast ultrasound imaging. *IEEE Transactions on Ultrasonics, Ferroelectrics, and Frequency Control*, 53, 1118–1129.

Averkiou, M.A., Juang, E.K., Gallagher, M.K., Cuevas, M.A., Wilson, S.R., Barr, R.G., Carson, P.L. (2020). Evaluation of the reproducibility of bolus transit quantification with contrast-enhanced ultrasound across multiple scanners and analysis software packages – A quantitative imaging biomarker alliance study. *Investigative Radiology*, 55, 643–656.

Baish, J.W. and Jain, R.K. (2000). Fractals and cancer. *Cancer Research*, 60, 3683–3688.

Bakas, S., Doulgerakis-Kontoudis, M., Hunter, G.J.A., Sidhu, P.S., Makris, D., Chatzimichail, K. (2019). Evaluation of indirect methods for motion compensation in 2-D focal liver lesion contrast-enhanced ultrasound (CEUS) imaging. *Ultrasound in Medicine & Biology*, 45, 1380–1396.

Bar-Zion, A.D., Tremblay-Darveau, C., Yin, M., Adam, D., Foster, F.S. (2015). Denoising of contrast-enhanced ultrasound cine sequences based on a multiplicative model. *IEEE Transactions on Biomedical Engineering*, 62, 1969–1980.

Bar-Zion, A.D., Solomon, O., Tremblay-Darveau, C., Adam, D., Eldar, Y.C. (2018). SUSHI: Sparsity-based ultrasound super-resolution hemodynamic imaging. *IEEE Transactions on Ultrasonics, Ferroelectrics, and Frequency Control*, 65, 2365–2380.

Barrois, G., Coron, A., Lucidarme, O., Bridal, S.L. (2015). Automatic motion estimation using flow parameters for dynamic contrast-enhanced ultrasound. *Physics in Medicine & Biology*, 60, 2117.

Bassingthwaighte, J.B., Ackerman, F.H., Wood, E.H. (1966). Applications of the lagged normal density curve as a model for arterial dilution curves. *Circulation Research*, 18, 398–415.

Bertolotto, M., Bucci, S., Valentino, M., Currò, F., Sachs, C., Cova, M.A. (2018). Contrast-enhanced ultrasound for characterizing renal masses. *European Journal of Radiology*, 105, 41–48.

Bogaard, J.M., Smith, S.J., Versprille, A., Wise, M.E., Hagemeijer, F. (1984). Physiological interpretation of the skewness of indicatordilution curves; theoretical considerations and a practical application. *Basic Research in Cardiology*, 79, 479–493.

Bogaard, J.M., Jansen, J.R.C., von Reth, E.A., Versprille, A., Wise, M.E. (1986). Random walk type models for indicator-dilution studies: Comparison of a local density random walk and a first passage times distribution. *Cardiovascular Research*, 20, 789–796.

Bouhlel, N., Coron, A., Barrois, G., Lucidarme, O., Bridal, S.L. (2014). Dual-mode registration of dynamic contrast-enhanced ultrasound combining tissue and contrast sequences. *Ultrasonics*, 54, 1289–1299.

Cai, W., Bin, Yang, H.L., Zhang, J., Yin, J.K., Yang, Y.L., Yuan, L.J., Zhang, L., Duan, Y.Y. (2015). The optimized fabrication of nanobubbles as ultrasound contrast agents for tumor imaging. *Scientific Reports*, 5, 13725.

Căleanu, C.-D., Simion, G., David, C., Gui, V., Moga, T., Popescu, A., Sirli, R., Sporea, I. (2014). A study over the importance of arterial phase temporal parameters in focal liver lesions CEUS based diagnosis. *11th International Symposium on Electronics and Telecommunications (ISETC)*. IEEE, 1–4.

Calliada, F., Campani, R., Bottinelli, O., Bozzini, A., Sommaruga, M.G. (1998). Ultrasound contrast agents: Basic principles. *European Journal of Radiology*, 27, 157–160.

Cantisani, V., Bertolotto, M., Weskott, H.P., Romanini, L., Grazhdani, H., Passamonti, M., Drudi, F.M., Malpassini, F., Isidori, A., Meloni, F.M. et al. (2015). Growing indications for CEUS: The kidney, testis, lymph nodes, thyroid, prostate, and small bowel. *European Journal of Radiology*, 84, 1675–1684 [Online]. Available at: https://doi.org/10.1016/j.ejrad.2015.05.008.

Cao, X.L., Bao, W., Zhu, S.G., Wang, L.H., Sun, M.H., Wang, L., Men, Y.M., Xue, J. (2014). Contrast-enhanced ultrasound characteristics of breast cancer: Correlation with prognostic factors. *Ultrasound in Medicine & Biology*, 40, 11–17.

Carr, C.L., Qi, Y., Davidson, B., Chadderdon, S., Jayaweera, A.R., Belcik, J.T., Benner, C., Xie, A., Lindner, J.R. (2011). Dysregulated selectin expression and monocyte recruitment during ischemia-related vascular remodeling in diabetes mellitus. *Arteriosclerosis, Thrombosis, and Vascular Biology*, 31, 2526–2533.

Carvalho, D.D.B., Akkus, Z., Bosch, J.G., Oord, S.C.H. van den Niessen, W.J., Klein, S. (2014). Nonrigid motion compensation in B-mode and contrast enhanced ultrasound image sequences of the carotid artery. *Proceedings of the SPIE*, 9034, 157–163 [Online]. Available at: https://doi.org/10.1117/12.2043549.

Charalampidis, D., Pascotto, M., Kerut, E.K., Lindner, J.R. (2006). Anatomy and flow in normal and ischemic microvasculature based on a novel temporal fractal dimension analysis algorithm using contrast enhanced ultrasound. *IEEE Transactions on Medical Imaging*, 25, 1079–1086.

Chen, C.C., Sirsi, S.R., Homma, S., Borden, M.A. (2012). Effect of surface architecture on in vivo ultrasound contrast persistence of targeted size-selected microbubbles. *Ultrasound in Medicine and Biology*, 38, 492–503.

Chen, F., Ma, M., Wang, J., Wang, F., Chern, S.-X., Zhao, E.R., Jhunjhunwala, A., Darmadi, S., Chen, H., Jokerst, J. (2017). Exosome-like silica nanoparticles: A novel ultrasound contrast agent for stem cell imaging. *Nanoscale*, 9, 402–411.

Christensen-Jeffries, K., Couture, O., Dayton, P.A., Eldar, Y.C., Hynynen, K., Kiessling, F., O'Reilly, M., Pinton, G.F., Schmitz, G., Tang, M.X. et al. (2020). Super-resolution ultrasound imaging. *Ultrasound in Medicine & Biology*, 46, 865–891.

Claudon, M., Dietrich, C.F., Choi, B.I., Cosgrove, D.O., Kudo, M., Nolsøe, C.P., Piscaglia, F., Wilson, S.R., Barr, R.G., Chammas, M.C. (2013). Guidelines and good clinical practice recommendations for contrast enhanced ultrasound (CEUS) in the liver – Update 2012. *Ultraschall in der Medizin-European Journal of Ultrasound*, 34, 11–29.

Cobbold, R.S.C. (2006). *Foundations of Biomedical Ultrasound*. Oxford University Press, Oxford.

Cobelli, C., Foster, D., Toffolo, G. (2007). *Tracer Kinetics in Biomedical Research: From Data to Model*. Springer Science & Business Media, Berlin.

Correas, J.-M., Bridal, L., Lesavre, A., Méjean, A., Claudon, M., Hélénon, O. (2001). Ultrasound contrast agents: Properties, principles of action, tolerance, and artifacts. *European Radiology*, 11, 1316–1328.

Cosgrove, D. (2006). Ultrasound contrast agents: An overview. *European Journal of Radiology*, 60, 324–330.

Couture, O., Fink, M., Tanter, M. (2012). Ultrasound contrast plane wave imaging. *IEEE Transactions on Ultrasonics, Ferroelectrics, and Frequency Control*, 59, 2676–2683.

Couture, O., Hingot, V., Heiles, B., Muleki-Seya, P., Tanter, M. (2018). Ultrasound localization microscopy and super-resolution: A state of the art. *IEEE Transactions on Ultrasonics, Ferroelectrics, and Frequency Control*, 65, 1304–1320.

Davenport, R. (1983). The derivation of the gamma-variate relationship for tracer dilution curves. *Journal of Nuclear Medicine: Official Publication, Society of Nuclear Medicine*, 24, 945–948.

Davis Jr, G.C. and Kutner, M.H. (1976). The lagged normal family of probability density functions applied to indicator-dilution curves. *Biometrics*, 32(3), 669–675.

Deshpande, N., Needles, A., Willmann, J.K. (2010). Molecular ultrasound imaging: Current status and future directions. *Clinical Radiology*, 65, 567–581.

Dietrich, C.F., Averkiou, M.A., Correas, J.-M., Lassau, N., Leen, E., Piscaglia, F. (2012). An EFSUMB introduction into dynamic contrast-enhanced ultrasound (DCE-US) for quantification of tumour perfusion. *Ultraschall in der Medizin – European Journal of Ultrasound*, 33, 344–351.

Dietrich, C.F., Averkiou, M., Nielsen, M.B., Barr, R.G., Burns, P.N., Calliada, F., Cantisani, V., Choi, B., Chammas, M.C., Clevert, D.-A. et al. (2018). How to perform contrast-enhanced ultrasound (CEUS). *Ultrasound International Open*, 4, E2–E15.

Dollet, B., van der Meer, S.M., Garbin, V., de Jong, N., Lohse, D., Versluis, M. (2008). Nonspherical oscillations of ultrasound contrast agent microbubbles. *Ultrasound in Medicine & Biology*, 34, 1465–1473.

El Kaffas, A., Sigrist, R.M.S., Fisher, G., Bachawal, S., Liau, J., Wang, H., Karanany, A., Durot, I., Rosenberg, J., Hristov, D. et al. (2017). Quantitative three-dimensional dynamic contrast-enhanced ultrasound imaging: First-in-human pilot study in patients with liver metastases. *Theranostics*, 7, 3745–3758.

El Kaffas, A., Hoogi, A., Zhou, J., Durot, I., Wang, H., Rosenberg, J., Tseng, A., Sagreiya, H., Akhbardeh, A., Rubin, D.L. et al. (2020a). Spatial characterization of tumor perfusion properties from 3D DCE-US perfusion maps are early predictors of cancer treatment response. *Scientific Reports*, 10, 1–11.

El Kaffas, A., Gong, R., Sridharan, S., Sigrist, R.M.S., Durot, I., Willmann, J.K., Hristov, D. (2020b). Clinical evaluation of real-time optical-tracking navigation and live time-intensity curves to provide feedback during blinded 4D contrast-enhanced ultrasound imaging. arXiv:2011.00744.

Erlichman, D.B., Weiss, A., Koenigsberg, M., Stein, M.W. (2020). Contrast enhanced ultrasound: A review of radiology applications. *Clinical Imaging*, 60, 209–215.

Errico, C., Pierre, J., Pezet, S., Desailly, Y., Lenkei, Z., Couture, O., Tanter, M. (2015). Ultrafast ultrasound localization microscopy for deep super-resolution vascular imaging. *Nature*, 527, 499.

Faez, T., Emmer, M., Kooiman, K., Versluis, M., van der Steen, A., de Jong, N. (2013). 20 years of ultrasound contrast agent modeling. *IEEE Transactions on Ultrasonics, Ferroelectrics, and Frequency Control*, 60, 7–20.

Feinstein, S.B. (2004). The powerful microbubble: From bench to bedside, from intravascular indicator to therapeutic delivery system, and beyond. *American Journal of Physiology. Heart and Circulatory Physiology*, 287, H450–H457.

Fidler, I.J. (2001). Angiogenic heterogeneity: Regulation of neoplastic angiogenesis by the organ microenvironment. *Journal of the National Cancer Institute*, 93(14), 1040–1041.

Folkman, J. (1984). Angiogenesis. In *Biology of Endothelial Cells. Developments in Cardiovascular Medicine*, vol 27, Jaffe, E.A. (ed.). Springer, Boston, MA [Online]. Available at: https://doi.org/10.1007/978-1-4613-2825-4_42.

Fox, I.J. (1962). History and developmental aspects of the indicator-dilution technic. *Circulation Research*, 10, 381–92.

Frinking, P.J.A., Bouakaz, A., Kirkhorn, J., ten Cate, F.J., de Jong, N. (2000). Ultrasound contrast imaging: Current and new potential methods. *Ultrasound in Medicine & Biology*, 26, 965–975.

Gauthier, T.P., Averkiou, M.A., Leen, E.L.S. (2011). Perfusion quantification using dynamic contrast-enhanced ultrasound: The impact of dynamic range and gain on time-intensity curves. *Ultrasonics*, 51, 102–106.

Gilmore, F.R. (1952). The growth or collapse of a spherical bubble in a viscous compressible liquid. Report no. 26-4, Hydrodynamics Laboratory, California Institute of Technology, Pasadena, CA [Online]. Available at: https://authors.library.caltech.edu/561/1/Gilmore_fr_26-4.pdf.

Hamilton, W.F., Moore, J.W., Kinsman, J.M., Spurling, R.G. (1928). Simultaneous determination of the pulmonary and systemic circulation times in man and of a figure related to the cardiac output. *American Journal of Physiology-Legacy Content*, 84, 338–344.

Harabis, V., Kolar, R., Mezl, M., Jirik, R. (2013). Comparison and evaluation of indicator dilution models for bolus of ultrasound contrast agents. *Physiological Measurement*, 34, 151–162.

Herbst, E., Unnikrishnan, S., Wang, S., Klibanov, A.L., Hossack, J.A., Mauldin Jr, F.W. (2017). The use of acoustic radiation force decorrelation-weighted pulse inversion (ADW-PI) for enhanced ultrasound contrast imaging. *Investigative Radiology*, 52, 95.

Herring, C. (1941). Theory of the pulsations of the gas bubble produced by an underwater explosion. Report C4-sr20-010, Columbia University Division of National Defense Research, New London, CT.

Huang, Q. and Zeng, Z. (2017). A review on real-time 3D ultrasound imaging technology. *BioMed Research International*, 6027029 [Online]. Available at: https://doi.org/10.1155/2017/6027029.

Huang-Wei, C., Bleuzen, A., Bourlier, P., Roumy, J., Bouakaz, A., Pourcelot, L., Tranquart, F. (2006). Differential diagnosis of focal nodular hyperplasia with quantitative parametric analysis in contrast-enhanced sonography. *Investigative Radiology*, 41, 363–368.

Hudson, J.M., Karshafian, R., Burns, P.N. (2009). Quantification of flow using ultrasound and microbubbles: A disruption replenishment model based on physical principles. *Ultrasound in Medicine & Biology*, 35, 2007–2020.

Hudson, J.M., Williams, R., Karshafian, R., Milot, L., Atri, M., Burns, P.N., Bjarnason, G.A. (2014). Quantifying vascular heterogeneity using microbubble disruption-replenishment kinetics in patients with renal cell cancer. *Investigative Radiology*, 49, 116–123.

Hwang, M., Back, S.J., Didier, R.A., Lorenz, N., Morgan, T.A., Poznick, L., Steffgen, L., Sridharan, A. (2020). Pediatric contrast-enhanced ultrasound: Optimization of techniques and dosing. *Pediatric Radiology*, 51, 2147–2160.

Jhanji, S., Dawson, J., Pearse, R.M. (2008). Cardiac output monitoring: Basic science and clinical application. *Anaesthesia*, 63, 172–181.

de Jong, N., Frinking, P.J.A., Bouakaz, A., ten Cate, F.J. (2000). Detection procedures of ultrasound contrast agents. *Ultrasonics*, 38, 87–92.

Kondo, S., Takagi, K., Nishida, M., Iwai, T., Kudo, Y., Ogawa, K., Kamiyama, T., Shibuya, H., Kahata, K., Shimizu, C. (2017). Computer-aided diagnosis of focal liver lesions using contrast-enhanced ultrasonography with perflubutane microbubbles. *IEEE Transactions on Medical Imaging*, 36, 1427–1437.

Kono, Y., Lyshchik, A., Cosgrove, D., Dietrich, C.F., Jang, H.J., Kim, T.K., Piscaglia, F., Willmann, J.K., Wilson, S.R., Santillan, C. et al. (2017). Contrast enhanced ultrasound (CEUS) liver imaging reporting and data system (LI-RADS®): The official version by the American College of Radiology (ACR). *Ultraschall in der Medizin*, 38, 85–86.

Krejcie, T.C., Jacquez, J.A., Avram, M.J., Niemann, C.U., Shanks, C.A., Henthorn, T.K. (1996). Use of parallel Erlang density functions to analyze first-pass pulmonary uptake of multiple indicators in dogs. *Journal of Pharmacokinetics and Biopharmaceutics*, 24, 569–588.

Krix, M., Kiessling, F., Farhan, N., Schmidt, K., Hoffend, J., Delorme, S. (2003). A multivessel model describing replenishment kinetics of ultrasound contrast agent for quantification of tissue perfusion. *Ultrasound in Medicine and Biology*, 29, 1421–1430.

Krix, M., Plathow, C., Kiessling, F., Herth, F., Karcher, A., Essig, M., Schmitteckert, H., Kauczor, H.-U., Delorme, S. (2004). Quantification of perfusion of liver tissue and metastases using a multivessel model for replenishment kinetics of ultrasound contrast agents. *Ultrasound in Medicine and Biology*, 30, 1355–1363.

Kuenen, M.P.J., Mischi, M., Wijkstra, H. (2011). Contrast-ultrasound diffusion imaging for localization of prostate cancer. *IEEE Transactions on Medical Imaging*, 30, 1493–1502.

Kuenen, M.P.J., Saidov, T.A., Wijkstra, H., de La Rosette, J.J.M.C.H., Mischi, M. (2013). Spatiotemporal correlation of ultrasound contrast agent dilution curves for angiogenesis localization by dispersion imaging. *IEEE Transactions on Ultrasonics, Ferroelectrics, and Frequency Control*, 60, 2665–2669.

Kuenen, M.P.J., Herold, I.H.F., Korsten, H.H.M., de La Rosette, J.J.M.C.H., Wijkstra, H., Mischi, M. (2014). Maximum-likelihood estimation for indicator dilution analysis. *IEEE Transactions on Biomedical Engineering*, 61, 821–831.

Lassau, N., Bonastre, J., Kind, M., Vilgrain, V., Lacroix, J., Cuinet, M., Taieb, S., Aziza, R., Sarran, A., Labbe-Devilliers, C. et al. (2014). Validation of dynamic contrast-enhanced ultrasound in predicting outcomes of antiangiogenic therapy for solid tumors: The French multicenter support for innovative and expensive techniques study. *Investigative Radiology*, 49, 794.

Lassau, N., Coiffier, B., Faivre, L., Benatsou, B., Bidault, S., Girard, E., Asselain, B., Pitre-Champagnat, S., Koscielny, S. (2017). Study of intrapatient variability and reproducibility of quantitative tumor perfusion parameters evaluated with dynamic contrast-enhanced ultrasonography. *Investigative Radiology*, 52, 148–154.

Leen, E., Averkiou, M., Arditi, M., Burns, P., Bokor, D., Gauthier, T., Kono, Y., Lucidarme, O. (2012). Dynamic contrast enhanced ultrasound assessment of the vascular effects of novel therapeutics in early stage trials. *European Radiology*, 22, 1442–1450.

Li, X., Li, Y., Zhu, Y., Fu, L., Liu, P. (2018). Association between enhancement patterns and parameters of contrast-enhanced ultrasound and microvessel distribution in breast cancer. *Oncology Letters*, 15, 5643–5649.

Lin, F., Shelton, S.E., Espíndola, D., Rojas, J.D., Pinton, G., Dayton, P.A. (2017). 3-D ultrasound localization microscopy for identifying microvascular morphology features of tumor angiogenesis at a resolution beyond the diffraction limit of conventional ultrasound. *Theranostics*, 7, 196.

Lindner, J.R. (2004). Microbubbles in medical imaging: Current applications and future directions. *Nature Reviews Drug Discovery*, 3, 527.

Liu, H., Jiang, Y., Dai, Q., Zhu, Q., Wang, L., Lu, J. (2014). Peripheral enhancement of breast cancers on contrast-enhanced ultrasound: Correlation with microvessel density and vascular endothelial growth factor expression. *Ultrasound in Medicine & Biology*, 40, 293–299.

Lowerison, M.R., Huang, C., Lucien, F., Chen, S., Song, P. (2020). Ultrasound localization microscopy of renal tumor xenografts in chicken embryo is correlated to hypoxia. *Scientific Reports*, 10, 1–13.

Lucidarme, O., Franchi-Abella, S., Correas, J.-M., Bridal, S.L., Kurtisovski, E., Berger, G. (2003). Blood flow quantification with contrast-enhanced US: "Entrance in the Section" phenomenon–phantom and rabbit study. *Radiology*, 228, 473–479.

Luo, W., Numata, K., Morimoto, M., Nozaki, A., Nagano, Y., Sugimori, K., Tanaka, K. (2009). Three-dimensional contrast-enhanced sonography of vascular patterns of focal liver tumors: Pilot study of visualization methods. *American Journal of Roentgenology*, 192, 165–173.

Mannaerts, C.K., Wildeboer, R.R., Postema, A.W., Hagemann, J., Budäus, L., Tilki, D., Mischi, M., Wijkstra, H., Salomon, G. (2018). Multiparametric ultrasound: Evaluation of greyscale, shear wave elastography and contrast-enhanced ultrasound for prostate cancer detection and localization in correlation to radical prostatectomy specimens. *BMC Urology*, 18, 98.

Marmottant, P., van der Meer, S., Emmer, M., Versluis, M., de Jong, N., Hilgenfeldt, S., Lohse, D. (2005). A model for large amplitude oscillations of coated bubbles accounting for buckling and rupture. *The Journal of the Acoustical Society of America*, 118, 3499.

Maxeiner, A., Fischer, T., Schwabe, J., Baur, A.D.J., Stephan, C., Peters, R., Slowinski, T., von Laffert, M., Marticorena Garcia, S.R., Hamm, B. et al. (2019). Contrast-enhanced ultrasound (CEUS) and quantitative perfusion analysis in patients with suspicion for prostate cancer. *Ultraschall in der Medizin*, 40, 340–348.

Mischi, M., Kalker, T., Korsten, E. (2003). Videodensitometric methods for cardiac output measurements. *EURASIP Journal on Applied Signal Processing*, 479–489.

Mischi, M., Jansen, A.H.M., Korsten, H.H.M. (2007). Identification of cardiovascular dilution systems by contrast ultrasound. *Ultrasound in Medicine & Biology*, 33, 439–451.

Mischi, M., den Boer, J.A., Korsten, H.H.M. (2008). On the physical and stochastic representation of an indicator dilution curve as a gamma variate. *Physiological Measurement*, 29, 281.

Mischi, M., Kuenen, M.P.J., Wijkstra, H. (2012). Angiogenesis imaging by spatiotemporal analysis of ultrasound contrast agent dispersion kinetics. *IEEE Transactions on Ultrasonics, Ferroelectrics, and Frequency Control*, 59, 621–629.

Mischi, M., Turco, S., Soliman, O.I., Folkert, J., Wijkstra, H., Schoots, I. (2018). *Quantification of Contrast Kinetics in Clinical Imaging*. Springer, Cham.

Molinari, F., Mantovani, A., Deandrea, M., Limone, P., Garberoglio, R., Suri, J.S. (2010). Characterization of single thyroid nodules by contrast-enhanced 3-D ultrasound. *Ultrasound in Medicine & Biology*, 36, 1616–1625.

Montaldo, G., Tanter, M., Bercoff, J., Benech, N., Fink, M. (2009). Coherent plane-wave compounding for very high frame rate ultrasonography and transient elastography. *IEEE Transactions on Ultrasonics, Ferroelectrics, and Frequency Control*, 56, 489–506.

Nolsøe, C.P. and Lorentzen, T. (2016). International guidelines for contrast-enhanced ultrasonography: Ultrasound imaging in the new millennium. *Ultrasonography (Seoul, Korea)*, 35, 89–103.

Paefgen, V., Doleschel, D., Kiessling, F. (2015). Evolution of contrast agents for ultrasound imaging and ultrasound-mediated drug delivery. *Frontiers in Pharmacology*, 6, 197.

Payen, T., Coron, A., Lamuraglia, M., Le Guillou-Buffello, D., Gaud, E., Arditi, M., Lucidarme, O., Bridal, S.L. (2013). Echo-power estimation from log-compressed video data in dynamic contrast-enhanced ultrasound imaging. *Ultrasound in Medicine and Biology*, 39, 1826–1837.

Perera, R.H., Hernandez, C., Zhou, H., Kota, P., Burke, A., Exner, A.A. (2015). Ultrasound imaging beyond the vasculature with new generation contrast agents. *Wiley Interdisciplinary Reviews: Nanomedicine and Nanobiotechnology*, 7, 593–608.

Piscaglia, F., Nolsøe, C., Dietrich, C.F., Cosgrove, D.O., Gilja, O.H., Bachmann Nielsen, M., Albrecht, T., Barozzi, L., Bertolotto, M., Catalano, O. et al. (2012). The EFSUMB guidelines and recommendations on the clinical practice of contrast enhanced ultrasound (CEUS): Update 2011 on non-hepatic applications. *Ultraschall in der Medizin*, 33, 33–59.

Pochon, S., Tardy, I., Bussat, P., Bettinger, T., Brochot, J., von Wronski, M., Passantino, L., Schneider, M. (2010). BR55: A lipopeptide-based VEGFR2-targeted ultrasound contrast agent for molecular imaging of angiogenesis. *Investigative Radiology*, 45, 89–95.

Pollard, R.E., Sadlowski, A.R., Bloch, S.H., Murray, L., Wisner, E.R., Griffey, S., Ferrara, K.W. (2002). Contrast-assisted destruction-replenishment ultrasound for the assessment of tumor microvasculature in a rat model. *Technology in Cancer Research & Treatment*, 1, 459–470.

Porter, T.R., Xie, F., Kricsfeld, D., Armbruster, R.W. (1996). Improved myocardial contrast with second harmonic transient ultrasound response imaging in humans using intravenous perfluorocarbon-exposed sonicated dextrose albumin. *Journal of the American College of Cardiology*, 27(6), 1497–1501.

Potdevin, T.C., Fowlkes, J.B., Moskalik, A.P., Carson, P.L. (2004). Analysis of refill curve shape in ultrasound contrast agent studies. *Medical Physics*, 31, 623–632.

Qian, H. and Bassingthwaighte, J.B. (2000). A class of flow bifurcation models with lognormal distribution and fractal dispersion. *Journal of Theoretical Biology*, 205, 261–268.

Quaia, E. (2007). Microbubble ultrasound contrast agents: An update. *European Radiology*, 17, 1995–2008.

von Reth, E.A. and Bogaard, J.M. (1983). Comparison of a two-compartment model and distributed models for indicator dilution studies. *Medical & Biological Engineering & Computing*, 21, 453–459.

Reyes, M., Meier, R., Pereira, S., Silva, C.A., Dahlweid, F.-M., von Tengg-Kobligk, H. Summers, R.M., Wiest, R. (2020). On the interpretability of artificial intelligence in radiology: Challenges and opportunities. *Radiology: Artificial Intelligence*, 2, e190043.

Rizzo, G., Tonietto, M., Castellaro, M., Raffeiner, B., Coran, A., Fiocco, U., Stramare, R., Grisan, E. (2017). Bayesian quantification of contrast-enhanced ultrasound images with adaptive inclusion of an irreversible component. *IEEE Transactions on Medical Imaging*, 36, 1027–1036.

Rognin, N.G., Frinking, P., Costa, M., Arditi, M. (2008). In-vivo perfusion quantification by contrast ultrasound: Validation of the use of linearized video data vs. raw RF data. *IEEE Ultrasonics Symposium*, 1690–1693.

Roux, E., Ramalli, A., Tortoli, P., Cachard, C., Robini, M.C., Liebgott, H. (2016). 2-D ultrasound sparse arrays multidepth radiation optimization using simulated annealing and spiral-array inspired energy functions. *IEEE Transactions on Ultrasonics, Ferroelectrics, and Frequency Control*, 63, 2138–2149.

Saidov, T., Heneweer, C., Kuenen, M., von Broich-Oppert, J., Wijkstra, H., de la Rosette, J.J.M.C.H., Mischi, M. (2016). Fractal dimension of tumor microvasculature by DCE-US: Preliminary study in mice. *Ultrasound in Medicine and Biology*, 42, 2852–2863.

Sboros, V. (2008). Response of contrast agents to ultrasound. *Advanced Drug Delivery Reviews*, 60, 1117–1136.

Schäfer, S., Nylund, K., Sævik, F., Engjom, T., Mézl, M., Jiřík, R., Dimcevski, G., Gilja, O.H., Tönnies, K. (2015). Semi-automatic motion compensation of contrast-enhanced ultrasound images from abdominal organs for perfusion analysis. *Computers in Biology and Medicine*, 63, 229–237.

Schalk, S.G., Demi, L., Smeenge, M., Mills, D.M., Wallace, K.D., de la Rosette, J.J., Wijkstra, H., Mischi, M. (2015). 4-D spatiotemporal analysis of ultrasound contrast agent dispersion for prostate cancer localization: A feasibility study. *IEEE Transactions on Ultrasonics, Ferroelectrics, and Frequency Control*, 62, 839–851.

Schalk, S.G., Demi, L., Bouhouch, N., Kuenen, M.P.J., Postema, A.W., de la Rosette, J.J.M.C.H., Wijkstra, H., Tjalkens, T.J., Mischi, M. (2017). Contrast-enhanced ultrasound angiogenesis imaging by mutual information analysis for prostate cancer localization. *IEEE Transactions on Biomedical Engineering*, 64, 661–670.

Schalk, S.G., Huang, J., Li, J., Demi, L., Wijkstra, H., Huang, P., Mischi, M. (2018). 3-D quantitative dynamic contrast ultrasound for prostate cancer localization. *Ultrasound in Medicine & Biology*, 44, 807–814.

de Senneville, B.D., Novell, A., Arthuis, C., Mendes, V., Dujardin, P., Patat, F., Bouakaz, A., Escoffre, J., Perrotin, F. (2018). Development of a fluid dynamic model for quantitative contrast-enhanced ultrasound imaging. *IEEE Transactions on Medical Imaging*, 37, 372–383.

Sheppard, C.W. (1962). Stochastic models for tracer experiments in the circulation: Parallel random walks. *Journal of Theoretical Biology*, 2, 33–47.

Shi, W.T., Forsberg, F., Liu, J.-B., Rawool, N.M., Goldberg, B.B. (2001). Blood flow estimation with harmonic flash echo imaging. *Ultrasonic Imaging*, 23, 161–170.

Sidhu, P.S., Cantisani, V., Deganello, A., Dietrich, C.F., Duran, C., Franke, D., Harkanyi, Z., Kosiak, W., Miele, V., Ntoulia, A. et al. (2017). Role of contrast-enhanced ultrasound (CEUS) in paediatric practice: An EFSUMB position statement. *Ultraschall in der Medizin*, 38, 33–43.

Sidhu, P.S., Cantisani, V., Dietrich, C.F., Gilja, O.H., Saftoiu, A., Bartels, E., Bertolotto, M., Calliada, F., Clevert, D.A., Cosgrove, D. et al. (2018). The EFSUMB guidelines and recommendations for the clinical practice of contrast-enhanced ultrasound (CEUS) in non-hepatic applications: Update 2017 (short version). *Ultraschall in der Medizin*, 39, 154–180.

Sirsi, S.R., Hernandez, S.L., Zielinski, L., Blomback, H., Koubaa, A., Synder, M., Homma, S., Kandel, J.J., Yamashiro, D.J., Borden, M.A. (2012). Polyplex-microbubble hybrids for ultrasound-guided plasmid DNA delivery to solid tumors. *Journal of Controlled Release*, 157, 224–234.

van Sloun, R.J.G., Demi, L., Postema, A.W., de la Rosette, J.J. Wijkstra, H., Mischi, M. (2017a). Entropy of ultrasound-contrast-agent velocity fields for angiogenesis imaging in prostate cancer. *IEEE Transactions on Medical Imaging*, 36(3), 826–837.

van Sloun, R.J.G., Demi, L., Postema, A.W., de la Rosette, J.J., Wijkstra, H., Mischi, M. (2017b). Ultrasound-contrast-agent dispersion and velocity imaging for prostate cancer localization. *Medical Image Analysis*, 35, 610–619.

van Sloun, R.J.G., Demi, L., Schalk, S.G., Caresio, C., Mannaerts, C., Postema, A.W., Molinari, F., van der Linden, H.C., Huang, P., Wijkstra, H. et al. (2018). Contrast-enhanced ultrasound tractography for 3D vascular imaging of the prostate. *Scientific Reports*, 8, 14640.

Smeenge, M., Tranquart, F., Mannaerts, C.K., de Reijke, T.M., van de Vijver, M.J., Laguna, M.P., Pochon, S., de la Rosette, J.J.M.C.H., Wijkstra, H. (2017). First-in-human ultrasound molecular imaging with a VEGFR2-specific ultrasound molecular contrast agent (BR55) in prostate cancer. *Investigative Radiology*, 52(7), 419–427.

Solomon, O., van Sloun, R.J.G., Wijkstra, H., Mischi, M., Eldar, Y.C. (2018). Exploiting flow dynamics for super-resolution in contrast-enhanced ultrasound. arXiv:1804.03134.

Stewart, G.N. (1921). Researches on the circulation time and on the influences which affect it V: The circulation time of the spleen, kidney, intestine, heart (coronary circulation) and retina, with some further observations on the time of the lesser circulation. *American Journal of Physiology-Legacy Content*, 58, 278–295.

Tang, M.-X., Mulvana, H., Gauthier, T., Lim, A.K.P., Cosgrove, D.O., Eckersley, R.J., Stride, E. (2011). Quantitative contrast-enhanced ultrasound imaging: A review of sources of variability. *Interface Focus*, 1, 520–539.

Taylor, G. (1953). Dispersion of soluble matter in solvent flowing slowly through a tube. *Proceedings of the Royal Society of London. Series A. Mathematical and Physical Sciences*, 219, 186–203.

Tigerstedt, R. (1921). *Die Physiologie Des Kreislaufes.* Vereinigung Wissensachaftlicher Verleger Walter de Gruyter, Berlin.

Turco, S., Wijkstra, H., Mischi, M. (2016). Mathematical models of contrast-agent transport kinetics for imaging of cancer angiogenesis: A review. *IEEE Reviews in Biomedical Engineering*, 9, 121–147.

Turco, S., Tardy, I., Frinking, P., Wijkstra, H., Mischi, M. (2017). Quantitative ultrasound molecular imaging by modeling the binding kinetics of targeted contrast agent. *Physics in Medicine and Biology*, 62(6), 2449.

Turco, S., El Kaffas, A., Zhou, J., Lutz, A.M., Wijkstra, H., Willmann, J.K., Mischi, M. (2018). Pharmacokinetic modeling of targeted ultrasound contrast agents for quantitative assessment of anti-angiogenic therapy: A longitudinal case-control study in colon cancer. *Molecular Imaging and Biology*, 21(4), 633–643.

Turco, S., Frinking, P., Wildeboer, R., Arditi, M., Wijkstra, H., Lindner, J.R., Mischi, M. (2020). Contrast-enhanced ultrasound quantification: From kinetic modeling to machine learning. *Ultrasound in Medicine and Biology*, 46(3), 518–543.

Vilana, R., Forner, A., Bianchi, L., Garcìa-Criado, Á., Rimola, J., de Lope, C.R., Reig, M., Ayuso, C., Brú, C., Bruix, J. (2010). Intrahepatic peripheral cholangiocarcinoma in cirrhosis patients may display a vascular pattern similar to hepatocellular carcinoma on contrast-enhanced ultrasound. *Hepatology*, 51(6), 2020–2029.

Villemain, O., Baranger, J., Friedberg, M.K., Papadacci, C., Dizeux, A., Messas, E., Tanter, M., Pernot, M., Mertens, L. (2020). Ultrafast ultrasound imaging in pediatric and adult cardiology: Techniques, applications, and perspectives. *JACC: Cardiovascular Imaging*, 13, 1771–1791.

Viti, J., Vos, H.J., Jong, N.D., Guidi, F., Tortoli, P. (2016). Detection of contrast agents: Plane wave versus focused transmission. *IEEE Transactions on Ultrasonics, Ferroelectrics, and Frequency Control*, 63, 203–211.

Wang, Y., Wang, D., Geng, N., Wang, Y., Yin, Y., Jin, Y. (2019). Stacking-based ensemble learning of decision trees for interpretable prostate cancer detection. *Applied Soft Computing*, 77, 188–204.

Wei, K., Jayaweera, A.R., Firoozan, S., Linka, A., Skyba, D.M., Kaul, S. (1998). Quantification of myocardial blood flow with ultrasound-induced destruction of microbubbles administered as a constant venous infusion. *Circulation*, 97, 473–483.

Wiencek, J.G., Feinstein, S.B., Walker, R., Aronson, S. (1993). Pitfalls in quantitative contrast echocardiography: The steps to quantitation of perfusion. *Journal of the American Society of Echocardiography*, 6, 395–416.

Wildeboer, R.R., van Sloun, R.J.G., Schalk, S.G., Mannaerts, C.K., van der Linden, J.C., Huang, P., Wijkstra, H., Mischi, M. (2018a). Convective-dispersion modeling in 3D contrast-ultrasound imaging for the localization of prostate cancer. *IEEE Transactions on Medical Imaging*, 37, 2593–2602.

Wildeboer, R.R., van Sloun, R.J.G., Mannaerts, C.K., van der Linden, J.C., Huang, P., Wijkstra, H., Mischi, M. (2018b). Probabilistic 3D contrast-ultrasound tractography based on a convective-dispersion finite-element scheme. *IEEE International Ultrasonics Symposium (IUS)*, October.

Wildeboer, R.R., van Sloun, R.J.G., Huang, P., Wijkstra, H., Mischi, M. (2019). 3-D multi-parametric contrast-enhanced ultrasound for the prediction of prostate cancer. *Ultrasound in Medicine & Biology*, 45, 2713–2724.

Wildeboer, R.R., Sammali, F., van Sloun, R.J.G., Huang, Y., Chen, P., Bruce, M., Rabotti, C., Shulepov, S., Salomon, G., Schoot, B.C. et al. (2020). Blind source separation for clutter and noise suppression in ultrasound imaging: Review for different applications. *IEEE Transactions on Ultrasonics, Ferroelectrics, and Frequency Control*, 67, 1497–1512.

Williams, R., Hudson, J.M., Lloyd, B.A., Sureshkumar, A.R., Lueck, G., Milot, L., Atri, M., Bjarnason, G.A., Burns, P.N. (2011). Dynamic microbubble contrast-enhanced US to measure tumor response to targeted therapy: A proposed clinical protocol with results from renal cell carcinoma patients receiving antiangiogenic therapy. *Radiology*, 260, 581–590.

Willmann, J.K., Bonomo, L., Carla Testa, A., Rinaldi, P., Rindi, G., Valluru, K.S., Petrone, G., Martini, M., Lutz, A.M., Gambhir, S.S. (2017). Ultrasound molecular imaging with BR55 in patients with breast and ovarian lesions: First-in-human results. *Journal of Clinical Oncology: Official Journal of the American Society of Clinical Oncology*, 35, 2133–2140.

Wu, K., Chen, X., Ding, M. (2014). Deep learning based classification of focal liver lesions with contrast-enhanced ultrasound. *Optik*, 125, 4057–4063.

Zhang, Q., Li, C., Han, H., Yang, L., Wang, Y., Wang, W. (2014). Computer-aided quantification of contrast agent spatial distribution within atherosclerotic plaque in contrast-enhanced ultrasound image sequences. *Biomedical Signal Processing and Control*, 13, 50–61.

Zhang, Q., Li, C., Han, H., Dai, W., Shi, J., Wang, Y., Wang, W. (2015). Spatio-temporal quantification of carotid plaque neovascularization on contrast enhanced ultrasound: Correlation with visual grading and histopathology. *European Journal of Vascular and Endovascular Surgery*, 50, 289–296.

Zhang, S., Du, H., Jin, Z., Zhu, Y., Zhang, Y., Xie, F., Zhang, M., Tian, X., Zhang, J., Luo, Y. (2020). A novel interpretable computer-aided diagnosis system of thyroid nodules on ultrasound based on clinical experience. *IEEE Access*, 8, 53223–53231.

Zhou, T., Cai, W., Yang, H., Zhang, H., Hao, M., Yuan, L., Liu, J., Zhang, L., Yang, Y., Liu, X. (2018). Annexin V conjugated nanobubbles: A novel ultrasound contrast agent for in vivo assessment of the apoptotic response in cancer therapy. *Journal of Controlled Release*, 276, 113–124.

7

Resolution Limits and Super-Resolution Imaging

Vincent HINGOT[1,2] and Olivier COUTURE[1]

[1] *CNRS, INSERM, Laboratoire d'Imagerie Biomédicale (LIB), Sorbonne Université, Paris, France*

[2] *ResolveStroke SAS, Paris, France*

7.1. Introduction

7.1.1. *Scales in biology and medicine*

We explore the surrounding world, from the microscopic to the astronomic scale, using a plethora of waves. Visible light allows us to describe cells in thin slices (Hooke 1665), but also deep space (Galilei 1610). The rest of the electromagnetic wave spectra help us communicate, sculpt fine electronic devices and explore the human body through the absorption of X-rays or the resonance of protons. Meanwhile, gravitational waves are providing new insight to astronomers. Mechanical waves, such as ultrasonic compression waves, are just another probe in our hands to understand the world, the body or diseases.

Each application leads to a specific choice of the wave type and wavelength imposed by trade-offs. It is just as unimaginable to explore a rotating neutron star with ultrasound as it would be to diagnose cancer with gravitational waves. More down to earth, the lack of transparency of the living human body has made in-depth

For a color version of all the figures in this chapter, see www.iste.co.uk/bridal/innovative.zip.

Innovative Ultrasound Imaging Techniques,
coordinated by S. Lori BRIDAL. © ISTE Ltd 2024.

optical observation particularly challenging, leading to the development of medical imaging modalities such as MRI, X-ray, PET and ultrasound.

These modalities are exploited differentially in the clinical context due to their various advantages and drawbacks. Selection criteria for the best imaging approach for any given application may include contrast, sensitivity to functional processes, cost, availability, penetration, user dependency, frame rate, etc. One of the main characteristics of comparison between imaging modality is their resolution. Resolution is the capacity to distinguish adjacent objects, which can be organelles, cells, tissues, vessels or organs depending on the scale of the observation. In wave-based imaging modalities, this resolution is linked to the probe and also to the properties of the exploited wave, in particular its wavelength. It is important to note here that resolution is not the capacity to localize a single isolated object, nor the apparent size of this object that can be modified through post-treatment. Indeed, resolution is a physical property that depends on the interference of the different waves originating from the adjacent objects.

Introduced originally in microscopy, but applicable to ultrasound, the Airy or Rayleigh criteria give a minimum distance between two objects necessary for them to be separable on the image. The Rayleigh criterion states that the limit of diffraction is attained when the first diffraction minimum of an object coincides with the maximum of the other (see Figure 7.1). Hence, the resolution of a wave-based imaging method is determined, in good part, by its wavelength λ or, as it more often stated in ultrasound, as the inverse of f, the ultrasonic frequency. The two are related by the speed of sound c, close to 1,500 m/s in most tissues as:

$$\lambda = \frac{c}{f} \tag{7.1}$$

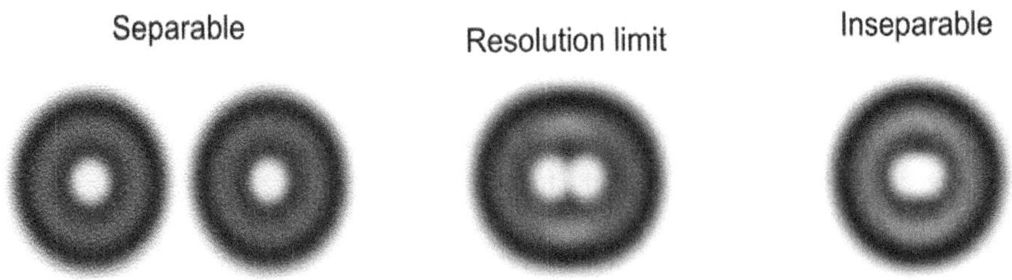

Figure 7.1. *Interference between two wave sources leads to the minimal distance at which they become indistinguishable from each other*

7.1.2. Resolution depends on wavelength and geometry

Ultrasound imaging is performed by arrays of finite transducers, which leads to diffraction processes that depend both on the ultrasound wavelength and on the geometry of the emitters and receivers. Diffraction can be seen as a low-pass filter. Due to interferences at the scale of the wavelength, fluctuations in the wave field at a smaller scale fade through propagation. For example, a collection of sources that are a tenth of the wavelength apart will be seen as a single emitter at a distance $d >> \lambda$. In the near field, resolution is not limited by the wavelength. Indeed, the high-frequency spatial fluctuations induced by the presence of small sources are retained and can be used to explore objects with a subwavelength resolution. In such cases, resolution is limited rather by the distance between the object and the probe (Fink and Tanter 2010). The far field of a piston transducer, for example, can be roughly defined as beyond (Foote 2014) the distance s, as defined in equation [7.2], where a is the radius of the piston and λ is the wavelength:

$$s = \frac{a^2}{\lambda} \quad [7.2]$$

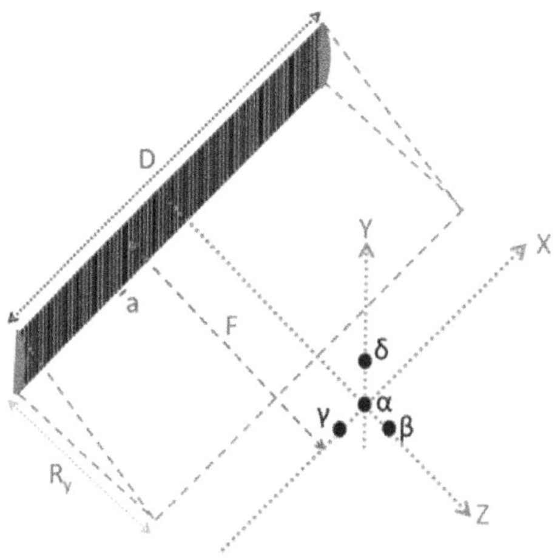

Figure 7.2. *Typical geometry of a linear array for performing 2D ultrasound scanning*

The typical geometry of a linear array used for ultrasound imaging is shown in Figure 7.2. An ultrasound array for imaging in 2D is formed by tens to hundreds of transducer elements with an inter-element distance (pitch) close to or smaller than the acoustic wavelength and a height which can be on the order of several wavelengths. **D** is the total width of the array. Focusing an ultrasonic pulse at a distance **F** is performed by optimizing electronic delays to ensure positive interference of the arrival of a pulse of duration n**T** at the focal point, where n is the number of periods in the pulse and T is the duration of a single period. The coordinates **(X, Z, Y)** describe the lateral, axial and elevation directions, respectively. Most probes are linear arrays with a fixed, physical focus in the elevation direction to a fixed distance **Ry**.

The resolution problem in ultrasound imaging refers to the determination of our ability to distinguish two points following the Rayleigh criterion. However, because ultrasound transducers do not encircle these points completely, the attainable resolution is not isotropic, i.e. axial and lateral resolutions differ. Moreover, we will see that the focusing capacity depends on the focal length with respect to the aperture size and, consequently, the resolution will also depend on the position of the points.

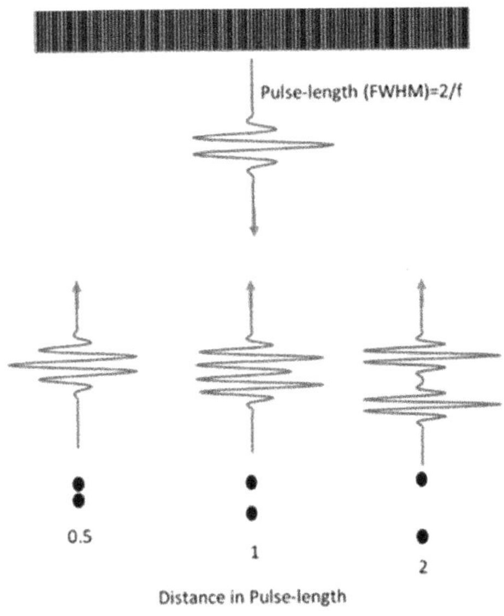

Figure 7.3. *Representation of the axial resolution problem whereby the length of the pulses determines the separability of two points at different depths. In this case, a Gaussian pulse with an FWHM of n = 2 periods is presented*

The axial resolution, which corresponds to the minimal separation distance necessary to distinguish points **α** (at z_1) and **β** (at z_2) in Figure 7.2, can be approximated in a straightforward manner. Indeed, the echoes from point beta must arrive after the end of the echo from point alpha, which is also determined by the duration of the pulse, **nT**. This is represented by equation [7.3] and Figure 7.3:

$$\frac{2z_2}{c_0} - \frac{2z_1}{c_0} > nT \; or \; \Delta z = z_2 - z_1 > n\frac{c_0 T}{2} \qquad [7.3]$$

Hence, the axial resolution is approximated to Δz. With the pulse duration being inversely proportional to the bandwidth, the axial resolution is optimized through physical improvements of the transducer itself. Modern transducers can generate ultrasound with bandwidths approximately 100%, which allows short pulses and consequently an axial resolution close to a few wavelengths. Typically, the length is comprised between n = 0.5 and n = 10 wavelengths.

In the lateral direction, the resolution is determined by the minimal distance between points **α** and **γ** that allows them to be distinguished (see Figure 7.2). To solve this case, it is appropriate to use the concept of the point-spread function, which is the response of the system to a point source. The general case is based on the decomposition of any aperture into infinitesimal small slits. The formalism of Fourier transforms simplifies the operation. The operation of diffraction through any aperture can be expressed as a convolution with the Fourier transform of the aperture. For imaging systems, this function is the spatial impulse response of the aperture, which is equal to the image of a punctual source through the aperture (Bamber and Dickinson 1980):

$$Im = Obj \otimes PSF \qquad [7.4]$$

This point spread function (PSF) can be understood as a spatial low-pass filter that therefore limits the resolution. The axial dimension of the PSF is directly proportional to the pulse duration and is a direct consequence of the principle illustrated in Figure 7.3. In the lateral and elevation directions, the width of the PSF, and therefore the resolution, depends on the ability to focus the ultrasound beam. In the lateral direction, a classical approach is to calculate the pressure field at a given depth **z**. For a linear array under typical conditions, the pressure field can be described with a sinc function (see equation [7.5]). The first zero-crossing occurs at a lateral position, Rx, that depends on the wavelength and the focusing parameter, f_{number}, that is usually between 0.5 and 2:

$$p(x) \sim sinc\left(\frac{\pi x D}{\lambda z}\right) \; where \; R_x = \frac{\lambda z}{D} = \lambda f_{number} \qquad [7.5]$$

In the elevation direction, linear arrays for 2D imaging are generally equipped with a focusing lens, for which the radius of curvature is fixed. Consequently, the question of the separability of points alpha and delta in Figure 7.2 becomes that of the PSF of a cylindrically focused beam (1). We can add a fourth dimension to the resolution problem by considering the frame rate. Regardless of the acquisition mode, conventional focused waves or plane-wave ultrafast imaging, for example, a key factor determining the frame rate is the time of flight to the deepest region from which returned echoes are detectable (and thus could interfere with echoes from the next pulse) (Tanter and Fink 2014). At 1,500 m/s, the ultrasound wave takes 133 microseconds to travel to a scatterer 10 cm away and back. Consequently, at this depth, a maximum of 7,500 pulse echoes can be performed per second. Although a single plane-wave acquisition over all transducer elements can yield data describing a full image plane within such a time, image quality is obtained either through the compounding of several plane waves or by focused imaging. If a hundred pulses are required to generate each image, then a frame rate of 75 Hz (7,500 pulse echoes divided by 100) will be attainable. This will effectively limit the time resolution for imaging to this depth more strongly than the simple pulse-echo time of flight. Time resolution can be increased if the number of pulse-echo sequences required to create each image can be reduced.

7.1.3. *The resolution penetration trade-off*

Due to the spatial resolution considerations described in section 7.1.2, the scale that can be observed with ultrasound is roughly defined by its wavelength. In water, a 1 GHz ultrasonic wave could theoretically distinguish structures as small as 1.5 microns, which is on the cellular scale. Acoustic microscopes exploit these very high frequencies to observe tissue at the microscopic scale (Briggs 1992). However, this resolution can only be attained for samples with a very limited thickness, like the thin tissue slices used in optical microscopy. Resolution improves with a shortened wavelength, but it is accompanied by an increase in attenuation because the attenuation, expressed in dB/cm, increases linearly or, in some cases, quadratically as a function of the frequency (Bamber 2004).

In the liver, the attenuation can be approximated to be 0.5 dB/cm around 1 MHz, with an $f^{1.2}$ dependency within the range of frequencies used to scan the liver in a clinical setting (Mast 2000; Cobbold 2006). For a 15 cm imaging depth at 3 MHz, this would lead to a 56 dB loss due to attenuation both ways, which is on the order of the dynamic range available with a clinical ultrasound scanner. However, the 880 dB attenuation loss that would be expected for the same 15 cm depth at 30 MHz would make imaging over the entire depth of the organ unattainable. Consequently, there is a general trade-off between accessible resolution and penetration (see Figure 7.4).

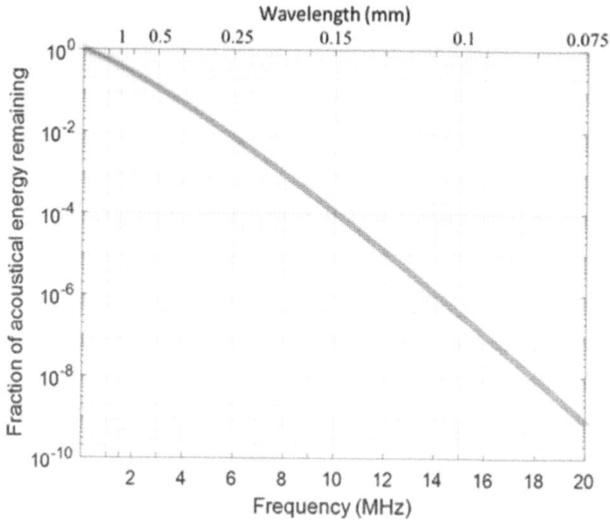

Figure 7.4. *There is a tradeoff between the resolution and penetration that can be obtained with ultrasound. For example, the attenuation in the liver depends on the depth and the frequency with an approximate value of 0.5 dB/cm/MHz. As the frequency increases, the wavelength is shorter and able to provide better spatial resolution. However, the fraction of acoustical energy remaining in the beam after 10 cm of propagation through the liver (as shown on the y-axis) is much lower at short wavelengths*

Cardiac, liver or transcranial Doppler are performed at lower frequencies (2–4 MHz), yielding a maximum resolution of approximately 500 microns to image the entire depth of the organ. On the contrary, superficial imaging of the thyroid, for example, can be performed at 8 MHz with a resolution closer to 200 microns. Because each transducer has a natural resonance, this trade-off also determines the ultrasonic probe used for each application.

In general, with respect to other imaging modalities, ultrasound displays a high spatial resolution (a few hundred microns) and time resolution (tens of images per second and up to thousands of images per second for ultrafast imaging).

7.1.4. *Surpassing the resolution penetration trade-off*

Because attenuation and resolution are both linked to the wavelength, the two processes appear inseparable, leading to an insurmountable trade-off between resolution and penetration. However, many approaches have been proposed to circumvent this limit. The most obvious approach to improve resolution is to increase the frequency, simply sacrificing penetration. Imaging at frequencies higher than 15 MHz has allowed great progress for small animal imaging, especially for longitudinal studies, and high frequencies are now being exploited for specific applications in humans (Foster et al. 1993, 2011; Lockwood et al. 1996). However, due to the penetration–resolution trade-off, these highly resolved images are limited to depths that do not extend beyond a few millimeters.

Tissue harmonic imaging also uses higher frequencies induced by nonlinear propagation to improve the resolution. Since the emitted frequencies are lower than those ultimately returned from scattering structures, part of the ultrasound propagation occurs under relatively low attenuation conditions (Tranquart et al. 1999). Another technique called ultrasound angiography bypasses some of the penetration issues by detecting the super-harmonics generated by injected microbubbles (Gessner et al. 2013). For example, microbubbles can be insonified at 3 MHz and their scattering observed with another probe at 15 MHz (Bouakaz et al. 2002). Contrary to tissue, microbubbles are highly nonlinear and can generate fifth-order harmonics. Not only does this technique provide high contrast between contrast agents and tissue, but it also benefits from the fact that the high-frequency waves must only propagate on their way back from the microbubbles so the high-frequency attenuation only increases signal loss along the return path.

True super-resolution imaging, however, can be defined as an imaging method that surpasses the classical diffraction limit in resolving power, generally for distinguishing two objects. The field of super-resolution ultrasound imaging has been discussed for several decades (Ikeda et al. 1979; Jones 1992). Such a feat was achieved for a limited number of sources by Prada and Thomas (2003) through the decomposition of the time-reversal operator. A priori information about the target source can also be exploited to enhance resolution, such as in the wire-imaging method proposed by Clement et al. (2005).

Most concepts introduced in this chapter concern the far field that lies several wavelengths away from the probe. In the near field, the diffraction limit does not apply, and the limiting distance becomes that between the object and the instrument. Near-field acoustic microscopy can achieve resolutions that are orders of magnitude better than the wavelength. These apparatuses are closer in principle to atomic force microscopy than they are to ultrasound scanners. Metamaterials such as phononic crystals can also be exploited to achieve near-field super-resolution (Page et al. 2016).

However, since medical imaging is performed at depths that are generally many wavelengths away from the transducer, we will restrict our further description to far-field super-resolution. Moreover, since medical imaging collects the signal originating from a combination of sources in each pixel, it is difficult to exploit super-resolution approaches that are designed for a limited number of known sources unless the distribution of sources can be carefully controlled, as in ultrasound localization microscopy (ULM). ULM (Couture et al. 2018; Christensen-Jeffries et al. 2020) was introduced in 2010 (Couture et al. patent 2010; IUS 2011) and then improved by several groups (Desailly et al. 2013; Viessmann et al. 2013; Christensen-Jeffries et al. 2014). The principles of this method will be covered thoroughly in this chapter.

In addition to ULM, several other approaches have also been proposed to attain super-resolution ultrasound, such as the acoustical version of super-resolution optical fluctuation imaging (SOFI) and structured insonification. SOFI (Dertinger et al. 2009) is a post-processing method that reduces the width of the PSF by collecting many realizations of decorrelating optical sources. It requires the injection of a contrast agent, but does not require long acquisition times. It is based on the temporal correlations of independently fluctuating sources. It relies on the calculation of cumulants or correlations over time. For the autocorrelation, the width of the PSF is reduced by a factor $\sqrt{2}$, thus improving the resolution of the image by this factor. This approach has been implemented using ultrafast ultrasound imaging. After clutter filtering, a series of beamformed data exhibit only moving features of the signal which correspond to flowing red blood cells. In fact, ultrasound power Doppler expresses autocorrelation and images image fluctuations without exogenous contrast agents. The high-order fluctuations of pixel intensity in time can be exploited to reduce the point-spread function in vascular imaging. Inspired by SOFI in optical microscopy, SUSHI can improve the resolution by a factor limited by noise fluctuations (Bar-Zion et al. 2018). Nevertheless, it can be exploited with high concentrations of contrast agents since it avoids localization limitations.

Another technique to achieve super-resolution in ultrasound is called structure insonification microscopy (Iovitsch et al. 2018). This approach was inspired by structured illumination microscopy (SIM) techniques (Gustafsson 2000). Upon crossing any aperture, diffraction acts as a low-pass filter that removes high-frequency content and limits resolution. The principle of SIM methods is to shape the emission patterns so that the frequency content is shifted in the Fourier space and higher frequency components will get through the diffraction window. For example, if the emission is a plane wave modulated by a sinus function in the lateral direction, the frequency spectrum will be shifted. After being diffracted by the aperture, high-frequency components are downshifted and can now be observed within the diffraction window. A reconstruction algorithm then reorganizes the original frequency content to form an image with a narrower PSF (see Figure 7.5).

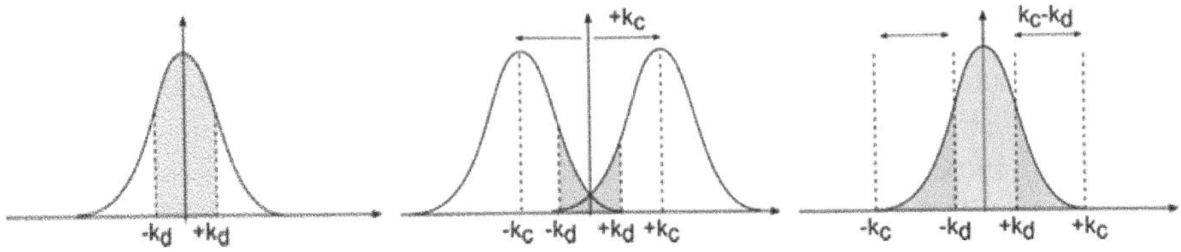

Figure 7.5. *Principle of structured insonification. The frequency components higher than kd are lost due to the low-pass filter (left). After modulation of the emitted amplitude, the pulse is shifted by kc (shifted within the diffraction window through grated insonification) and the higher frequencies fall within the observable range (middle). A reconstruction step recombines high and low frequencies (right)*

7.1.5. *Super-resolution with single-molecule localization microscopy*

The marvels of current medicine are deeply indebted to optical microscopy. For example, microscopic observation of histological slices remains one of the dominant diagnostic tools of medicine. As in ultrasound imaging, optical microscopy is also limited in resolution by its wavelength. The wavelengths used in optical microscopy are in the range of hundreds of nanometers. The resolution limit in microscopy is generally described as the Abbe diffraction limit:

$$Res = \frac{\lambda}{2NA} \qquad [7.6]$$

where *Res* is the resolution (the smallest resolvable distance between two objects), *NA* is a general term for the microscope numerical aperture (often approximately 1.5) and λ is the imaging wavelength. Until recently, Abbe's limit only allowed the resolution of larger organelles under the optical microscopy. Higher resolution could be obtained using shorter wavelengths with higher energy photons or electrons that fall outside the visible range. However, molecular biology is still heavily reliant on visible light microscopy. For example, many fluorescent reporter molecules and genes used to describe cellular mechanisms are emitting in the visible spectrum, even though the size of the marked molecules is often more than a hundred times smaller than the detected optical wavelengths.

Multiple techniques were proposed to move beyond the diffraction limit in optical microscopy. Near-field, structured illumination, nonlinear response of fluorescent labels and metamaterials have all permitted microscopy to achieve resolution beyond the wavelength.

One revolutionary early achievement was the observation of the fluorescence of a single molecule (Moerner and Kador 1989; Betzig and Chichester 1993). An individual molecule with a nanometer in size, emitting light with a hundred-nanometer wavelength, could be observed, linking scales on several orders of magnitude. Interestingly, the localization of the center of an isolated source is not limited by diffraction since the resolving power is limited only by the interference between sources. Rather, the localization precision is limited by the signal-to-noise ratio of the source as described by Betzig.

Although individual sources can be localized with a boundless precision, interaction of light with biological samples results in a collection of wave sources that interfere with one another. This interference occurs on the scale of the wavelength, which mixes the contribution of each source, making them indistinguishable. However, sources that are not present in the same image cannot interfere with each other. Thus, by separating emission events through multiple acquisition, it is possible to isolate and localize sources separately.

Single-molecule localization microscopy (SMLM) techniques such as PALM, STOM or FPALM rely on this approach (Hell and Wichmann 1994; Hess et al. 2006; Betzig et al. 2006). In SMLM, fluorescent labels can switch between a bright and a dark state. In each image, only a subset of them can be observed due to the switching mechanism. Waves from the limited number of sources do not interfere, and the individual emissions resemble that of individual and separated point-spread functions. By deconvolving the obtained images of sparse sources from this PSF, it becomes possible to determine the center point of each fluorescent label with a subwavelength resolution.

After a collection of different localization positions of fluorescent labels obtained from thousands of acquisitions, these detected points can be accumulated onto a single image to create a super-resolved image that can have a resolution of a few nanometers. An example is shown in Figure 7.6 with the conventional, diffraction-limited image on the left, and the progressive accumulation of subwavelength localization to reconstruct a super-resolution image.

Betzig et al. (2006) stated that the error in positioning these sources is inversely correlated with the square root of the number of detected photons. For 10,000 photons per fluorescent label, a number close to typical observations with SMLM, a 100-fold improvement in precision with respect to the wavelength is attainable.

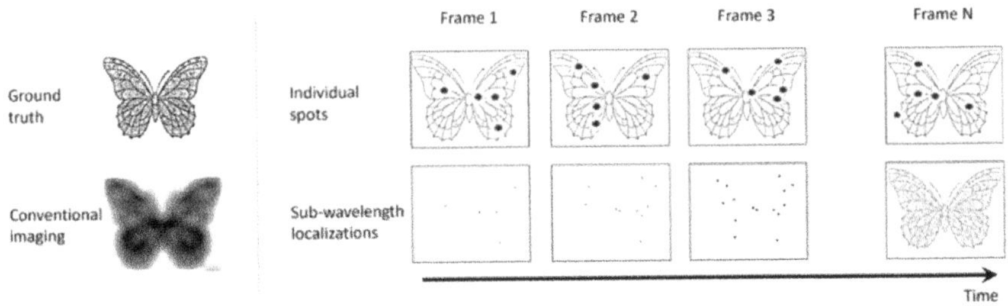

Figure 7.6. *Principles of SMLM techniques. Figure reproduced with permission from Hingot (2019)*

7.2. Ultrasound localization microscopy

7.2.1. *Microbubbles as contrast sources for localization microscopy*

In SMLM, fluorescent labels are used to link two scales: the nanometric one of the molecules that attach to the cellular structure and the submicron one of the wavelengths they emit. This is essential to super-resolution imaging since the precise localization of a collection of sources must be used to reconstruct a meaningful subwavelength structure.

In ultrasound imaging, we readily have access to a label that connects two different scales through its size and wavelength emission. Since the discovery by Gramiak and Shah (1968), it has been known that microbubbles are small enough to circulate within capillaries and that they can be detected with ultrasound imaging in the MHz frequency range. These micrometric agents remain in the blood flow and increase its contrast due to several effects. First, contrast is induced by the difference in acoustical impedance between the gaseous microbubble and the surrounding blood (Leighton 2012). Due to their compressibility and surrounding liquid mass, microbubbles are also resonant at certain frequencies that fortunately fall within the frequency range of ultrasound imaging. Moreover, microbubbles oscillate nonlinearly, and this nonlinear response can be specifically detected either by detecting the generated harmonics or by using contrast-specific imaging sequences (pulse inversion, amplitude modulation, see Figure 7.7). Finally, microbubbles can be disrupted by the ultrasound pulses themselves, allowing a measurement of reperfusion time.

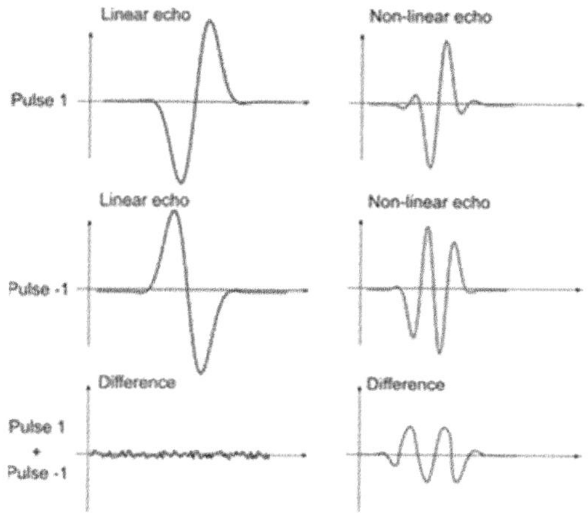

Figure 7.7. *Nonlinear sequences for the detection of microbubbles*

Due to these contrast mechanisms, a single microbubble, smaller than a red blood cell, can be detected at several centimeters in depth. This makes ultrasound one of the most sensitive imaging techniques for the detection of its contrast agent (Klibanov et al. 2002). Even though the microbubbles are smaller than capillaries, they appear on the ultrasound images as the point-spread function of the system itself, which can be several wavelengths wide.

From a wave physics point of view, ultrasound and optic share many similarities. Yet, when considering the translation of localization microscopy from optics to ultrasound, a major difference that has important implications for the imaging techniques is the source of contrast. In SMLM, fluorophores are molecules that bind to proteins. This has the great advantage to offer flexible imaging options and the ability to target different structures. This flexible marking comes with the disadvantage that the fluorophore is fixed to the target. Activating the light from only a fraction of the fluorophores to make them blink on and off while maintaining good spatial sampling has been the main difficulty to overcome with SMLM.

Ultrasound contrast agents are substantially different from bound fluorophores and come with a different set of challenges. Ultrasound contrast agents are micron-sized gas bubbles in water, stabilized with a lipid shell. Their size is comparable to that of red blood cells, which are among the smallest of human cells. Due to their size, they are not able to cross the endothelial membrane of vessels. Therefore, they are mainly used as a vascular contrast agent. This has two major consequences on the resulting imaging. Since they are intravascular, microbubbles are washed out of the imaging plane rapidly. This eliminates the need to make them blink. Unfortunately, this also implies that they struggle to tag other structures than those inside of blood vessels. ULM has also been described with nanoparticles that could potentially populate other tissues (Zhang et al. 2018; Riemer et al. 2022), but their clinical application remains a challenge. Nanobubbles are also being developed without a current aim to develop them towards super-resolution imaging applications (Wang et al. 2010).

As conventional microbubbles are gaseous, there is a large impedance mismatch at the water–gas interface, causing a large scattered signal from any impinging ultrasound wave. Furthermore, microbubbles also resonate at frequencies in the range of clinical insonification. A single microbubble has a relatively sharp resonance peak, determined by its size and shell properties. However, commercial formulations for microbubbles are usually fairly polydisperse, ensuring that a good contrast can be maintained over the entire clinical range of ultrasonic frequencies.

Moreover, since the microbubble concentration must be kept low to ensure sparse microbubble distribution on the images, a new trade-off between spatial resolution and spatial sampling is imposed. In SMLM, this trade-off is driven by the blinking/bleaching pattern operated by the system, whereas in ULM, this trade-off is driven by microvascular flow refreshing microbubbles in and out of the imaging field. It will be described later in this chapter.

7.2.2. *The process of ultrasound localization microscopy*

The concept of ULM is based on SMLM but requires additional steps due to the specificity of ultrasound and microbubbles. We will describe these steps in further detail in the next sections, but in summary, super-resolution ultrasound images can be obtained by 1) acquiring many images of a tissue perfused with an optimized concentration of microbubbles, 2) separating signals from the microbubbles from those returned by tissue, 3) localizing the center of each of the detected microbubbles, 4) tracking their motion, 5) collecting tracks of sequential detections and finally, 6) visualizing the cumulative image.

In ultrasound imaging, the incident wave is backscattered by all tissues. Differentiating individual contrast sources from the overall received wave is not as straightforward as in SMLM, where the excited fluorescent frequencies are different from the other light sources in the image and can be filtered out specifically. Similar imaging paradigms exist for contrast-enhanced ultrasound, but they require the use of two ultrasound transducers that generally have a narrow bandwidth (Gessner et al. 2013). Other schemes have also been developed to separate microbubbles from the surrounding clutter noise.

The most widespread method to highlight the individual microbubble response relies on their nonlinear properties when insonified at high enough amplitudes near the resonance frequencies (Averkiou et al. 2020). Under these conditions, the microbubbles oscillate at higher order modes and generate harmonics. This will slightly deform the received echo originating from the microbubbles. While tissues do not exhibit this type of harmonic generation at low amplitude, a microbubble specific image can be reconstructed by summation of two pulses with opposite polarity. Tissue echoes will cancel out, while the microbubbles' nonlinear components will add.

These methods are particularly efficient close to the resonant frequency, which is typically around 3 MHz. Most contrast enhancement modes on clinical scanners were designed with this type of sequence and work best in this frequency range. However, for research purposes in small animals, the frequencies are usually beyond 10 MHz and fall outside the typical resonance of microbubbles (Deffieux et al. 2018). Other more efficient methods for these conditions have been developed.

For animal experiments, high-frequency probes are used to increase the frequency to observe smaller organs. They often have dense arrangements of elements with a small pitch. For example, the probe used by Errico et al. (2015) had a 15 MHz central frequency and a 100 μm pitch. Fine spatial sampling, coupled with good temporal sampling, offered by ultrafast ultrasound scanners, have made it possible to suppress clutter using temporal filtering.

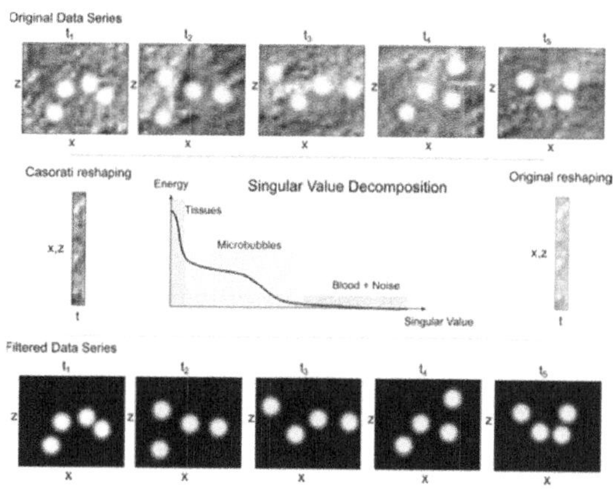

Figure 7.8. *Removing clutter with singular value decomposition (SVD) clutter filters*

These filters assume that any movement of tissues between sequential frames is very slow while microbubbles are moving fast compared to the acquisition frame rate. Therefore, microbubbles can be identified based on their temporal frequency content. Clutter suppression is no longer done on individual images, but on a temporal series of images comprising hundreds or thousands of consecutive frames (Demené et al. 2015) (see Figure 7.8).

Better filtering strategies can be developed by relying on the spatial coherence of objects, since echoes from tissues have very low spatial frequency compared to microbubble signals because microbubbles are smaller objects. The most frequently used of these spatio-temporal filters is based on a singular value decomposition (Demené et al. 2015; Desailly et al. 2017). A 3D matrix composed of a temporal series of frames (2D+t) is rearranged in a Casorati matrix with only one dimension for space and one dimension for time. Then, the decomposition is performed to express this matrix as a product of three submatrices corresponding to the temporal singular vectors, the spatial singular vectors and a diagonal matrix of their energies. When ordered by decreasing intensities, the order of the singular values corresponds to the structures present in the image. The highest singular values correspond to slow-moving and intense structures, like tissues, while the lowest singular values correspond to fast-moving components in blood and noise. In the middle, microbubbles have their own spatio-temporal coherence. A Casorati matrix is reformed after zeroing the singular values of tissue and noise before a filtered data series can be reconstructed without tissue and noise signals.

Although spatio-temporal filtering is very effective in high-frame-rate and high spatial sampling settings (high frequency and small pitch), it has several drawbacks. First, it tends to eliminate slow-flowing microbubbles. Since the clutter suppression is mostly based on motion, the components originating from slow microbubbles are hard to discriminate from the residual clutter. Moreover, this filtering is further degraded in the presence of motion (e.g. moving tissue), which tends to widen the range of singular values from the tissue and impact the efficiency of the filtering.

7.2.3. *Localization of individual and punctual sources*

After clutter filtering, microbubbles appear as bright spots emerging from the noise and residual clutter level. A standard procedure to detect and select individual objects is to search for the local maxima. Most search methods will detect many more local maxima than there are microbubbles, and an additional thresholding condition is often added.

The original idea in SMLM and ULM is to isolate and localize a single punctual source with a precision higher than the diffraction limit. This can be achieved by understanding the relation between the intensity repartition from an isolated source on beamformed images and its actual position (Couture et al. 2018). Theoretically, this is a resolution of an inverse problem, where the intensity repartition is a spatial sampling of the PSF, and the solution is the coordinate of the source. Unfortunately, this problem is often ill-posed due to insufficient spatial sampling, or a poor signal-to-noise ratio. Still, indirect methods have been used to approach the localization of the source without a direct deconvolution.

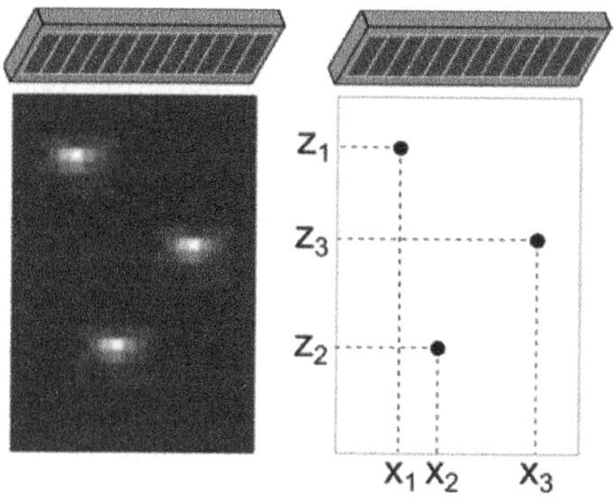

Figure 7.9. *Localization of individual scatterers on contrast-enhanced images*

The capacity of localization methods can depend on the beamforming method that was used, and in particular on the spatial grid size chosen to reconstruct the images. As the resolution is usually on the order of the imaging wavelength and pitch, images are most often beamformed on grids with pixel sizes in these ranges.

A straightforward method for source localization is to interpolate the original dataset so that it is resampled on a finer grid. The choice of the interpolation kernel is crucial and should aim to replicate the original shape of the PSF. Main candidates are Gaussian, Spline and Lanczos kernels. On this fine grid size, the position of the microbubble is simply the position of the maximum intensity. The precision of the measurement is determined by the choice of the grid size and the signal-to-noise ratio (Desailly et al. 2015). However, the accuracy of the measurement, which is the distance to the ground truth, depends primarily on the localization kernel (Heiles et al. 2022).

A more robust method for estimating the position of the maximum of intensity is to fit a function on the intensity repartition. A classical fit function is a simple Gaussian that should represent the shape of the PSF. This fit can be performed independently of the grid size, although the robustness of fit is usually better with well-sampled data.

Both interpolation and Gaussian fitting methods are relatively costly from a computing perspective, which adds up for data with a lot of microbubbles. For 3D ULM, the localization algorithms need to handle a third dimension, as well as a larger field of view containing a lot more sources. Therefore, lighter computing methods are needed, such as a weighted average, which simply computes the position as an average of the neighboring pixel positions, weighted by their respective intensities.

However, the weighted average method performs relatively poorly in low signal-to-noise conditions and tends to suffer from strong biases. A more robust algorithm has therefore been used, based on the radial symmetry of the PSF. It is still based on a direct calculation of the position from the intensity distribution, but exploits the symmetry of the PSF in all the radial directions.

A thorough comparison between these algorithms was performed on simulated and in vivo data and showed that the weighted average method was the fastest to compute, but lacked precision and sensitivity compared to the other algorithms (Heiles et al. 2022). While Gaussian fitting and interpolation methods have great sensitivity and precision, they are computationally heavy, and the conclusion of the study was that the radial symmetry-based algorithms had similar performance while being significantly faster.

7.2.4. *Inter-frame tracking of moving microbubbles*

As microbubbles flow through the blood circulation, an individual microbubble will move according to the local blood velocity. If the imaging frame rate is high enough to ensure that the inter-frame displacement of the microbubble remains small, this means that a single source can be followed and therefore be used to sample the velocity of the blood that carries it. Microbubbles act as small probes for the blood velocity field.

To follow the course of an individual source, the main method used initially was based on a frame-to-frame assignment (see Figure 7.10). This operation consists of finding the corresponding links in two sets of microbubble coordinates in two consecutive frames. The first step is usually performed by calculating the interdistance matrix between the two sets of points. Then, different algorithms have been used, either using a nearest neighbor approach or the Kuhn–Munkres algorithm for assignment, which minimizes the total sum of distances (Tinevez 2017; simpletracker, see: https://github.com/tinevez/simpletracker). Finally, a linking step connects all the assigned points together to form a track, which is a list of all the coordinates of an individual microbubble.

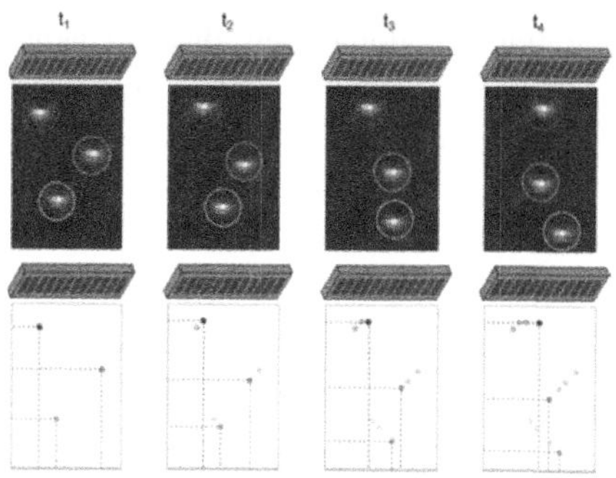

Figure 7.10. *Inter-frame tracking of individual moving microbubbles*

The Kuhn–Munkres algorithm for assignment is a simple method to track microbubbles, but does not exploit the whole richness of ULM data. Because microbubbles flow in blood vessels, their behavior tends to remain relatively linear and smooth. More advanced tracking methods have been implemented to exploit a priori information on microbubble behavior using Markov chains (Opacic et al. 2018) or bipartite graphs (Song et al. 2017). These methods are particularly useful for low frame rates or high microbubble concentrations, in order to compensate for a larger distance between two consecutive positions or for the crossing of multiple microbubble trajectories. However, specific tracks of microbubbles such as those in glomeruli do not correspond to the a priori of linearity and smoothness (Denis et al. 2023).

7.2.5. *Visualization of ultrasound localization microscopy data*

At this stage, the data are not images, but rather lists of coordinates of points corresponding to microbubble tracks. To become an image, they must undergo a few additional steps. Some analysis of the tracks can be applied to remove very short courses or very tortuous ones that are more susceptible to be artifacts. An additional resampling step can be added to populate the entire track on a chosen grid size so that every pixel of the final image will count one and only one microbubble detection.

The most common type of image reconstructed in ULM is a density map, counting the number of microbubbles detected in every subpixel. A common hypothesis is that microbubbles are evenly distributed in the bloodstream, and therefore the number of microbubbles should be related to the blood volume. This hypothesis has yet to be nuanced by the lack of sensitivity to the slowest flow that accounts for an important fraction of the total blood volume.

As microbubbles are tracked along their displacement in blood, each track contains instantaneous velocity information. Therefore, an image of the velocity can be represented by assigning to each pixel the average velocity of the microbubbles that passed through it. This representation is usually complemented with the up/down direction of the microbubble to mimic the color Doppler representation. In some organs, the arteriovenous organization is well described with this representation.

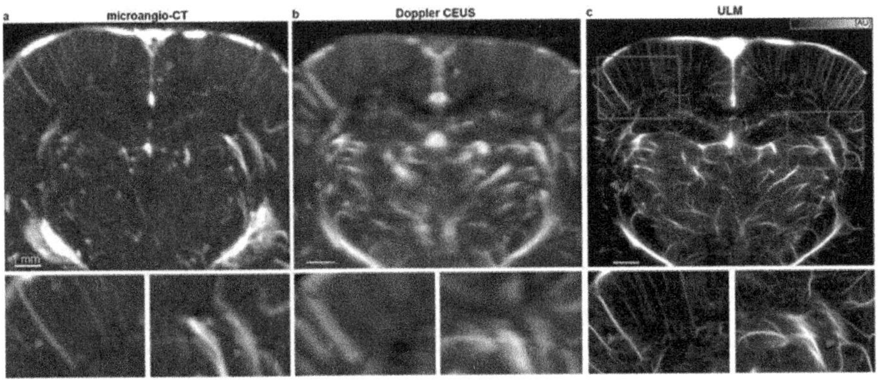

Figure 7.11. *Comparison of images from the same animal in vitro. CT enhanced with X-ray contrast agent on the left, ultrasensitive power Doppler in the middle and 2D ULM on the right. Reproduced in accordance with the policies for supplementary information published in Nature Biomedical Engineering from Heiles et al. (2022)*

7.2.6. *Comparison with micro-CT for ground truth*

The major limit of ULM today is the lack of validation of the imaging method compared to the ground truth. Indeed, no other imaging method offers a similar type of imaging at such depths. Optical methods are more resolved but cannot image a similar field of view or depth, while the quality of blood vessel detection in small animals with CT scanners and MRI of blood vessels remains limited. A basic comparison can be performed when the vascularization is superficial and under conditions where optical macroscopy and ultrasound can be coplanar. For example, the chorioallantoic membrane in an ex ovo model was used to measure ULM resolution and optimize its methodology (Huang et al. 2020; Lowerison et al. 2020; Tang et al. 2020). In humans, ULM images have been compared with contrast-enhanced CT angiography (Demené et al. 2021).

Post-mortem microscopy based on tissue clearing reconstructs beautiful images of whole organs in animals with very high resolution, but introduces strong deformations in tissues during the clearing step. To validate the results of ULM in the rat brain, the most convincing result obtained so far has been the comparison of images from the same animal obtained with 2D ULM and with ex vivo micro- and nano-CT, enhanced using X-ray contrast agent injection, as shown in Figure 7.11.

7.3. Topics in ultrasound localization microscopy

7.3.1. *Topics in ultrasound localization microscopy*

In the previous section, we exposed the basic principles behind image formation in ULM. In this section, we will discuss four different topics that present key technical challenges for ULM in the near future.

7.3.2. *Definition and measurement of the resolution*

In the imaging community, the term resolution can have different meanings. Intuition may suggest that resolution is the level of detail present in an image. Unfortunately, there are several definitions of the term that are not entirely satisfactory. Another misleading definition relates resolution to the size of the pixels of the final image. This can be highly biased because the number of pixels has more to do with the formation of the image than with the actual structures that have to be separated. Another definition is based on the ability to separate two close sources based on the width of the PSF. For conventional gray scale images, this definition accurately depicts the level of details revealed in an image, but does not apply to SMLM and ULM, where the width of the PSF is no longer correlated with the final image. Moreover, concepts such as sharpness and contrast resolution bring additional information on image "resolution", but are not included in any of the above-mentioned definitions.

For ULM, confusion regarding what is meant by resolution comes from a new trade-off that originates from the imaging method itself. In order to have punctual sources, only a few microbubbles should be present in every imaged frame. This amounts to a dilution of the sources in space. To reconstruct the object, many localized sources need to be accumulated over a long time. Instead of having all sources present in one frame, they are diluted in time. This new trade-off can be formalized using the Nyquist dimension, a typical length that describes the adequate spatial sampling of the final image. The resolution (R_{ULM}) of a ULM image can be thought of as the quadratic sum of the localization error δ_loc and the Nyquist dimension δ_Nyq (equation [7.7]), where the Nyquist dimension is a characteristic length depicting microbubble density ρ adjusted with respect to the dimension of the image κ to be adimensional (Hingot et al. 2021):

$$\delta_{Nyq} = \frac{2}{\rho^{\kappa}} \; and \; R_{ULM} = \sqrt{\delta_{loc}^2 + \delta_{Nyq}^2} \qquad [7.7]$$

From this equation, it can be understood that, when correctly sampled, ULM resolution saturates to a localization precision determined by the acquisition system and its signal-to-noise ratio (Desailly et al. 2015). It also shows that higher resolution can only be obtained by accumulating more samples, and therefore requires a longer acquisition time (Viessman et al. 2013; Christensen-Jeffries et al. 2019; Hingot et al. 2019, 2021; Huang et al. 2020). The link between the acquisition time and the number of detected samples depends mainly on the intravascular microbubble contrast agents and the speed at which new microbubbles are brought to the smallest vessels. This is directly linked to the physiology of the microcirculation.

These considerations are merely theoretical and pose two main questions. The first one is a methodological question. How can we define and measure the resolution in settings adapted to ULM? The second one is a more practical question. Given a set of imaging conditions, how do we choose the final grid size that is most appropriate for data representation in ULM?

A wide set of methods have been proposed to answer these questions. Some are based on direct comparison of the imaged structures with the ground truth. Such comparisons have provided significant information on the overall quality of the ULM imaging method and its ability to accurately describe objects. However, this approach is not adaptable to general imaging conditions where ground truth is unknown. Other methods to assess ULM resolution are based on the localization precision of individual sources. Unfortunately, these methods do not account for the appropriate spatial sampling, and therefore fail to describe the resolution of the final image. Still other methods rely on the extraction of features from an image. For example, vessels are extracted and the separation between neighboring vessels or the shape of a flow profile is measured. Although such evaluations yield precious information about how well structures can be separated, they depend on a selection step that is very user dependent and therefore fails to be generalizable.

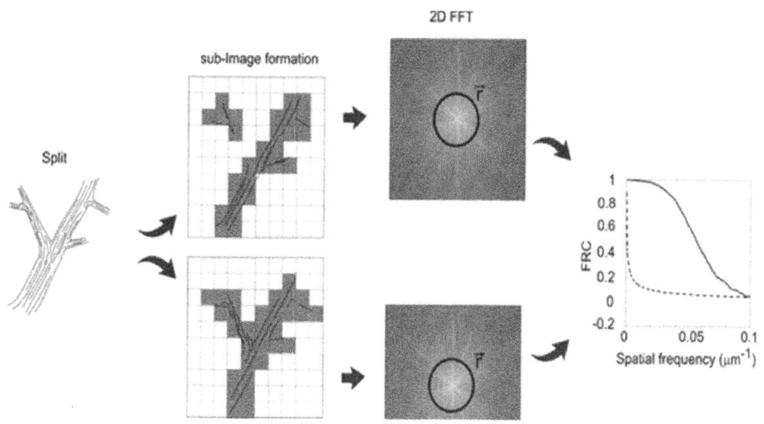

Figure 7.12. *Principle of Fourier ring correlation as a resolution measurement in ultrasound localization microscopy*

A potential answer to the problem of ULM resolution characterization could be found by using the Fourier ring correlation method (see Figure 7.12). This is a very general method that derives the relevant, maximum spatial frequency from an image, independently of the imaging conditions and/or the operator. The 2D Fourier transform from two images is computed and used to calculate their correlation along iso-frequency rings (van Heel et al. 2005; Banterle et al. 2013; Nieuwenhuizen et al. 2013). For each spatial frequency, this method gives a value between 0 and 1 that represents the consistency of the information at that frequency. The consistency of the information is 1 for the lowest frequencies and drops to around zero for the highest frequencies that do not contain valuable information. The "resolution" is then measured by applying different sets of thresholds. For example, fixed thresholds have been easy to use and implement; the resolution corresponds to the maximum frequency that yields a correlation higher than said threshold.

7.3.3. *Common artifacts and compensation methods*

Because of the long acquisition times imposed by the resolution-to-acquisition time trade-off, obtaining super-resolution images from moving organs is no easy task. When imaging abdominal organs, such as the kidneys or the liver, the imaging sequence can be strongly affected by motions, mostly caused by breathing. These motions can be several orders of magnitude larger than the targeted resolution, thus drastically degrading image quality (Foiret et al. 2017; Hingot et al. 2017; Harput et al. 2019).

To maintain a good image quality, the most straightforward method is to physically limit the impact of motion on the imaging conditions. This can be done in animals by triggering the acquisitions outside of the active respiratory phases or by using surgery to physically restrain the organ. Adult human patients can be asked to hold their breath and remain still for some time.

Still, these methods can only limit motions, and not eliminate them, especially on a scale below 100 µm. For small motions, some methods can be used to compensate acquired data for the presence of motion. One simple solution is based on the calculation of the correlation coefficient with respect to a reference frame. All frames that do not have a satisfactory correlation are discarded before microbubble detection and tracking. For slow motions, displacements can be measured to correct the positions of the microbubbles so that all the detections are displayed on a static grid. For fast-moving motions that degrade the quality of spatio-temporal clutter filters, registration can be used on every frame to realign tissues before clutter filtering. Registration strategies and algorithms vary strongly between research teams, and the identification of the best method remains an open question in ULM (Hingot et al. 2017; Foiret et al. 2018; Harput et al. 2018) (see Figure 7.13). Most often, some type of motion estimation is performed on B-mode-like images, and then used to register microbubble positions.

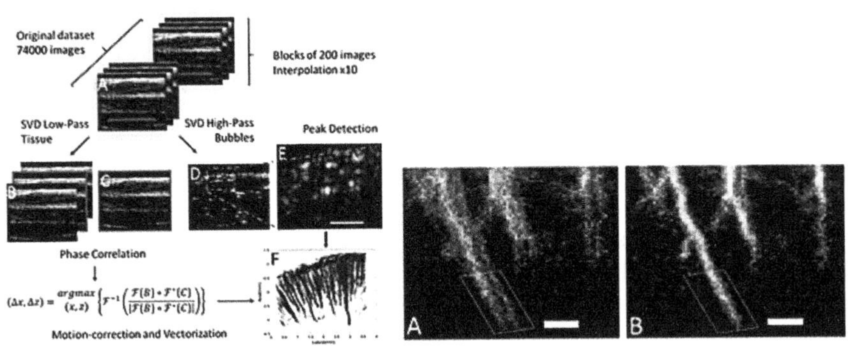

Figure 7.13. *Motion correction strategy in the rat brain using phase correlation to estimate tissue motion to correct the relative image positions before registering microbubble positions. Figures reused from Hingot et al. (2017) in accordance with the journal's open access author's rights*

Another source of distortion for microbubble localization is due to the aberration from layers of tissue between the imaged zone and the transducer. When imaging abdominal organs or the brain, the ultrasound wave must pass through a thick layer of fat or bone, respectively. Unlike most soft tissues, fat and bone are not mainly composed of water, and the velocity of ultrasound in these media (1,400 m/s for fat, >2,000 m/s for bone) is very different from that in water. This can introduce some strong artifacts in the image because the wavefront will be delayed and distorted by the aberrating layers (see Figure 7.14).

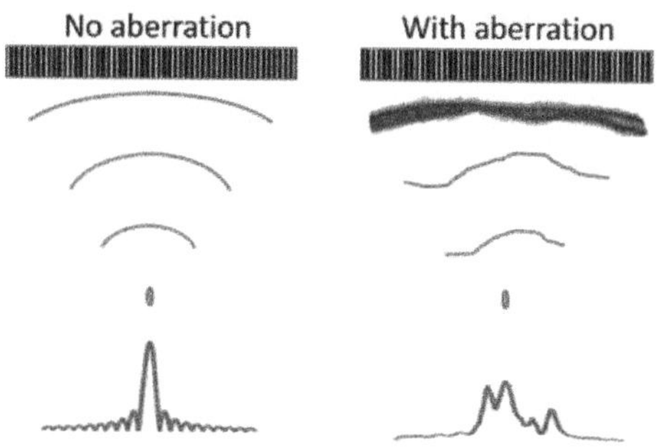

Figure 7.14. *Aberration causes distortion in the propagation path of the ultrasound beam, hence modifying the point-spread function of the system*

To compensate for this artifact, one solution is to estimate the additional delay law introduced by the propagation through the layers of tissue. This is best performed using an exogenous source, such as an individual microbubble, but can also be performed through the creation of a non-physical punctual source from speckle noise, or simply by estimating the thickness and speed of sound of the aberrating layer. This delay law can then be used to realign the data before the beamforming step, thus removing the impact of the aberrating material on the image.

The main limitation of this method is that it works best when the delay law is homogeneous in space and can be estimated based on a single point alone. A more thorough method proposes a description of the propagation in the entire ensemble of media using a matrix formalism and decomposes the propagation in the different media. The aberration compensation can then be performed at all points of space.

7.3.4. *From 2D to 3D ultrasound localization microscopy*

Imaging in 2D is standard practice in ultrasound but has several strong drawbacks. Because the field of view is limited, finding the relevant structure of interest requires extensive training and skill, and makes the examination very dependent on the operator. Moreover, imaging of blood flow in 2D, like color Doppler or ULM, is only sensitive to flow within the imaged plane and is blind to flow in vessels crossing the plane. Finally, since motion compensation strategies used to correct motion artifacts (see section 7.3.3) rely on the estimation of displacements that are detectable in the imaged plane, they are not able to compensate for any out-of-plane motions.

Achieving 3D imaging with ultrasound is challenging. For conventional systems relying on sweeping focused beams over the entire imaging field, an increased field of view can only be obtained at the price of much reduced frame rates. Thus, these imaging strategies are only performed for specific indications, such as cardiac imaging. For the latest generation of ultrasound scanners, with which an entire imaging plane can be insonified simultaneously at a very high frame rate, 3D imaging has been implemented with a complex acquisition system comprised of four ultrafast systems with 256 received channels each (Heiles et al. 2019, 2021), and the complete ULM pipeline was adapted from 2D to 3D. Since these initial innovations, methods to perform 3D ULM have been designed, which require less sophisticated hardware by using sparse or row–column arrays or a fully populated probe with a 4:1 multiplexer (Chavignon et al. 2021) (see Figure 7.15). Cardiac and brain applications have since been described in 3D (Demeulenaere et al. 2022a, 2022b).

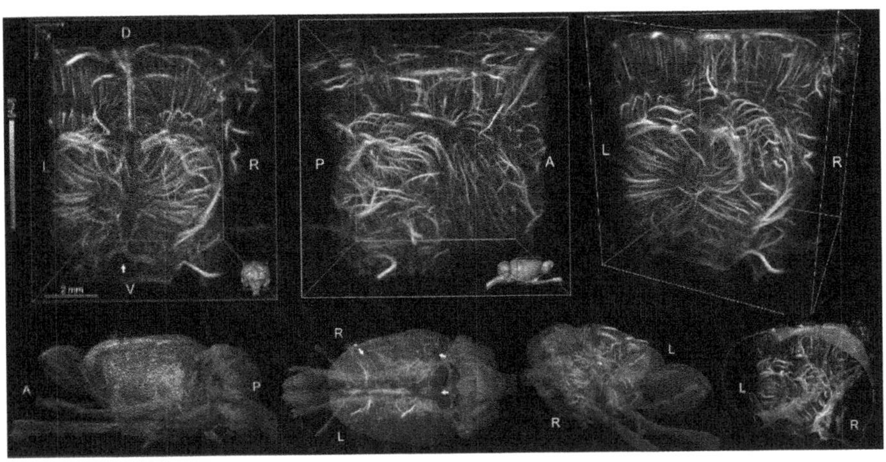

Figure 7.15. *Volumetric imaging of the vascularization in the rat brain. Republished with permission from Chavignon (2021)*

7.3.5. *Artificial intelligence*

Two main challenges associated with ULM today are the improvement of the imaging quality and the reduction in acquisition and computing times. Artificial intelligence and, in particular, the use of convolutional neural networks are an interesting option to improve the rapidity of analysis algorithms and their robustness when confronted with noise and high microbubble concentrations. This has the potential not only to improve image quality, but also to reduce data acquisition times because a higher microbubble concentration allows faster acquisition of a larger number of microbubble detections.

The main key to integrating machine learning strategies for ULM is the ability to train the models with realistic data so that the model can be generalized to a wide range of situations. Since the true position of microbubbles is required to train the models, most models under development have been working with simulated data and this limits their generalization to in vivo situations. A more practical framework has been introduced based on the simulation of sources in a realistic medium, and the machine learning approach called Deep-stULM has been shown to perform better than the current expert ULM method in high microbubble concentration acquisitions (see Figure 7.16). However, it still has to be tested under a larger range of experimental conditions.

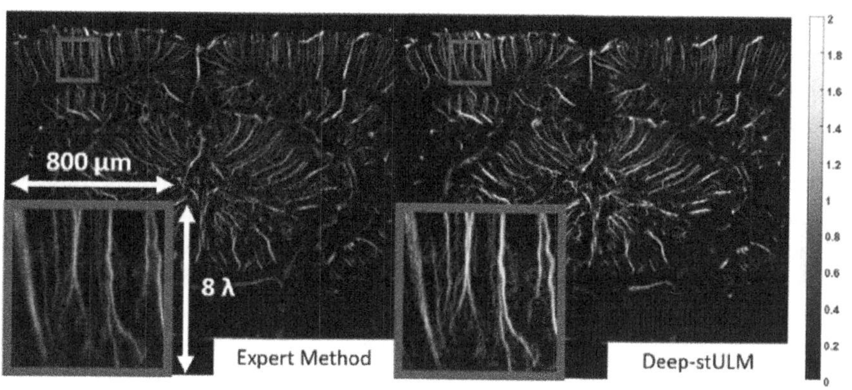

Figure 7.16. *Deep learning approach for ULM of brain vasculature. © (2021) IEEE. Reprinted with permission from Milecki et al. (2021)*

7.4. Perspectives and challenges

7.4.1. *Applications of super-resolution ultrasound*

In 2022, super-resolution ultrasound and, in particular, ULM remain a research subject with no recognized clinical applications. Several convincing demonstrations have been made in animals and humans, but the diagnostic interest is still unproven. Research efforts are currently concentrated on several applications: the brain and nervous systems, abdominal organs, tumors, peripheral imaging and a few other systems.

In 2015, a landmark study was published using ULM in the rat brain (Errico et al. 2015). Beyond a proof of concept, the interest of studying super-resolution in the brain is profound. Indeed, cerebral microcirculation impacts both the brain physiology and many other pathologies. With an average perfusion of 50 mL of blood per 100 grams of brain tissue per minute, the brain requires 15% of the cardiac output for only 2% of the body mass. This is required to feed the metabolism of 86 billion neurons, providing an estimated 1 exaflop of calculation power. For comparison, the exaflop computer Frontier still in development in 2021 is expected to use 20 megawatts of power. In this context, the brain remains the most eco-friendly source of calculation, as proposed in the classic movie series *The Matrix*.

The microcirculation of the brain is far from passive. The activity of neurons and blood flow within the vessels is linked through the neurovascular complex. An increase in brain activity in a specific zone is linked to an increase in blood flow, which is the foundation of functional imaging techniques such as fMRI (Rosen et al. 1998) and functional ultrasound imaging (Deffieux et al. 2018).

Other medical imaging techniques are already providing an exquisite window to the brain. For example, MRI displays not only proton density, but also water diffusion, fat content, large vessels and perfusion (Nishimura 2010). With CT and PET scans, MRI is used for most diagnostic techniques, while the use of transcranial ultrasound Doppler remains limited. However, resolving the microcirculation remains a challenge, even in animal models. Shallow imaging can be performed on live tissue with optical techniques such as confocal or two-photon microscopy. Meanwhile, the microcirculation of the entire brain can be observed through micro-CT or tissue clearing, which involves very invasive or terminal approaches (Ueda et al. 2020; Zhu et al. 2020).

Several pathologies affecting the brain could be explored with ULM. Leading to six million deaths every year, stroke is one of the main causes of death in the world. Brain cancer kills hundreds of thousands each year. Dementias such as Alzheimer's disease lead to an additional two million deaths. Each of these diseases involves, at least partly, a modification of the microcirculation, which highlights the importance of microvascular imaging in both animal models and humans.

Ultrasound is not a common brain imaging technique. The main reason for this is that the skull attenuates ultrasound at a level of approximatively 10–20 dB/cm around 1 MHz (Pichardo et al. 2010). Moreover, the speed of sound in the skull can be more than twice as high as that in brain tissue. The thickness of the skull also varies between individuals and between different regions of the head. This can lead to aberrations, which need to be corrected for both ultrasonic imaging and therapy. Several approaches have been proposed for the correction of aberration due to the skull, including phase conjugation (Hynynen and Clement 2007), time-reversal (Pernot et al. 2007) or focal correction (Soulioti et al. 2019). However, the skull can also be an advantage for ULM. Since this technique requires the accumulation of many microbubble tracks to obtain micrometric resolution, it is highly impacted by small motions during data acquisition. The skull stabilizes the brain, which improves ULM results.

The brain had been targeted early on as an application for ULM, using a spherical array originally designed for therapy, in order to observe a spiral tubing thinner than the wavelength (O'Reilly et al. 2013). Errico et al. (2015) demonstrated that ULM could detect microvessels on the scale of the micron in a rat brain following craniotomy. This paper also showed a possibility of distinguishing vessels separated by 16 micrometers or 1/6 of the ultrasonic wavelength. Furthermore, the study demonstrated that contrast agent tracking could be used for velocimetry with a precision down to 1 millimeter per second.

For ULM, the brain cortex is an excellent model since the vessels are arranged in a structured planar pattern. The brains of rats and mice have been used to demonstrate the technical evolution of ULM. For example, Hardy et al. (2021) described the interest of using sparse channel sampling in ULM by imaging the craniotomized rat brain. The same group demonstrated their deep learning framework on the rat brain (Milecki et al. 2021), as well as a novel sensitivity to the pulsatility of microvascular flow (Bourquin et al. 2022). The chicken embryo brain was exploited by Huang et al. (2020) to introduce their novel microbubble separation algorithm. Finally, Heiles et al. (2021) demonstrated the potential of 3D ULM on a craniotomized rat brain model. They applied a matrix transducer piloted with four ultrafast ultrasound systems to acquire data from seven different regions of the brain and obtain volumetric vascular imaging over the entire organ on a scale of a few tens of microns. A further improvement was introduced by Chavignon et al. (2022) who described 3D ULM with a multiplexed matrix transducer that could provide volumetric imaging with a much simpler ultrasound scanner.

Disease models in the brain are also beginning to be studied with ULM. Hingot et al. (2020) used ULM to characterize the evolution of ischemic stroke in the first 24 hours. A more general study on the differentiation of the hemorrhagic and ischemic stroke in 3D was recently published by Chavignon et al. (2022). Lowerison et al. (2020a) have now proposed the use of ULM in an aging mouse model to establish biomarkers of the evolution of disease.

Meanwhile, transcranial 3D ULM and super-resolved functional imaging have been demonstrated in murine models (Demeulenaere et al. 2022a, 2022b; Renaudin et al. 2022). Finally, the use of 2D ULM on human patients was demonstrated in a clinic, highlighting abnormal blood flow in aneurysm transcranially (Demené et al. 2021).

Beyond the brain, the spinal cord has also been studied with ULM. A study on spinal nociceptive circuits in rats has exploited ULM to characterize the microvascular network implicated in this functional response (Rahal et al. 2020). Deep learning-aided spinal cord ULM imaging was demonstrated by van Sloun et al. (2020).

Recently, Huang et al. (2021) exploited ULM to image several abdominal organs in human subjects. Based on their previous development to reduce imaging time, they demonstrated the possibility of obtaining rapid ULM images of the healthy human liver and kidney. Moreover, they demonstrated the possibility of observing the microcirculation generated within pancreatic and breast tumors.

Before this important transfer of ULM to the clinic, several groups have published ULM developments in abdominal imaging, especially in the kidney. Foiret et al. (2017) assessed the microvasculature of the rat kidney with ULM. The kidney model was also used to demonstrate nonlinear motion-independent ULM (Kierski et al. 2020), as well as 3D imaging of the organ. ULM of the kidney has been shown to compare favorably well with CT by Anderson et al. (2021).

The diabetic kidney is of primary importance due to the impact of the disease on its microcirculation. Chronic kidney disease was shown to impact ULM-extracted parameters in the kidney (Zhang et al. 2021). In models of hypertensive nephrosclerosis, it was demonstrated that flow speeds derived from ULM were different with respect to control (Qiu et al. 2022).

Beyond abdominal organ imaging, ULM has also been applied to cardiac imaging. Coronary flow was mapped through 3D ULM by Demeulenaere et al. (2022).

Tumor imaging is one of the primary targets of super-resolution ultrasound. In a foundational presentation at the IEEE International Ultrasound Symposium, Siepmann et al. (2011) showed that the accumulation of centroid detection of dilute microbubbles flowing in a tumor mouse model could yield images with much higher resolution than conventional Doppler or contrast-enhanced ultrasound. Lin et al. (2017) presented plane-by-plane ULM imaging of tumor angiogenesis (see Figure 7.17).

Tumor imaging with ULM was implemented in humans by Opacic et al. (2018; Dencks et al. 2018). The particularity of this study was to use conventional frame rate imaging scanners, generalizing ULM to the thousands of ultrasound scanners available in hospitals. They exploited novel tracking methods to compensate for the lack of time resolution.

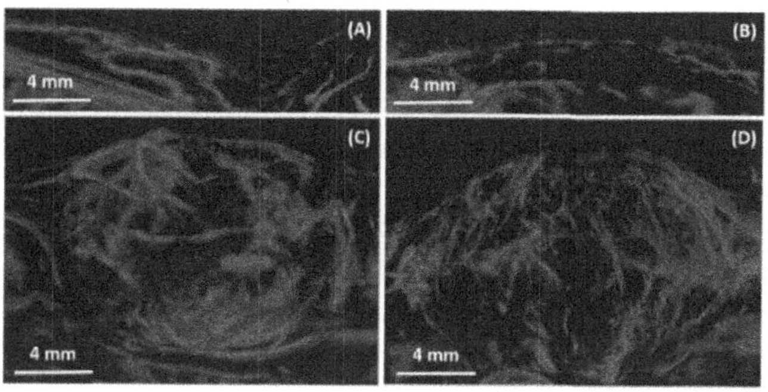

Figure 7.17. *Sections of maximum intensity projection ULM reveal the heterogeneous nature of the microvascular architecture in a rat tumor. Reproduced from Lin et al. (2017), copyright © Ivyspring International Publisher*

7.4.2. *Upcoming challenges and perspectives*

In the last 12 years, ULM has evolved drastically. From being demonstrated simply in microvessel channels, it has become a modality that can be implemented in patients in the clinical setting. Most of the publications in the field of ultrasonic super-resolution are still centered on ULM; however, some non-localization modalities have also been presented. ULM is currently the only medical imaging modality that can resolve the microcirculation in deep tissue. Nevertheless, it remains far from integration in the clinical routine.

The first hurdle of SRUS is to demonstrate its applicability for human diagnosis. Indeed, since the observation of the microcirculation is insufficient, it is necessary for this technique to modify patients' path to recovery for it to be considered in the medical toolbox. ULM tends to yield impressive images in both 2D and 3D, but a key consideration is to convert these beautiful images into imaging biomarkers to contribute to medical decisions. Moreover, ULM needs to show that additional information can be obtained with respect to perfusion imaging, which is already standard in ultrasound, CT and MRI. Hence, additional benefits of resolving the smallest vessels need to be demonstrated.

Several studies have given hints concerning potential biomarkers obtainable from ULM. For example, bubble velocities appear to be modified in the small vessels of the hippocampus in a murine Alzheimer's model (Lowerison et al. 2022b). Providing a way to follow or even predict the impact of Alzheimer's disease on the brain microvasculature in human subjects would be of great importance.

Ultrasound imaging in the brain is severely impacted by the compromise between resolution and penetration. Because skull attenuation is high, it forces the use of lower frequencies and longer wavelengths to image the brain relative to frequencies that can be used for similar depths in other regions of the body. This significantly impacts the quality of ultrasonic imaging of the brain. ULM holds the key to retrieving image resolution in the brain, even in the clinic. Because of the portability of ultrasound imaging, a portable brain scanner for emergency stroke diagnosis can potentially be designed using ULM. This approach would help distinguish ischemic and hemorrhagic stroke and allow the former to be treated in the ambulance. If successful, such an approach could quite significantly reduce the mortality and morbidity of stroke, which is very dependent on the time required to select the appropriate treatment.

The microcirculation observed by ULM could also become a biomarker for angiogenesis in tumors. Beyond simple perfusion, the structure, shape and heterogeneity of vessels at the smallest scale could contribute to determining the aggressiveness of tumors. However, single-plane ULM would probably be insufficient to truly describe the vascular network since the vessels are not as nicely organized as in the cortex of the brain or the kidney.

Deficits of the microcirculation can also be described with ULM, and such an approach could help highlight the effect of diabetes in the periphery circulation or in the kidneys. Again, to be beneficial with respect to perfusion imaging, ULM will need to demonstrate that the microstructure of vessels needs to be revealed to modify medical decisions. Heterogeneities in perfusion smaller than the wavelength could be observed by ULM and give a better prediction of the lack of oxygenation in tissue.

Even though multiple applications demanding ULM are identified and demonstrated, many other issues remain to be solved. A key aspect is the time resolution, which is lost due to the acquisition time of ULM. Part of the acquisition time can be retrieved by increasing the number of microbubbles that can be localized in any single frame. ULM images with sufficient quality for diagnostic use are already being obtained within a few seconds of acquisition. However, physiology also limits the number of vessels visited by microbubbles at any time. Resolution at 30 frames per seconds will remain difficult to attain at subwavelength resolution.

Another approach would be to circumvent the time resolution issue by moving away from the handheld approach of ultrasound scanning. Currently, ultrasound imaging remains user dependent because volumetric imaging is reconstructed in the echographist's head from a succession of 2D plane. Moreover, plane selection requires significant expertise since poor selection can annul the benefit of the entire exam. The evolution of ultrasound towards 3D imaging could help shift the imaging paradigm closer to that of MRI and CT. Ultrasonic volumetric data acquisition allows physicians to study the dataset offline and better guarantee the diagnosis. Placing the probe is also made easier because the plane under consideration can be found afterwards from a larger dataset. Finally, if user dependency is reduced during acquisition, ultrasound can be made compatible with remote diagnosis, which would be particularly beneficial for stroke imaging.

ULM has been demonstrated to benefit strongly from 3D imaging. The latter solves projection issues, biased velocimetry and lack of motion correction in the elevation direction. Moreover, it allows the interception and tracking of many more microbubbles since they are detected throughout the volume. Furthermore, if volumes are acquired rather than planes, a lower time resolution has less relative impact because, among other medical imaging modalities, it is typical to scan for several minutes to obtain 3D image stacks.

The field of ULM appears to be on the path towards more systematic volumetric data acquisition. Any improvement in the number of microbubbles intercepted per volume will have an important impact on image quality and improve calculation time. Currently, 3D ULM is most often performed with short data acquisition times but with long post-treatment of the data. The acquisition and analysis intervals should become more equivalent over the next few years.

In this context, we can foresee ULM as a method whereby wide matrix transducers will be placed over the organ of interest before beginning the acquisition of injected microbubbles. This can be made compatible with transcranial acquisitions, and also with abdominal or even cardiac imaging if motion correction algorithms are correctly put in place.

As many chronic diseases, such as cancer, stroke, arteriosclerosis and dementia, have a microvascular component, we believe that ULM can provide a wide spectrum of new biomarkers that could strongly impact the diagnosis of these diseases. However, while achieving micrometric resolution, ultrasound imaging will need to preserve its portability and accessibility so that most of the world's population can access this emerging imaging technique.

7.5. References

Andersen, S.B., Taghavi, I., Kjer, H.M., Søgaard, S.B., Gundlach, C., Dahl, V.A., Nielsen, M.B., Dahl, A.B., Jensen, J.A., Sørensen, C.M. (2021). Evaluation of 2D super-resolution ultrasound imaging of the rat renal vasculature using ex vivo micro-computed tomography. *Scientific Reports*, 11, 1–13.

Averkiou, M.A., Bruce, M.F., Powers, J.E., Sheeran, P.S., Burns, P.N. (2020). Imaging methods for ultrasound contrast agents. *Ultrasound in Medicine & Biology*, 46(3), 498–517.

Bamber, J.C. (2004). Attenuation and absorption. In *Physical Principles of Medical Diagnosis*, 2nd edition, Hill, C.R., Bamber, J.C., ter Haar, G.R. (eds). Wiley, Chichester.

Bamber, J.C. and Dickinson R.J. (1980). Ultrasonic B-scanning: A computer simulation. *Physics in Medicine and Biology* 25, 463–479. https://doi.org/10.1088/0031-9155/25/3/006.

Banterle, N., Bui, K.H., Lemke, E.A., Beck, M. (2013). Fourier ring correlation as a resolution criterion for super-resolution microscopy. *Journal of Structural Biology*, 183, 363–367. https://doi.org/10.1016/j.jsb.2013.05.004.

Bar-Zion, A., Solomon, O., Tremblay-Darveau, C., Adam, D., Eldar, Y.C. (2018). SUSHI: Sparsity-based ultrasound super-resolution hemodynamic imaging. *IEEE Transactions on Ultrasonics, Ferroelectrics, and Frequency Control*, 65, 2365–2380. https://doi.org/10.1109/TUFFC.2018.2873380.

Betzig, E. and Chichester, R.J. (1993). Single molecules observed by near-field scanning optical microscopy. *Science*, 262, 1422–1425. https://doi.org/10.1126/science.262.5138.1422.

Betzig, E., Patterson, G.H., Sougrat, R., Lindwasser, O.W., Olenych, S., Bonifacino, J.S., Davidson, M.W., Lippincot-Schwartz, J., Hess, H.F. (2006). Imaging intracellular fluorescent proteins at nanometer resolution. *Science*, 313, 1642–1645.

Bouakaz, A., Frigstad, S., Ten Cate, F.J., de Jong, N. (2002). Super harmonic imaging: A new imaging technique for improved contrast detection. *Ultrasound in Medicine & Biology*, 28, 59–68. https://doi.org/10.1016/S0301-5629(01)00460-4.

Bourquin, C., Poree J., Lesage, F., Provost, J. (2022). In vivo pulsatility measurement of cerebral microcirculation in rodents using dynamic ultrasound localization microscopy. *IEEE Transactions on Medical Imaging*, 41, 782–792. https://doi.org/10.1109/TMI.2021.3123912.

Briggs, A. (1992). *Acoustic Microscopy*. Oxford University Press, Oxford.

Chavignon, A. (2021). Microscopie par localisation ultrasonore dans les modèles d'accidents vasculaires cérébraux. Doctoral dissertation, ESPCI Paris, Université PSL.

Chavignon, A., Heiles, B., Hingot, V., Orset, C., Vivien, D., Couture, O. (2021). 3D transcranial ultrasound localization microscopy in the rat brain with a multiplexed matrix probe. *IEEE Transactions on Biomedical Engineering*, 69, 2132–2142.

Chavignon, A., Hingot, V., Orset, C., Vivien, D., Couture, O. (2022). 3D transcranial ultrasound localization microscopy for discrimination between ischemic and hemorrhagic stroke in early phase. *Scientific Reports*, 12(1), 14607.

Christensen-Jeffries, K., Browning, R.J., Tang, M.X., Dunsby, C., Eckersley, R.J. (2014). In vivo acoustic super-resolution and super-resolved velocity mapping using microbubbles. *IEEE Transactions on Medical Imaging*, 34, 433–440.

Christensen-Jeffries, K., Brown, J., Harput, S., Zhang, G., Zhu, J., Tang, M.-X., Dunsby, C., Eckersley, R.J. (2019). Poisson statistical model of ultrasound super-resolution imaging acquisition time. *IEEE Transactions on Ultrasonics Ferroelectrics and Frequency Control*, 66, 1246–1254. https://doi.org/10.1109/TUFFC.2019.2916603.

Christensen-Jeffries, K., Couture, O., Dayton, P.A., Eldar, Y.C., Hynynen, K., Kiessling, F., O'Reilly, M.A., Pinton, G., Schmitz, G., Tang, M.X. et al. (2020). Super-resolution ultrasound imaging. *Ultrasound in Medicine & Biology*, 46, 865–891.

Clement, G.T., Huttunen, J., Hynynen, K. (2005). Superresolution ultrasound imaging using back-projected reconstruction. *Journal of the Acoustical Society of America*, 118, 3953–3960.

Cobbold, R.S. (2006). *Foundations of Biomedical Ultrasound*. Oxford University Press, Oxford.

Couture, O., Tanter, M., Fink, M. (2010). Method and device for sound imaging. Patent, FR1060633A.

Couture, O., Besson, B., Montaldo, G., Fink, M., Tanter, M. (2011). Microbubble ultrasound super-localization imaging (MUSLI). *IEEE International Ultrasonics Symposium (IUS)*, 797, 1285–1287.

Couture, O., Hingot, V., Heiles, B., Muleki-Seya, P., Tanter, M. (2018). Ultrasound localization microscopy and super-resolution: A state of the art. *IEEE Transactions on Ultrasonics, Ferroelectrics, and Frequency Control*, 65, 1304–1320. https://doi.org/10.1109/TUFFC.2018.2850811.

Deffieux, T., Demene, C., Pernot, M., Tanter, M. (2018). Functional ultrasound neuroimaging: A review of the preclinical and clinical state of the art. *Current Opinion in Neurobiology*, 50, 128–135.

Demené, C., Deffieux, T., Pernot, M., Osmanski, B.F., Biran, V., Gennisson, J.-L., Sieu, L.-A., Bergel, A., Franqui, S., Correas, J.-M. et al. (2015). Spatiotemporal clutter filtering of ultrafast ultrasound data highly increases Doppler and Ultrasound sensitivity. *IEEE Transactions on Medical Imaging*, 34, 2271–2285.

Demené, C., Robin, J., Dizeux, A., Heiles, B., Pernot, M., Tanter, M., Perren, F. (2021). Transcranial ultrafast ultrasound localization microscopy of brain vasculature in patients. *Nature Biomedical Engineering*, 5, 219–228.

Demeulenaere, O., Bertolo, A., Pezet, S., Ialy-Radio, N., Osmanski, B., Papadacci, C., Tanter, M., Deffieux, T., Pernot, M. (2022a). In vivo whole brain microvascular imaging in mice using transcranial 3D ultrasound localization microscopy. *EBioMedicine*, 79, 103995.

Demeulenaere, O., Sandoval, Z., Mateo, P., Dizeux, A., Villemain, O., Gallet, R., Ghaleh, B., Deffieux, T., Demènè, C., Tanter, M. (2022b). Coronary flow assessment using 3-dimensional ultrafast ultrasound localization microscopy. *JACC: Cardiovascular Imaging*, 15, 1193–1208.

Dencks, S., Piepenbrock, M., Opacic, T., Krauspe, B., Stickeler, E., Kiessling, F., Schmitz, G. (2018). Clinical pilot application of super-resolution US imaging in breast cancer. *IEEE Transactions on Ultrasonics, Ferroelectrics, and Frequency Control*, 66, 517–526.

Denis, L., Bodard, S., Hingot, V., Chavignon, A., Battaglia, J., Renault, G., Lager, F., Aissani, A., Hélénon, O., Correas, J.-M. et al. (2023). Sensing ultrasound localization microscopy for the visualization of glomeruli in living rats and humans. *Ebiomedicine*, 91. https://doi.org/10.1016/j.ebiom.2023.104578.

Dertinger, T., Colyer, R., Iyer, G., Weiss, S., Enderlein, J. (2009). Fast, background-free, 3D super-resolution optical fluctuation imaging (SOFI). *Proceedings of the National Academy of Sciences*, 106, 22287–22292.

Desailly, Y., Couture, O., Fink, M., Tanter, M. (2013). Sono-activated ultrasound localization microscopy. *Applied Physics Letters*, 103, 174107.

Desailly, Y., Pierre, J., Couture, O., Tanter, M. (2015). Resolution limits of ultrafast ultrasound localization microscopy. *Physics in Medicine & Biology*, 60, 8723.

Desailly, Y., Tissier, A.M., Correas, J.-M., Wintzenrieth F., Tanter M., Couture, O. (2017). Contrast enhanced ultrasound by real-time spatiotemporal filtering of ultrafast images. *Physics in Medicine and Biology*, 62, 31–42. https://doi.org/10.1073/pnas.0907866106.

Errico, C., Pierre, J., Pezet, S., Desailly, Y., Lenkei, Z., Couture, O., Tanter, M. (2015). Ultrafast ultrasound localization microscopy for deep super-resolution vascular imaging. *Nature*, 527, 499–502.

Fink, M. and Tanter, M. (2010). Multiwave imaging and super resolution. *Physics Today*, 63, 28–33.

Foiret, J., Zhang, H., Ilovitsh, T., Mahakian, L., Tam, S., Ferrara, K.W. (2017). Ultrasound localization microscopy to image and assess microvasculature in a rat kidney. *Scientific Reports*, 7, 1–12.

Foote, K.G. (2014). Discriminating between the nearfield and the farfield of acoustic transducers. *The Journal of the Acoustical Society of America*, 136(4), 1511–1517.

Foster, F.S., Lockwood, G.R., Ryan, L.K., Harasiewicz, K.A., Berube, L., Rauth, A.M. (1993). Principles and applications of ultrasound backscatter microscopy. *IEEE Transactions on Ultrasonics, Ferroelectrics and Frequency Control*, 40, 608–617. https://doi.org/10.1109/58.238115.

Foster, F.S., Hossack, J., Adamson, S.L. (2011). Micro-ultrasound for preclinical imaging. *Interface Focus*, 1, 576–601. https://doi.org/10.1098/rsfs.2011.0037.

Galilei, G. (1610). *Sidereus Nuncius*. Thomas Baglioni, Venice.

Gessner, R.C., Frederick, C.B., Foster, F.S., Dayton, P.A. (2013). Acoustic angiography: A new imaging modality for assessing microvasculature architecture. *International Journal of Biomedical Imaging*, 9. https://doi.org/10.1155/2013/936593.

Gramiak, R., and Shah, P.M. (1968). Echocardiography of the aortic root. *Investigative Radiology*, 3(5), 356–366.

Gramiak, R., Shah, P.M., Kramer, D.H. (1969). Ultrasound cardiography: Contrast studies in anatomy and function. *Radiology*, 92, 939–948.

Gustafsson, M.G. (2000). Surpassing the lateral resolution limit by a factor of two using structured illumination microscopy. *Journal of Microscopy*, 198, 82–87.

Hardy, E., Porée, J., Belgharbi, H., Bourquin, C., Lesage, F, Provost, J. (2021). Sparse channel sampling for ultrasound localization microscopy (SPARSE-ULM). *Physics in Medicine & Biology*, 66, 095008. https://doi.org/10.1088/1361-6560/abf1b6.

Harput, S., Christensen-Jeffries, K., Brown, J., Li, Y., Williams, K.J., Davies, A.H., Eckersley, R.J., Dunsby, C., Tang, M.-X. (2018). Two-stage motion correction for super-resolution ultrasound imaging in human lower limb. *IEEE Transactions on Ultrasound, Ferroelectrics and Frequency Control*, 65, 803–814. https://doi.org/10.1109/TUFFC.2018.2824846.

van Heel, M. and Schatz, M. (2005). Fourier shell correlation threshold criteria. *Journal of Structural Biology*, 151, 250–262. https://doi.org/10.1016/j.jsb.2005.05.009.

Heiles, B., Correia, M., Hingot, V., Pernot, M., Provost, J., Tanter, M., Couture, O. (2019). Ultrafast 3D ultrasound localization microscopy using a 32 x 32 matrix array. *IEEE Transactions on Medical Imaging*, 38, 2005–2015.

Heiles, B., Chavignon, A., Bergel, A., Hingot, V., Serroune, H., Maresca, D., Pezet, S., Pernot, M., Tanter, M., Couture, O. (2021). Volumetric ultrasound localization microscopy of the whole brain microvasculature. *bioRxiv*. https://doi.org/10.1101/2021.09.17.460797.

Heiles, B., Chavignon, A., Hingot, V., Lopez, P., Teston, E., Couture, O. (2022). Performance benchmarking of microbubble-localization algorithms for ultrasound localization microscopy. *Nature Biomedical Engineering*, 6, 605–616.

Hell, S.W. and Wichmann, J. (1994). Breaking the diffraction resolution limit by stimulated emission: Stimulated-emission-depletion fluorescence microscopy. *Optics Letters*, 19, 780.

Hess, S.T., Girirajan, T.P.K., Mason, M.D. (2006). Ultra-high resolution imaging by fluorescence photoactivation localization microscopy. *Biophysical Journal*, 91, 4258–4272.

Hingot, V. (2019). Development of ultrasound localization microscopy to measure cerebral perfusion during stroke: A study in mouse models prior to its translation in humans. Doctoral dissertation, Sorbonne Université, Paris.

Hingot, V., Errico, C., Tanter, M., Couture, O. (2017). Subwavelength motion-correction for ultrafast ultrasound localization microscopy. *Ultrasonics*, 77, 17–21. https://doi.org/10.1016/j.ultras.2017.01.008.

Hingot, V., Errico, C., Heiles, B., Rahal, L., Tanter, M., Couture, O. (2019). Microvascular flow dictates the compromise between spatial resolution and acquisition time in ultrasound localization microscopy. *Scientific Reports*, 9, 2456. https://doi.org/10.1038/s41598-018-38349-x.

Hingot, V., Brodin, C., Lebrun, F., Heiles, B., Chagnot, A., Yetim, M., Gaubert, M., Orset, C., Tanter, M., Couture, O. et al. (2020). Early ultrafast ultrasound imaging of cerebral perfusion correlates with ischemic stroke outcomes and responses to treatment in mice. *Theranostics*, 10, 7480.

Hingot, V., Chavignon, A., Heiles, B., Couture, O. (2021). Measuring image resolution in ultrasound localization microscopy. *IEEE Transactions on Medical Imaging*, 40, 3812–3819. https://doi.org/10.1109/TMI.2021.3097150.

Hooke, R. (1665). *Micrographia*. Royal Society, London.

Huang, C., Lowerison, M.R., Trzasko, J.D., Manduca, A., Bresler, Y., Tang, S., Gong, P., Lok, U.-W., Song, P., Chen, S. (2020). Short acquisition time super-resolution ultrasound microvessel imaging via microbubble separation. *Scientific Reports*, 10, 1–13.

Huang, C., Zhang, W., Gong, P., Lok, U.-W., Tang, S., Yin, T., Zhang, X., Zhu, L., Sang, M., Song, P. et al. (2021). Super-resolution ultrasound localization microscopy based on a high frame-rate clinical ultrasound scanner: An in-human feasibility study. *Physics in Medicine & Biology*, 66, 08NT01.

Hynynen, K. and Clement, G. (2007). Clinical applications of focused ultrasound – The brain. *International Journal of Hyperthermia*, 23, 193–202.

Ikeda, O., Sato, T., Suzuki, K. (1979). Super-resolution imaging system using waves with a limited frequency bandwidth. *Journal of the Acoustical Society of America*, 65, 75–81.

Ilovitsh, T., Ilovitsh, A., Foiret, J., Fite, B.Z., Ferrara, K.W. (2018). Acoustical structured illumination for super-resolution ultrasound imaging. *Communications Biology*, 1, 3. https://doi.org/10.1038/s42003-017-0003-5.

Jones, H.W. (1992). Superresolution in ultrasonic imaging. In *Acoustical Imaging*, Ermert, H. and Harjes, H.-P. (eds). Springer, Boston, MA.

Kierski, T.M., Espindola, D., Newsome, I.G., Cherin, E., Yin, J., Foster, F.S., Demore, C.E.M., Pinton, G.F., Dayton, P.A. (2020). Superharmonic ultrasound for motion-independent localization microscopy: Applications to microvascular imaging from low to high flow rates. *IEEE Transactions on Ultrasonics, Ferroelectrics, and Frequency Control*, 67, 957–967.

Klibanov, A.L., Rasche, P.T., Hughes, M.S., Wojdyla, J.K., Galen, K.P., Wible, J.H., Brandenburger, G.H. (2002). Detection of individual microbubbles of an ultrasound contrast agent. *Academic Radiology*, 9, S279–S281. https://doi.org/10.1016/S1076-6332(03)80203-9.

Leighton, T. (2012). *The Acoustic Bubble*. Academic Press, London.

Lin, F., Shelton, S.E., Espíndola, D., Rojas, J.D., Pinton, G., Dayton, P.A. (2017). 3-D ultrasound localization microscopy for identifying microvascular morphology features of tumor angiogenesis at a resolution beyond the diffraction limit of conventional ultrasound. *Theranostics*, 7, 196–204. https://doi.org/10.7150/thno.16899.

Lockwood, G.R., Turnball, D.H., Christopher, D.A., Foster, F.S. (1996). Beyond 30 MHz (applications of high-frequency ultrasound imaging). *IEEE Engineering in Medicine and Biology Magazine*, 15, 60–71.

Lowerison, M.R., Huang, C., Lucien, F., Chen, S., Song, P. (2020). Ultrasound localization microscopy of renal tumor xenografts in chicken embryo is correlated to hypoxia. *Scientific Reports*, 10, 1–13.

Lowerison, M.R., Sekaran, N.V.C., Zhang, W., Dong, Z., Chen, X., Llano, D.A., Song, P. (2022a). Aging-related cerebral microvascular changes visualized using ultrasound localization microscopy in the living mouse. *Scientific Reports*, 12, 1–11.

Lowerison, M.R., Sekaran, N.V.C., Dong, Z., Chen, X., You, Q., Llano, D.A., Song, P. (2022b). Super-resolution ultrasound imaging of cerebrovascular impairment in a mouse model of Alzheimer's disease. *bioRxiv*. https://doi.org/10.1101/2022.10.05.511008.

Mast, T.D. (2000). Empirical relationships between acoustic parameters in human soft tissues. *Acoustics Research Letters*, 1, 37–42.

Milecki, L., Poree, J., Belgharbi, H., Bourquin, C., Damseh, R., Delafontaine-Martel, P., Lesage, F., Gasse, M., Provost, J. (2021). A deep learning framework for spatiotemporal ultrasound localization microscopy. *IEEE Transactions on Medical Imaging*, 40, 1428–1437. https://doi.org/10.1109/TMI.2021.3056951.

Moerner, W. and Kador, L. (1989). Optical detection and spectroscopy of single molecules in a solid. *Physical Review Letters*, 62, 2535–2538.

Nieuwenhuizen, R.P.J., Lidke, K.A., Bates, M., Puig, D.L., Grunwald, D., Stallinga, S., Rieger, B. (2013). Measuring image resolution in optical nanoscopy. *Nature Methods*, 10, 557–562. https://doi.org/10.1038/nmeth.2448.

Nishimura, D.G. (2010). *Principles of Magnetic Resonance Imaging*. Standford University, Palo Alto, CA.

Opacic, T., Dencks, S., Theek, B., Piepenbrock, M., Ackermann, D., Rix, A., Twan, L., Stickler, E., Delorme, S., Schmitz, G. et al. (2018). Motion model ultrasound localization microscopy for preclinical and clinical multiparametric tumor characterization. *Nature Communications*, 9, 1–13.

O'Reilly, M.A. and Hynynen, K. (2013). A super-resolution ultrasound method for brain vascular mapping. *Medical Physics*, 40, 110701.

Page, J.H. (2016). Focusing of ultrasonic waves by negative refraction in phononic crystals. *AIP Advances*, 6(12), 121606.

Pernot, M., Aubry, J.-F., Tanter, M., Boch, A.-L., Marquet, F., Kujas, M., Seilhean, D., Fink, M. (2007). In vivo transcranial brain surgery with an ultrasonic time reversal mirror. *Journal of Neurosurgery*, 106, 1061–1066. https://doi.org/10.3171/jns.2007.106.6.1061.

Pichardo, S., Sin, V.W., Hynynen, K. (2010). Multi-frequency characterization of the speed of sound and attenuation coefficient for longitudinal transmission of freshly excised human skulls. *Physics in Medicine & Biology*, 56, 219–250.

Prada, C. and Thomas, J.-L. (2003). Experimental subwavelength localization of scatterers by decomposition of the time reversal operator interpreted as a covariance matrix. *Journal of the Acoustical Society of America*, 114, 235–243.

Qiu, L., Zhang, J., Yang, Y., Zhang, H., Lee, F.F., He, Q., Huang, C., Huang, L., Qian, L., Luo, J. (2022). In vivo assessment of hypertensive nephrosclerosis using ultrasound localization microscopy. *Medical Physics*, 49, 2295–2308.

Rahal, L., Thibaut, M., Rivals, I., Claron, J., Lenkei, Z., Sitt, J.D., Tanter, M., Pezet, S. (2020). Ultrafast ultrasound imaging pattern analysis reveals distinctive dynamic brain states and potent sub-network alterations in arthritic animals. *Scientific Reports*, 10, 1–17.

Renaudin, N., Demené, C., Dizeux, A., Ialy-Radio, N., Pezet, S., Tanter, M. (2022). Functional ultrasound localization microscopy reveals brain-wide neurovascular activity on a microscopic scale. *Nature Methods*, 19, 1004–1012.

Riemer, K., Toulemonde, M., Yan, J., Lerendegui, M., Stride, E., Weinberg, P.D., Dunsby, C., Tang, M.-X. (2022). Fast and selective super-resolution ultrasound in vivo with acoustically activated nanodroplets. *IEEE Transactions on Medical Imaging*, 42(4), 1056–1067.

Rosen, B.R., Buckner, R.L., Dale, A.M. (1998). Event-related functional MRI: Past, present, and future. *Proceedings of the National Academy of Sciences*, 95, 773–780.

Siepmann, M., Schmitz, G., Bzyl, J., Palmowski, M., Kiessling, F. (2011). Imaging tumor vascularity by tracing single microbubbles. *2011 IEEE International Ultrasonics Symposium*, 19069.

van Sloun, R.J., Solomon, O., Bruce, M., Khaing, Z.Z., Wijkstra, H., Eldar, Y.C., Mischi, M. (2020). Super-resolution ultrasound localization microscopy through deep learning. *IEEE Transactions on Medical Imaging*, 40, 829–839.

Song, P., Trzasko, J.D., Manduca, A., Huang, R., Kadirvel, R., Kallmes, D.F., Chen, S. (2017). Improved super-resolution ultrasound microvessel imaging with spatiotemporal nonlocal means filtering and bipartite graph-based microbubble tracking. *IEEE Transactions on Ultrasonics, Ferroelectrics, and Frequency Control*, 65(2), 149–167.

Soulioti, D.E., Espíndola, D., Dayton, P.A., Pinton, G.F. (2019). Super-resolution imaging through the human skull. *IEEE Transactions on Ultrasonics, Ferroelectrics, and Frequency Control*, 67, 25–36.

Tang, S., Song, P., Trzasko, J.D., Lowerison, M., Huang, C., Gong, P., Lok, U.-W., Manduca, A., Chen, S. (2020). Kalman filter-based microbubble tracking for robust super-resolution ultrasound microvessel imaging. *IEEE Transactions on Ultrasonics, Ferroelectrics and Frequency Control*, 67, 1738–1751.

Tanter, M. and Fink, M. (2014). Ultrafast imaging in biomedical ultrasound. *IEEE Transactions on Ultrasonics, Ferroelectrics, and Frequency Control*, 61, 102–119.

Tinevez, J.-Y., Perry, N., Schindelin, J., Hoopes, G.M., Reynolds, G.D., Laplantine, E., Bednarek, S.Y., Shorte, S.L., Eliceiri, K.W. (2017). TrackMate: An open and extensible platform for single-particle tracking. *Methods*, 115, 80–90.

Tranquart, F., Grenier, N., Eder, V., Pourcelot, L. (1999). Clinical use of ultrasound tissue harmonic imaging. *Ultrasound in Medicine & Biology*, 25, 88994.3.

Ueda, H.R., Ertürk, A., Chung, K., Gradinaru, V., Chédotal, A., Tomancak, P., Keller, P.J. (2020). Tissue clearing and its applications in neuroscience. *Nature Reviews Neuroscience*, 21, 61–79.

Viessmann, O.M., Eckersley, R.J., Christensen-Jeffries, K., Tang, M.X., Dunsby, C. (2013). Acoustic super-resolution with ultrasound and microbubbles. *Physics in Medicine & Biology*, 58, 6447.

Wang, Y., Li, X., Zhou, Y., Huang, P., Xu, Y. (2010). Preparation of nanobubbles for ultrasound imaging and intracelluar drug delivery. *International Journal of Pharmaceutics*, 384, 148–153.

Zhang, G., Harput, S., Lin, S., Christensen-Jeffries, K., Leow, C.H., Brown, J., Dunsby, C., Eckersley, R.J., Tang, M.-X. (2018). Acoustic wave sparsely activated localization microscopy (AWSALM): Super-resolution ultrasound imaging using acoustic activation and deactivation of nanodroplets. *Applied Physics Letters*, 113, 014101.

Zhang, J., Zhang, H., Yang, Y., He, Q., Qiu, L., Qian, L., Luo, J. (2021). In vivo assessment of diabetic kidney disease using ultrasound localization microscopy. *IEEE International Ultrasonics Symposium (IUS)*, 1–3.

Zhu, J., Yu, T., Li, Y., Xu, J., Qi, Y., Yao, Y., Ma, Y., Wan, P., Chen, Z., Li, X. et al. (2020). MACS: Rapid aqueous clearing system for 3D mapping of intact organs. *Advanced Science*, 7, 1903185.

8

Sources of Image Degradation and their Correlation in Single-sided Ultrasound Imaging of Heterogeneous Tissues

Guillaume RENAUD[1], Danai E. SOULIOTI[2] and Gianmarco PINTON[2]

[1] *Department of Imaging Physics, Delft University of Technology, The Netherlands*
[2] *Joint Department of Biomedical Engineering, University of North Carolina at Chapel Hill and North Carolina State University, USA*

8.1. Introduction

The generation of an ultrasound image, or echography, is based on determining the time it takes for a wave to propagate from a ultrasound transducer to a target (forward propagation) and the time for the resulting echo to return to the probe (backward propagation). Approaches for image reconstruction rely on assumptions of wave propagation in the region of interest that convert the travel time from the transducer to a target and from a target to the transducer into spatial maps or images from the echoes. These simplifying assumptions can be divided into three categories:

1) uniformity of the wave speed;

For a color version of all the figures in this chapter, see www.iste.co.uk/bridal/innovative.zip.

2) uniformity of attenuation;

3) absence of multiple scattering.

Even though complex heterogeneous media, such as the soft tissue in the human body, clearly violate these assumptions, ultrasound scanners are capable of producing exquisite images. Obtaining high-quality images depends on approaches that are either insensitive to these sources of image degradation or capable of correcting them.

With the continuous improvement of the quality of electronics, transducer sensitivity and image processing for optimizing display, the flaws in ultrasound images resulting from simplifying assumptions made during image reconstruction become more and more noticeable. Over the past 20 years, the development of software-based image reconstruction and large-bandwidth, high-frame-rate imaging hardware has enabled new imaging approaches (e.g. imaging of tissue stiffness with shear-wave elastography, ultrafast imaging of blood flow) and greatly improved the versatility of ultrasound imaging. Sophisticated image sequence design, such as synthetically focused ultrasound imaging, which stores digitized raw echo signals in computer memory and uses unfocused transmit beams instead of focused transmit beams, is straightforward to implement in a modern scanner. By lowering these technological barriers, there is a renewed focus on understanding and overcoming the underlying physical sources of image degradation that occur from the wave propagation physics and how it applies to the wide variety of image formation approaches.

Understanding and accounting for these physical sources of degradation remains a critical challenge in many applications of ultrasound imaging. Transcranial imaging, for example, remains a highly challenging environment for ultrasound imaging due to the strong acoustical barrier presented by the skull. Even in transabdominal imaging, a significant portion of patients are difficult to image due to thick layers of subcutaneous fat which obscure the underlying anatomy.

The potential offered due to the greater performance and increased versatility of ultrasound provides new arms with which to combat effects such as aberration or reverberation that can degrade ultrasound images. The objective of this chapter is to review the current state of knowledge on physical sources of image degradation within the medium and give possible future research directions to further improve image quality in medical ultrasound imaging. The architecture and performances of modern ultrasound systems provide us with a versatile technology that can be used to revisit pioneering work, improve it and perhaps even go far beyond it.

8.2. Sources of image degradation

Among all sources of image degradation, side lobes and grating lobes are well known. Their origin pertains to the finite size of the transducer aperture and the periodicity of the transducer array, respectively. Because their cause is not the heterogeneity of the scanned region, this issue will not be addressed in this chapter. For detailed information about the origin of side lobes and grating lobes, and solutions to reduce them, we refer the readers to Szabo (2013) and Shung (2015). This chapter concentrates on the sources of image degradation arising from the heterogeneity of the scanned region.

The focus will also be on conventional, i.e. single-sided ultrasound imaging, which relies on:

1) the transmission of a set of pulsed ultrasound beams in the region of interest with an array transducer;

2) the recording (for each transmission) of ultrasound waves scattered by heterogeneities in the region of interest, typically with the same array transducer;

3) the use of an algorithm for image reconstruction that processes the recorded scattered echo signals.

Tissue inhomogeneities create a variety of image artifacts. Some of them, in particular the edge shadowing artifact, the mirror-image artifact and the comet tail artifact, have been well described in the literature (see, for example, Chapter 5 in Hoskins et al. (2019)) and therefore will not be treated in this chapter.

8.2.1. *Aberration and aberrators*

8.2.1.1. *Definitions*

An aberration refers to a defect in the ultrasound image that is caused by an inaccurate description of ultrasound propagation. An aberrator refers to any sub-region in the scanned region of interest that causes an aberration. An aberrator typically engenders ultrasound wave phenomena that are more complex than the physics modeled in the algorithm for image reconstruction.

Aberrations are often studied in terms of amplitude aberration and phase aberration. Amplitude aberration refers to a departure of the performance of the ultrasound imaging system caused by an altered amplitude (compared to amplitude expected with the three major assumptions) of recorded ultrasound wavelets. Phase aberration refers to a departure of the performance of the ultrasound imaging system caused by the altered arrival time (or phase) of recorded ultrasound wavelets.

8.2.1.2. *Aberration in weakly and highly heterogeneous regions*

The wave speed in the region between the ultrasound transducer and the region of interest is always unknown in medical ultrasound imaging. Fortunately, the range of variation of the ultrasound wave speed in biological soft tissues is well known (1,400–1,700 m/s). An ultrasound scanner typically uses a constant value of 1,540 m/s during image reconstruction because this value is generally accepted as the average speed of sound in biological soft tissues. However, the actual average wave speed in the scanned region never equals 1,540 m/s. Even if the scanned region is weakly heterogeneous, using an incorrect average wave speed during image reconstruction leads to phase aberration, which leads to sub-optimal image reconstruction.

The situation becomes far more complicated if the scanned region is highly heterogeneous. The sub-region with the most atypical properties would be called the aberrator. It can be a layer (e.g. a fat layer under the skin or the bone layer of the skull) or a circumscribed area (e.g. a fat inclusion in the breast or a cyst). Two tissue types are responsible for most severe aberrations:

– fat, which has a low wave speed and a low mass density (1,400 m/s and 900 kg/m^3, respectively);

– bone, which has a high wave speed and a high mass density (1,600–4,200 m/s and 1,100–2,000 kg/m^3, exact values are highly dependent on porosity).

Typical situations where strong aberration can occur are:

– ultrasound imaging of organs in the abdomen due to adipose tissue beneath the skin (subcutaneous fat) and around organs (visceral fat);

– breast ultrasound imaging because breast tissue contains a large amount of adipose tissue (subcutaneous fat);

– transcranial ultrasound imaging of the brain due to the skull;

– intraosseous ultrasound imaging.

8.2.1.3. *Phase aberration: orders of magnitude and characterization*

An extended plane or spherical wavefront propagates in a homogeneous, non-attenuating medium without local distortion of its phase or amplitude. However, when propagating through a few centimeters of heterogeneous biological tissue, an extended wavefront experiences local distortion of its phase because its travels across regions with different wave speeds.

Figure 8.1 illustrates these effects with synthetic data generated numerically by propagating in a two-dimensional space the wavefront emitted by a point source located in the medium and received by a transducer array (128 elements, pitch equals 0.3 mm, center ultrasound frequency equals 5 MHz). This is equivalent to studying only the return trip of backscattered echoes (from targets to the transducer array) during pulse-echo ultrasound imaging. The aberration caused by a model of abdominal wall tissue is simulated.

A wavefront scattered by a target and recorded by a transducer array contains a geometric delay component that has a large curvature compared to the fluctuations caused by tissue heterogeneities. After geometric correction of the recorded wavefront, it is possible to extract the arrival time fluctuations caused by tissue heterogeneities, i.e. phase aberration (see Figure 8.1(e) and (f)).

Several research groups (Sumino and Waag 1991; Trahey et al. 1991; Freiburger et al. 1992; Liu and Waag 1995) have proposed to characterize the phase aberration by measuring the amplitude of the arrival time fluctuations and the spatial variation of wavefront distortion in the array aperture. The amplitude of the arrival time fluctuations is measured with the root-mean-square (rms) value, which characterizes the strength of the phase aberration. The spatial variation of wavefront distortion in the array aperture is measured with a correlation length defined as the full width at half-maximum of the autocorrelation function (in space) of the arrival time fluctuations, which characterizes the complexity of the phase aberration. It is possible to correct for the phase aberration (section 8.3.2) only if the transducer array can properly sample the spatial variation of the wavefront distortion. More specifically, the spatial period in the transducer array (pitch) must be smaller than the spatial correlation length of the aberration profile.

In the case shown in Figure 8.1, the rms value of the arrival time fluctuations is 56 ns and the spatial correlation length of the aberration profile is 4 mm. It is also worth noting that there exists an offset error in the arrival times with the abdominal wall, since all arrival times are larger than that expected in a uniform medium with a sound speed of 1,540 m/s. This means that the average sound speed in the abdominal wall model is slightly less than 1,540 m/s.

Experimental studies have reported arrival time fluctuations up to 100 ns as an ultrasound wave propagates through a 2 cm-thick layer of abdominal wall or breast (abdominal/body wall (O'Donnell and Flax 1988b; Sumino and Waag 1991; Hinkelman et al. 1994), breast (Trahey et al. 1991; Hinkelman et al. 1995)), with a root-mean-square value over the transducer aperture in the range 30–70 ns. The skull generates larger phase aberrations, up to 1 μs where the skull is the thickest (Marquet et al. 2009; Marsac et al. 2017). For diagnostic ultrasound, the temporal region of the skull is often used because it is thinner and the root-mean-square phase aberration over the transducer aperture is in the range of 50–150 ns for this region (Phillips et al. 1975b; Tanter et al. 1998; Lindsey and Smith 2013; Soulioti et al. 2020).

The correlation length measured for the abdominal wall or the breast was reported between 3 and 11 mm (Freiburger et al. 1992; Hinkelman et al. 1994). For the temporal bone of the skull, the correlation length was measured between 1 and 4 mm (Vignon et al. 2008; Lindsey and Smith 2013).

Thus, the phase aberration is most often stronger when imaging through the temporal bone of the skull than when imaging the breast or through the abdominal wall.

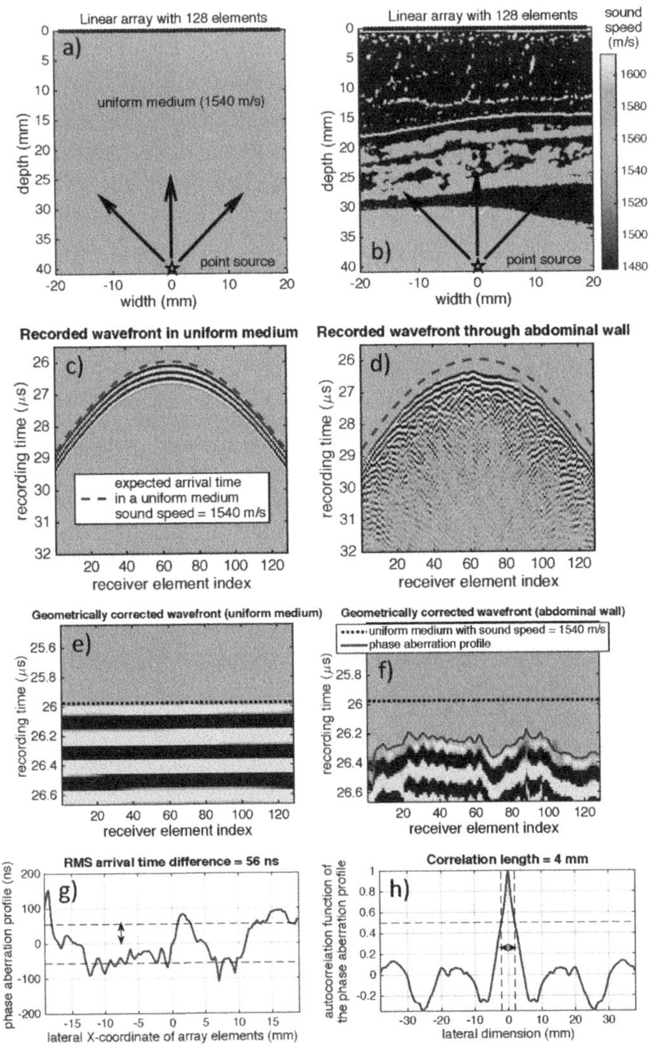

Figure 8.1. *Illustration of phase aberration during the return trip only (simulating backscattering from a point target is analogous to placing a point source in the medium). Synthetic signals were generated with a time-domain wave propagation solver through a) a uniform medium and b) an abdominal wall model. The wavefronts recorded by a transducer array are shown in c) and d). After geometric correction, the wavefront is perfectly flat in the uniform medium (e), while arrival time fluctuations remain as a result of phase aberration caused by the abdominal wall (f). The phase aberration profile is characterized by the rms value of the arrival time fluctuations (g) and the spatial correlation length (h)*

8.2.1.4. *Consequences of phase aberration on beam focusing, beam steering and image reconstruction*

It has been shown that the quality of in vivo liver scans is degraded when phase aberrations are strong (O'Donnell and Flax 1988b).

Traditional ultrasound imaging relies on the transmission of focused ultrasound beams. Beam focusing and steering is generated by delaying the emission of individual elements of the transducer array. The specific transmit delays are calculated such that all wavelets emitted by individual elements arrive at the same instant at the desired focal point. The accurate calculation of these transmit delays requires knowing the wave speed in the scanned area. Current medical ultrasound scanners assume a uniform wave speed of 1,540 m/s when calculating transmit delays. In the presence of strong aberrators (fat or bone), the calculation of transmit delays is obviously erroneous and leads to sub-optimal beam focusing and steering and hence poor image quality.

Phase aberration also has an important impact on image reconstruction. The most widely used algorithm for image reconstruction is delay-and-sum. Each image pixel is considered as a hypothetical scattering point. The reconstruction algorithm operates as a summation over the receive aperture of the transducer array of the recorded echo signals evaluated at the calculated round-trip travel times (see Chapter 2 of this book). For each image pixel, the calculated round-trip travel time is the sum of the forward travel time (from the transducer to the image pixel) and the return travel times (from the image pixel to each individual element of the transducer array). Current medical ultrasound scanners assume a uniform wave speed of 1,540 m/s to calculate the forward travel time and return travel times. As for transmit delays, in the presence of strong aberrators (fat or bone), the calculation of the forward travel time and return travel times is obviously incorrect and leads to sub-optimal image reconstruction.

8.2.1.5. *Amplitude aberration*

In addition to arrival time fluctuations (phase aberration), amplitude fluctuations are observed in a wavefront that traveled through heterogeneous tissue. They are created by the spatial variation of ultrasonic attenuation magnitude because different tissue types have different attenuation strengths. These amplitude fluctuations are also due to refraction and diffraction by tissue heterogeneities, which results in constructive or destructive phase interferences.

Experimental studies in soft tissues (through a 2 cm-thick abdominal wall) reported small-amplitude aberration (about 2–4 dB (O'Donnell and Flax 1988b; Hinkelman et al. 1994)). In contrast, the skull can produce large-amplitude aberrations of up to 20 dB (Tanter et al. 1998).

However, in recent work, it was shown that the correction of amplitude aberration results in a small improvement in image quality (Soulioti et al. 2020) compared to the correction of phase aberration. Most work in the literature is indeed focused on the correction of phase aberration. For this reason, this chapter will not discuss methods for the correction of amplitude aberration.

8.2.2. *Multiple scattering (reverberation)*

Wave speed and mass density heterogeneities can cause multiple scattering (or reverberation). In fact, aberrations and multiple scattering share the same cause, and they most often coexist. Multiple scattering is typically ignored during image reconstruction. Indeed, traditional image reconstruction assumes that echo signals are generated by a single interaction between the ultrasound pulse transmitted by a probe and scatterers in the medium. As a result, echoes arising from multiply scattered waves appear as clutter in the ultrasound image. A region made of multiple layers of different tissue types is often favorable to the generation of multiple scattering.

In a heterogeneous medium comprising various interfaces with large impedance mismatches, such as between fat and muscle, strong reflections may occur. Media with a layered structure, such as connective tissue, tend to trap acoustic energy, causing it to reverberate between layers. A portion of the trapped energy is transmitted back to the ultrasonic transducer, where it overlays acoustic noise onto its received signals.

When the tissue layers are nearly normal to the direction of wave propagation, the noise is visible in the ultrasonic image as bright bands that occur at integer multiples of the spatial period, or thickness, of the tissue layers. If the layers are not normal to the direction of propagation, the resulting reverberation is less coherent and appears as a haze overlaid on the B-mode (Brightness-mode) image. This behavior would be expected in higher body mass index patients where there are many connective tissue layer boundaries within the increased thickness of fat tissue (Pinton et al. 2011).

8.2.3. *Importance of the ultrasound frequency*

In general, the highest ultrasound frequency is desired to achieve the best spatial resolution in the ultrasound image. However, ultrasound attenuation increases with the ultrasound frequency. As a result, superficial imaging can use rather high frequencies (up to 15 MHz), while deep imaging is restricted to lower frequencies (close to 3 MHz). Besides the challenge of attenuation, increasing the ultrasound frequency may also further degrade image quality in heterogeneous tissues. While arrival time fluctuations are measured in nano- or microseconds, the impact of the phase aberration on image degradation depends on the ultrasound frequency. The magnitude of the phase aberration can also be expressed in radians or as a fraction of an ultrasound temporal period. Phase aberration causing arrival time fluctuations of T/10 or less, where T is the temporal period of the ultrasound wave, does not result in significant image degradation. Thus, imaging with a low ultrasound frequency is less impacted by phase aberration than imaging with a higher ultrasound frequency.

The ultrasound frequency also determines the magnitude of single and multiple diffuse scattering, i.e. scattering by small inhomogeneities. Indeed, diffuse scattering increases with the ultrasound frequency, particularly if the ultrasound wavelength becomes close to the mean size of the small inhomogeneities. For example, in transcranial imaging at 3 MHz, the ultrasound wavelength is close to 1 mm in cortical bone and the mean pore diameter in cortical bone was reported close to 90 μm in human skulls (Alexander et al. 2019). This means that the inhomogeneities in the dense bone tissue type of the skull are 10 times smaller than the wavelength. Using a higher ultrasound frequency for transcranial imaging would likely lead to enhanced clutter in the image due to enhanced multiple diffuse scattering.

8.2.4. *Illustration of the impact of aberration and multiple scattering on image quality with numerical simulations*

It is common practice to evaluate the performance of an imaging system using the point-spread function (PSF), i.e. the spatial impulse response of the imaging system. The PSF is obtained by producing a B-mode (Brightness-mode) image of a point target (sub-wavelength object). The PSF can be described as:

– a main central component, which determines axial and lateral spatial resolution in the ultrasound image;

– secondary components expanding from the main component with smaller amplitude, which determine contrast resolution in the ultrasound image.

Image quality is optimal if the spatial extent of the main central component is as small as possible and if the amplitude of secondary components is as weak as possible.

A schematic of typical PSFs in different media, as well as transmit and receive wavefronts for a plane or focused transmit beam are shown in Figure 8.2. In a homogeneous medium (left column), the wave is transmitted and received by the transducer without any disturbance; thus, an ideal PSF is produced. If we consider a hypothetical medium where aberration is present, but multiple scattering is absent (isoimpedance medium), the effects in the middle column are seen. Refraction causes distortion of the wavefront on transmit and receive; thus, the final PSF is degraded in shape and size and may also present registration errors in both directions. Lastly, when multiple scattering is present, but sound speed inhomogeneity is artificially absent (isovelocity medium), the PSF is no longer distorted in shape; however, a hazing effect is introduced due to multipath reverberations caused by reflections of the pulse at different medium layers (right column). Some portion of the energy is reflected towards the transducer, but a portion is also reflected towards the point target, causing the transmit waveform to become elongated, which causes trailing clutter to appear behind the main component of the PSF.

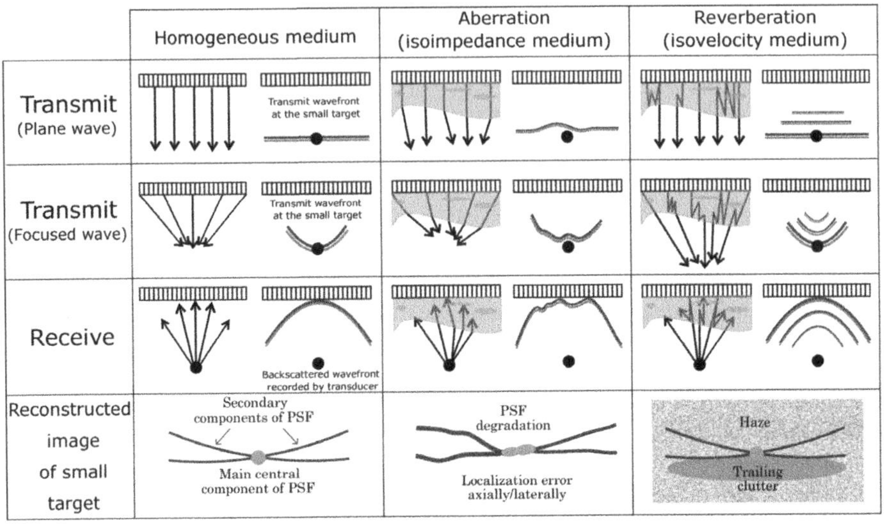

Figure 8.2. *Schematic representation of wave propagation in a homogeneous, isoimpedance and isovelocity medium. Two different transmit schemes, plane wave and focused wave, are shown. The transmit wavefront reaching the point target and the wavefront received at the transducer array are depicted for all cases. The reconstructed image of the small target in different media is shown in the bottom row*

Figure 8.3 illustrates transabdominal sound speed maps and B-mode images simulated using the Fullwave (Pinton et al. 2009a) numerical solver for a curved transducer at 3.7 MHz. Figure 8.3(A) is the input sound speed map used in the simulation which is segmented from the Visible Human Project optical dataset (see: https://www.nlm.nih.gov/research/visible/visible_human.html) and processed by assigning tabulated values to known structures such as fat, muscle and connective tissue. To simulate compression typically exerted by the sonographer during abdominal imaging, an arc following the shape of the transducer has been introduced to the maps. To accurately simulate tissue response, random scatterers are placed throughout the abdomen. Figure 8.3(B)–(E) all use a 3.7 MHz, two-cycle single-transmit emission focused at the depth of a point target, marked in red in Figure 8.3A. Image reconstruction is performed using a conventional delay-and-sum algorithm. Figure 8.3(B) shows an emission in a homogeneous medium, while Figure 8.3(C) shows the same target through the abdominal wall. The effects of aberration can be seen on the target. Reverberation has a more localized effect, mainly affecting the first 40 mm of the B-mode image. In Figure 8.3(D), in order to remove phase aberration, the sound speed maps of the abdominal wall are set to be constant, while the density maps remain unchanged. This results in an isovelocity B-mode image showing the effects of reverberation. To obtain an isoimpedance B-mode image, where the effects of reverberation are diminished, we performed a linear subtraction of the image obtained with an additional simulation through the abdominal wall, but without the target (not shown) from the image shown in Figure 8.3(C). This results in Figure 8.3(E), where multiple reverberations except trailing clutter are removed, but the effects of aberration are still intact.

A very similar process, as described for Figure 8.3, was used when generating Figure 8.4. A human skull was scanned with X-ray computed tomography and then converted to speed of sound, density and attenuation maps through a linear Hounsfield to density transformation (Lagravere et al. 2006). Figure 8.4(A) shows the sound speed map used in the full-wave simulations. A point target was placed at 50 mm and a full-aperture, single-transmit focused emission was used. The transmit frequency in this case is 2.5 MHz. As described before, homogeneous (see Figure 8.4(B)), heterogeneous (see Figure 8.4(C)), isovelocity (see Figure 8.4(D)) and isoimpedance (see Figure 8.4(E)) B-mode images show the effects of aberration and reverberation collectively and separately. In transcranial imaging, aberration is well known and extensively characterized as a source of image distortion. Reverberation also degrades image quality, and it reduces the target amplitude and compromises spatial resolution. Reverberation effects are more pronounced at shallower depths, but their contribution persists even at depths larger than 6 cm, as shown in Figure 8.4(C).

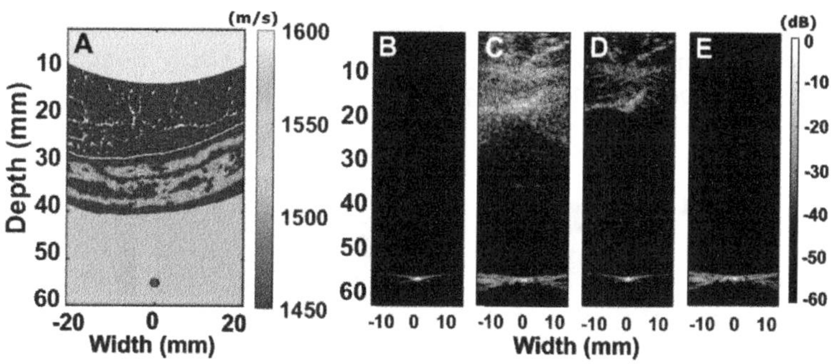

Figure 8.3. *(A) Speed of sound map for the human abdominal wall. (B)–(E) B-mode images for a target 55 mm from the transducer normalized by the maximum amplitude of the homogeneous case. The transducer was apodized at half the aperture. (B) is the B-mode image obtained through a homogeneous medium. (C) is the B-mode image obtained through the heterogeneous abdominal wall. (D) is the isovelocity B-mode image. (E) is the isoimpedance B-mode image obtained through clutter subtraction*

To illustrate the depth dependency of reverberation and its effect on image quality, a point target was placed at three different depths, namely 30, 50 and 70 mm, for the same map shown in Figure 8.5(A). At the shallow depth in Figure 8.5(B), reverberation completely compromises the target, whereas at 70 mm (Figure 8.5(D)), aberration is practically the sole degrading mechanism. At 50 mm, both mechanisms appear to contribute to the degradation. Trailing clutter is the result of the pulse lengthening with propagation and is independent of depth; thus, it persists in all cases.

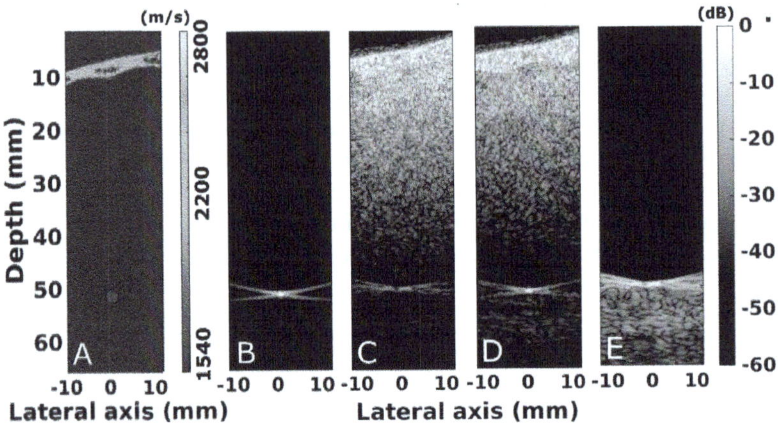

Figure 8.4. *(A) Speed of sound map for a CT-derived human skull slice. (B)–(E) B-mode images for a target at 50 mm from the transducer normalized by the maximum amplitude of the homogeneous case. (B) is the homogeneous B-mode. (C) is the heterogeneous B-mode through the skull. (D) is the isovelocity B-mode. (E) is the isoimpedance B-mode obtained through clutter subtraction*

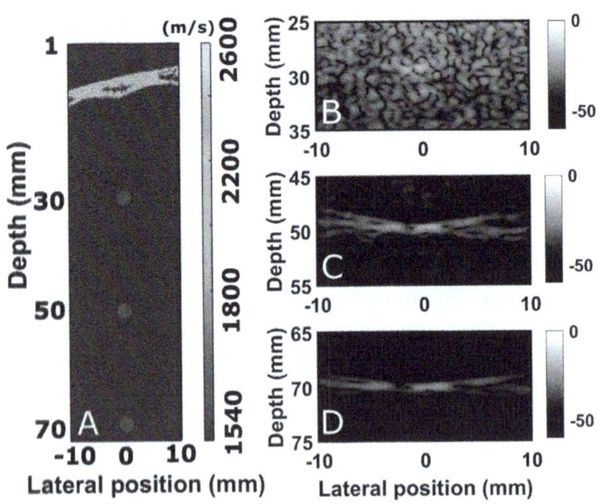

Figure 8.5. *(A) Illustration of sound speed maps for imaging point targets through the human skull at three different depths, namely: (B), at 3 cm; (C), at 5 cm and (D), at 7 cm. No aberration correction has been applied. Gray scale units are in normalized dB*

8.2.5. *Anisotropic elasticity in bone*

Ultrasound imaging of structures within bones or behind bones is very challenging, in particular because of the large wave speed difference between mineralized bone tissue and soft tissues. In addition to this, the elasticity of bone tissue is anisotropic, which results in wave speed anisotropy. The least porous type of bone tissue, called compact or cortical bone, has been the most studied (Yoon and Lawrence Katz 1976; Ashman et al. 1984; Peterson and Dechow 2003; Granke et al. 2011). The anisotropic elasticity of cortical bone is well approximated by a model of transverse isotropy. For the diaphysis of a long bone, the symmetry axis is nearly aligned with the bone axis (see Figure 8.6), it corresponds to the direction of maximum compressional wave speed. In any direction normal to the symmetry axis, the compressional wave speed is about 20% smaller. Transcranial ultrasound imaging is performed through the squamous part of the temporal bone of the skull, which is often a single layer of cortical bone. The elasticity of this region of the temporal bone can be approximated with transverse isotropy; however, the symmetry axis (which corresponds to the direction of maximum compressional wave speed) was shown to be inconsistent among specimens (Peterson and Dechow 2003).

In a medium with elastic anisotropy, the wave speed is described by two parameters, the phase velocity and the group velocity. A compressional wave has a quasi-longitudinal polarization and its phase velocity v_P is determined by four parameters α_0, β_0, ε and δ^* (Thomsen 1986):

$$v_P(\theta) = \alpha_0 \left[1 + \varepsilon \cos^2(\theta) + D^*\Big(\theta, \alpha_0, \beta_0, \varepsilon, \delta^*\Big)\right]^{1/2} \quad [8.1]$$

$$D^* = \frac{1}{2}\left(1 - \frac{\beta_0^2}{\alpha_0^2}\right) \times \left[\left(1 + \frac{4\delta^* \cos^2(\theta)\sin^2(\theta)}{(1-\beta_0^2/\alpha_0^2)^2} + \frac{4(1-\beta_0^2/\alpha_0^2+\varepsilon)\varepsilon}{(1-\beta_0^2/\alpha_0^2)^2}\cos^4(\theta)\right)^{1/2} - 1\right] \quad [8.2]$$

$$\alpha_0 = \sqrt{\frac{C_{33}}{\rho}} \quad [8.3]$$

$$\beta_0 = \sqrt{\frac{C_{44}}{\rho}} \quad [8.4]$$

$$\varepsilon = \frac{C_{11} - C_{33}}{2C_{33}} \quad [8.5]$$

$$\delta^* = \frac{1}{2C_{33}^2}\Big(2(C_{13}+C_{44})^2 - (C_{33}-C_{44})(C_{11}+C_{33}-2C_{44})\Big) \quad [8.6]$$

α_0 and β_0 are the phase velocities of a compression wave and a shear wave with vertical polarization, respectively, in the direction of the symmetry axis. ε and δ^* are two parameters of anisotropy. These four parameters are determined by the elastic stiffnesses C_{ij} and the mass density ρ. θ is the phase angle between the wave vector and the plane of isotropy (i.e. a plane perpendicular to the axis of symmetry, see Figure 8.6).

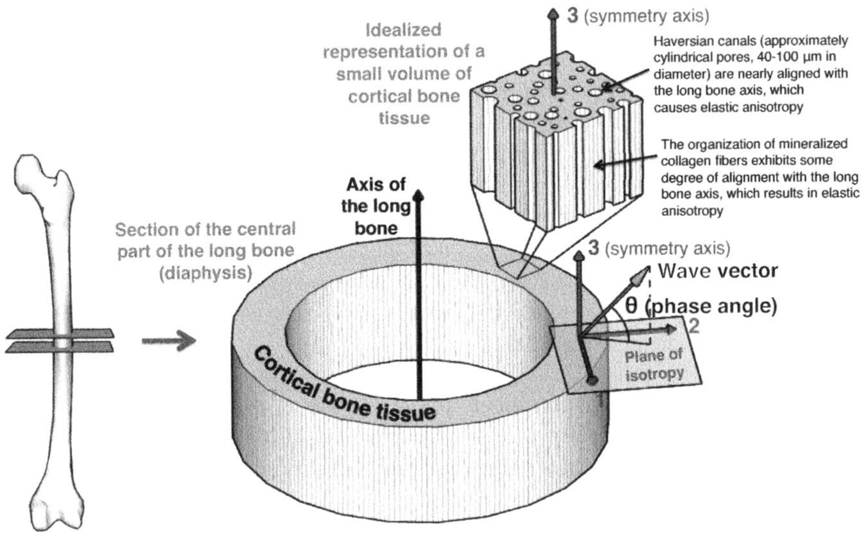

Figure 8.6. *Simplified representation of a section of the central part (diaphysis) of a long bone (e.g. humerus, radius, femur, tibia bones). The local symmetry axis of the cortical bone tissue (coordinate axis 3) is nearly aligned with the long bone axis. The plane (1,2) (or any plane perpendicular to the symmetry axis) is a plane of wave speed isotropy. θ is the phase angle between the wave vector and the plane of isotropy*

During ultrasound image reconstruction, we need the group velocity V (or ray velocity) and group angle ϕ (or ray angle). These can be calculated as follows (Thomsen 1986):

$$\tan\Big(\phi(\theta)\Big) = \left(\tan\theta + \frac{1}{v}\frac{\partial v}{\partial \theta}\right) \Big/ \left(1 - \frac{\tan\theta}{v}\frac{\partial v}{\partial \theta}\right) \qquad [8.7]$$

$$V^2\Big(\phi(\theta)\Big) = v^2(\theta) + \left(\frac{\partial v}{\partial \theta}\right)^2 \qquad [8.8]$$

where v is the phase velocity of a shear or a compression wave (equation [8.1]) and θ is the corresponding phase angle.

Equation [8.1] can be used for image reconstruction, but a weak-anisotropy simplification proposed by seismologists (Thomsen 1986) is advantageous because it reduces computation time. If $|\delta^*| \ll 1$ and $|\varepsilon| \ll 1$, after full linearization of equations [8.1] and [8.2], the group velocity of a compression wave V_P can be approximated as:

$$V_P(\phi) = V_P^{axial} - (V_P^{axial} - V_P^{radial}) \times \left[\xi \sin^2(\phi)\cos^2(\phi) + \cos^4(\phi)\right] \quad [8.9]$$

ϕ is the group angle. $V_P^{radial} = \sqrt{C_{11}/\rho}$ is the compression wave speed in the plane of isotropy of cortical bone. $V_P^{axial} = \alpha_0 = \sqrt{C_{33}/\rho}$ is the compression wave speed in the direction of the symmetry axis of cortical bone. It is worth noting that $V_P^{radial} = V_P(\phi = 0) = v_P(\theta = 0)$ and $V_P^{axial} = V_P(\phi = \pi/2) = v_P(\theta = \pi/2)$. ξ is an anisotropy form parameter. Even though the conditions $|\delta^*| \ll 1$ and $|\varepsilon| \ll 1$ are not properly fulfilled in bone, it was shown that equation [8.9] allows ultrasound image reconstruction of the bone cortex with satisfying accuracy (Renaud et al. 2018), and it is computationally efficient for real-time imaging.

Figure 8.7 illustrates the wave speed anisotropy of a compressional wave (or P-wave) in cortical bone.

Typical properties for human cortical bone (Bernard et al. 2016) were used to compute the wave speed anisotropy. It is seen that the compressional wave speed reaches a maximum value close to 4 mm/µs in the direction of the symmetry axis (i.e. approximately oriented along the main axis of a long bone for cortical bone tissue at the central part of the long bone). In a direction normal to the symmetry axis (i.e. a direction approximately perpendicular to the outer surface of a long bone at its midsection), the compressional wave speed exhibits a minimum value close to 3 mm/µs. For an oblique direction, unlike in a medium with isotropic elasticity, a plane wavefront generated by a planar transducer does not propagate in a direction normal to the surface of the transducer.

8.2.6. *Attenuation heterogeneity (shadowing and enhancement)*

Traditional B-mode imaging assumes that the backscattered echo amplitude (and thus brightness in the image) is determined by the target reflectivity. However, the backscattered echo amplitude is also influenced by the intrinsic attenuation of the tissues. During image reconstruction, the amplitude of echo signals is corrected assuming a uniform intrinsic attenuation, using an average value for biological soft tissue (0.5–1 dB/cm/MHz). If the ultrasound wave propagates through an inclusion with different intrinsic attenuation, the image brightness of the tissue surrounding this inclusion will not be constant. More specifically, the region deeper than the inclusion but right behind it will appear with a different brightness when it should not since the inclusion is surrounded with the same tissue type. This situation is often encountered due to the presence of a fluid-filled cyst, which exhibits much lower intrinsic attenuation compared to soft tissues. As a result, the region right behind the cyst shows enhanced brightness and can be misleading.

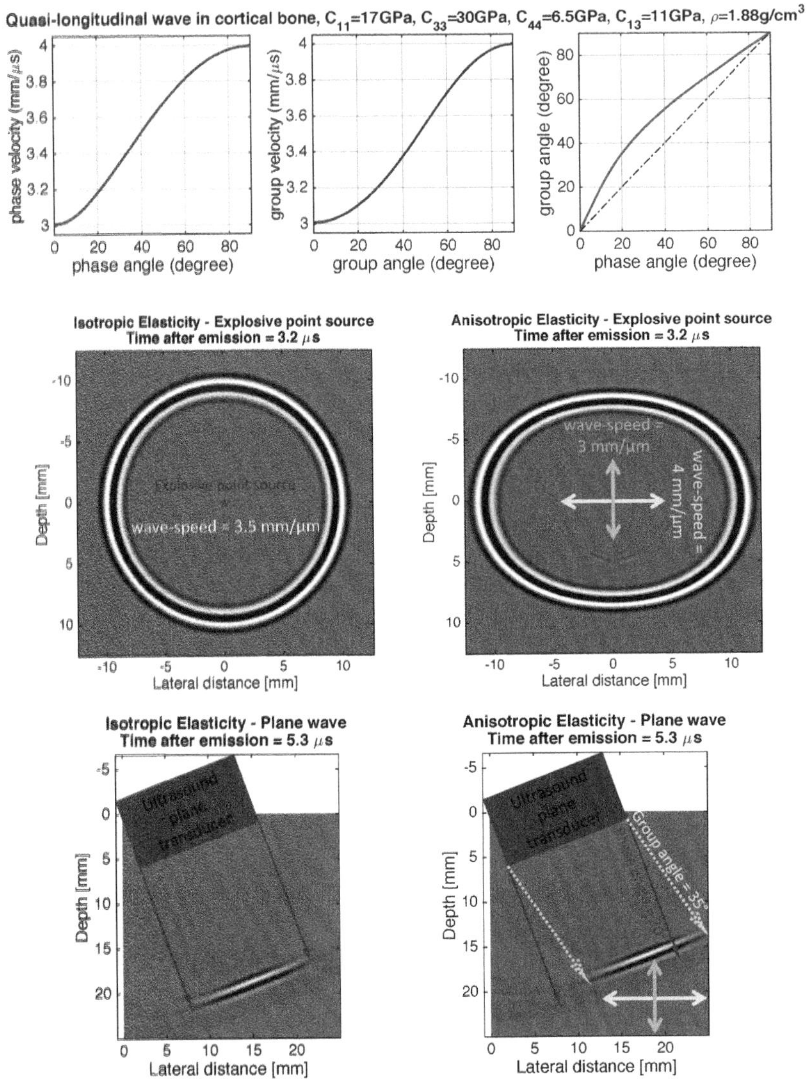

Figure 8.7. *Illustration of wave speed anisotropy for a compressional wave in human cortical bone. Top: phase and group velocities as functions of phase and group angles (phase angle $\theta = 90^o$ or group angle $\phi = 90^o$ corresponds to the direction of the symmetry axis). Middle: propagation of a wavefront generated by an explosive point source in a medium with isotropic and anisotropic elasticity. Bottom: propagation of a plane wavefront generated by a plane ultrasound transducer in a medium with isotropic and anisotropic elasticity*

Conversely, a small region of calcified tissue (atherosclerotic plaque calcification, tendon calcification or bone) causes large reflection and attenuation loss. As a result, the deeper region just beyond the calcification shows highly reduced brightness. Although image reading is not possible in this strongly shadowed area, this artifact is useful to detect a calcification. An example using simulations is shown in Figure 8.8. An anechoic lesion containing a lossless fluid is present in homogeneously attenuating tissue (1 dB/cm/MHz), as shown in image (A). In image (B), the calcification-like structure creates a shadow, making structures right behind the calcification indiscernible.

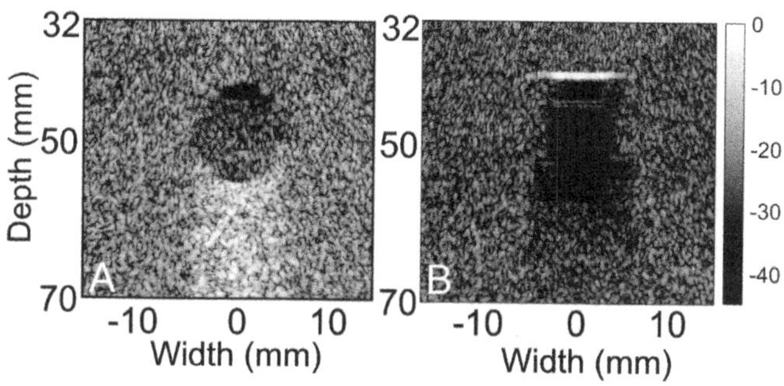

Figure 8.8. *B-mode image generated from a 5.5 MHz plane-wave emission of (A) a 10 mm diameter anechoic, lossless lesion in a homogeneously attenuating medium (1 dB/cm/MHz) and (B) a calcification-like structure with an attenuation value of 10 dB/cm/MHz. Gray scale unit is in normalized dB*

8.3. Correction methods

8.3.1. *Need for correction techniques in diagnostic ultrasound*

The problem of phase aberration was extensively studied with the development of therapeutic applications of ultrasound, in particular for transcranial high-intensity focused ultrasound. Several solutions have been proposed to efficiently correct phase aberrations caused by the skull, for example, the use of a 3D scan of the skull made with X-ray computed tomography or magnetic resonance imaging to estimate, and subsequently correct for, phase aberrations.

Transcranial diagnostic ultrasound is, in fact, more challenging than transcranial therapeutic high-intensity focused ultrasound, for the following reasons:

– While a low ultrasound frequency (1 MHz) is considered optimal for transcranial therapeutic ultrasound, a higher ultrasound frequency ($\geq$ 3 MHz) is desired for transcranial diagnostic ultrasound in order to achieve satisfying spatial resolution.

– In transcranial therapeutic ultrasound, only forward propagation is considered and hence ultrasound traverses the skull once. In contrast, for transcranial diagnostic ultrasound, ultrasound waves experience phase aberrations twice, during both forward and backward propagation.

– Transcranial therapeutic ultrasound typically uses a highly focused beam. As a result, reverberation has low impact. In contrast, transcranial diagnostic ultrasound uses weakly focused beams and relies on the processing of small-amplitude echo signals. In this situation, reverberation caused by the skull becomes an important problem.

Diagnostic transcranial ultrasound imaging is routinely performed in hospitals. Unfortunately, image quality achieved with current clinical ultrasound scanners is poor because the effect of the skull is ignored during image reconstruction. Several solutions have been investigated in the past four decades, but none of them have reached implementation in a clinical ultrasound scanner so far, for diagnostic transcranial ultrasound imaging. With the advent of ultrafast ultrasound imaging, which relies on the use of unfocused transmit beams and synthetic focusing, new achievements have recently been made for cerebral blood flow measurements (Demené et al. 2021). In addition, ultrasound imaging of the cortex of long bones (Renaud et al. 2018) and ultrasound quantification of intraosseous blood flow (Salles et al. 2021) was recently demonstrated.

Several manufacturers of clinical ultrasound systems offer some degree of correction of the effect of the lower sound speed in fat in abdominal and breast exams. Many machine vendors also offer a technique that reduces multiple scattering occurring near the transducer, called tissue harmonic imaging (see section 8.15). Unfortunately, despite these dedicated developments, a significant number of patients remain difficult to scan (Philips-Healthcare 2008).

8.3.2. *Correction of phase aberration*

8.3.2.1. *Uniform sound speed correction*

Several modern ultrasound scanners offer automatic determination of the sound speed in the region of interest (Napolitano et al. 2006; Treeby et al. 2011; Gyöngy and Kollár 2015). This provides optimal image reconstruction if the scanned region is nearly homogeneous (i.e. weak aberration). One approach consists of reconstructing the image for different values of sound speed. The estimate of the sound speed is the value that provides the image with the largest sharpness. There exist multiple metrics of sharpness, for example, the normalized variance of the pixel intensity in the image or metrics based on spatial gradients (Treeby et al. 2011).

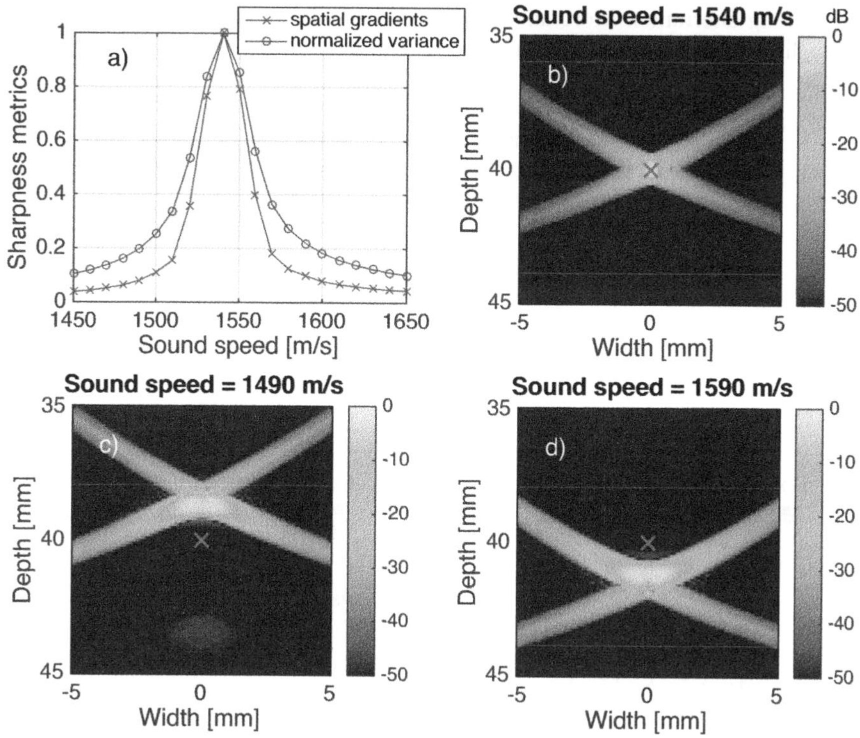

Figure 8.9. *Illustration of a method for estimating the sound speed in a homogeneous medium (same data as in Figure 8.1). (a) The sharpness metrics (normalized variance of the pixel intensity and spatial gradients in the image) as a function of the sound speed are shown. They peak for a sound speed of 1,540 m/s, which is the true sound speed in this numerical model. (b)–(d) The reconstructed images for three different values of sound speed are shown. The cross indicates the true position of the point source*

The synthetic data set for a uniform medium obtained with a numerical wave propagation solver shown in Figure 8.1(a) and (c) is used to illustrate the use of metrics of image sharpness to estimate the sound speed. The true sound speed in this numerical model is 1,540 m/s. Figure 8.9 shows that if the sound speed is larger or smaller than this value, the two metrics of image sharpness decrease.

When using the synthetic data set for the abdominal wall model (see Figure 8.1(b) and (d)), the two metrics of image sharpness show multiple peaks, as shown in Figure 8.10. The optimal image sharpness is found for a sound speed of 1,490 m/s. However, the image quality obtained with a sound speed of 1,490 m/s (see Figure 8.10(c)) is not significantly improved, compared to the image reconstructed with a default sound speed of 1,540 m/s. Therefore, the approach fails in medium with rather strong aberration. More advanced techniques are required to improve image quality, like those described in the following sections.

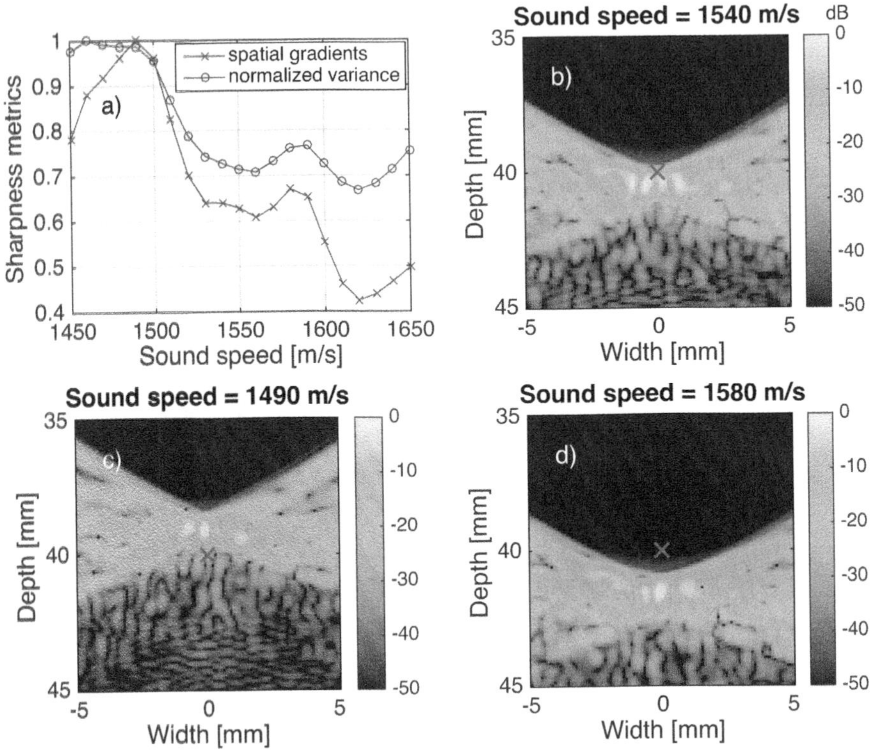

Figure 8.10. *Illustration of a method for estimating the average sound speed with the abdominal wall model (same data as in Figure 8.1). (a) The sharpness metrics (normalized variance of the pixel intensity and spatial gradients in the image) as a function of the sound speed are shown. Multiple peaks are found. (b)–(d) The reconstructed images for three different values of sound speed are shown. The cross indicates the true position of the point source*

8.3.2.2. *"Blind" methods, not trying to describe the medium geometry or estimate a sound speed map*

The only approaches for aberration correction that reached real-time implementation on an ultrasound scanner use a near-field phase screen model (Trahey et al. 1990; Liu et al. 2000; Rigby et al. 2000; Dahl et al. 2006). This model is simple, and it assumes that the distortion of the received wavefront is predominantly caused by a thin aberrating layer very near the transducer surface. This approach was very recently released on a clinical system, without any reduction of imaging rate (Masoy et al. 2022).

Early studies proposed to estimate arrival time fluctuations in the receiving aperture (after geometric correction of the arrival time) by means of two techniques:

– cross-correlations between raw echo signals recorded by individual elements of the transducer array (O'Donnell and Flax 1988a);

– iterative adjustment of the transmit and receive phasing of individual or groups of elements in order to reach maximum brightness of the speckle in a region of interest (Nock et al. 1989).

The two approaches and another one that used a waveform similarity factor as a quality factor (instead of the regional speckle brightness) (Liu et al. 2000) are in fact equivalent since they all try to realign the arrival times of the echo signals in the receive aperture (Ng et al. 1994).

It is interesting to note that the techniques can be applied to the wavefront arising from a small bright target (e.g. a small calcification) or from the focal region in tissue (with sub-wavelength heterogeneities) with transmit beam focusing (van Cittert–Zernike theorem (Mallart and Fink 1994)).

The synthetic data sets obtained with the numerical wave propagation solver shown in Figure 8.1 are now used to illustrate the cross-correlation technique, as described in Rigby et al. (2000). The method correlates individual element signals with a common reference signal, called the beamsum, obtained by summing all echo signals in the receive aperture (after geometric correction of the arrival time). Once the arrival time fluctuations are estimated, element-based time shifting of the echoes improves focusing, as shown in Figure 8.11. Traditional ultrasound imaging relies on the transmission of focused beams. Phase aberration correction improves focusing both in transmit and receive. Because phase aberration correction improves the shape of the transmit focused beam, the technique can be implemented iteratively in order to improve the estimation of the arrival time fluctuations (Rigby et al. 2000). A limitation of this technique is that the resulting image may be linearly translated to some unknown amount from its correct position, as shown in Figure 8.11(d) (Rachlin 1990).

The acoustic inhomogeneities (mass density and wave speed) are often not only located near the array transducer, but also distributed in the region of interest. As a result, the received wavefront is not only distorted by local time-shifting, its amplitude and shape are also distorted through diffraction, refraction and multiple scattering. Applying a near-field phase screen model to a medium with distributed aberration provides optimal phase aberration correction only in a limited region, called the isoplanatic patch. Because the size of the isoplanatic patch is often smaller than the size of the scanned volume, phase aberration correction must be applied to multiple sub-regions of the scanned volume (Lindsey and Smith 2013). Generally, the stronger the aberration, the smaller the size of the isoplanatic patch.

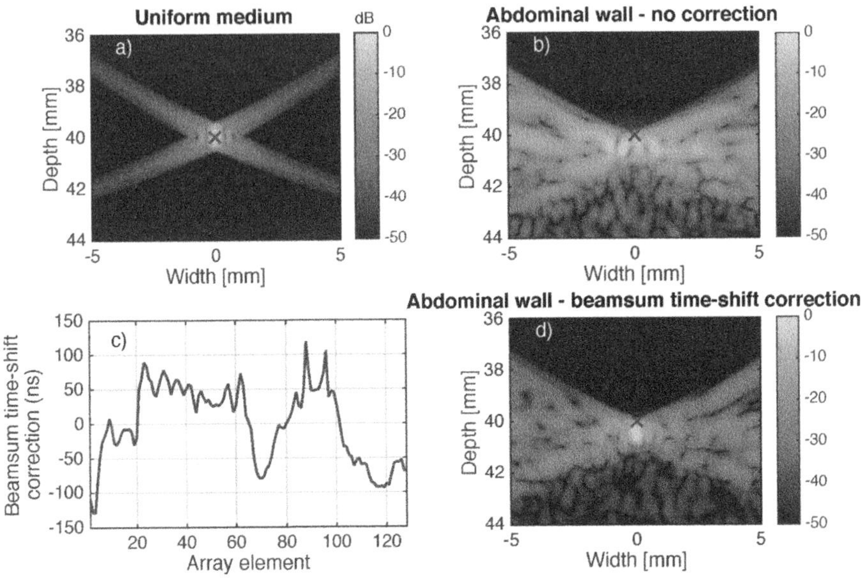

Figure 8.11. *Illustration of a phase aberration correction method, called the cross-correlation method. (a) and (b) The reconstructed images of a point source are shown using the same synthetic data sets shown in Figure 8.1, in a perfectly homogeneous medium and behind an abdominal wall model. (c) The aberration profile obtained with a cross-correlation method called beamsum is shown (Rigby et al. 2000). (d) The improvement of the reconstructed image of the point source behind the abdominal wall model is shown when element-based time shifting of the echoes is applied using the aberration profile shown in (c). The cross indicates the true position of the point source*

An improvement of the near-field phase screen model was proposed by Liu and Waag (1994). It consists of moving the phase screen in depth by backpropagating the echo signals recorded by the transducer array. The optimal depth of the phase screen is obtained by maximizing a waveform similarity factor.

Perhaps the most advanced technique is based on time-reversal acoustics (Montaldo et al. 2011). An iterative procedure relying on the broadcasting of the time-reversed version of echo signals recorded by individual transducer elements is capable of retrieving the Green's function between a point in the scanned volume and the transducer array in a heterogeneous medium. However, the technique requires sophisticated equipment since the ultrasound scanner must be able to send a time-reversed version of echo signals back to the medium. This approach allows for correction of all sources of aberration (diffraction, refraction and multiple scattering); however, optimal aberration correction is still restricted to a limited region (isoplanatic patch). Nonetheless, very recent work has proposed a method to estimate pixel-based optimal focusing delays, therefore potentially reducing the size of the isoplanatic patch to a single image pixel (Lambert et al. 2020). It relies on the construction of a distortion matrix and its time-reversal analysis, which enables the estimation of a transmission matrix between each array element and each image pixel.

Transcranial ultrasound imaging through the temporal bone of the skull is very challenging because the skull generates strong aberration. The near-field phase screen approach was investigated for transcranial ultrasound imaging with limited success (Ivancevich et al. 2008). Another approach using two transducers placed over opposing temporal acoustic windows was proposed (Phillips et al. 1975a; Vignon et al. 2006; Lindsey and Smith 2013). In this approach, the aberration profile can be learned near the receiving transducer one-way, through transmission between the two transducers. Nonetheless, the phase aberration correction remained optimal in a sub-region of the image. Therefore, the phase aberration correction had to be performed in multiple sub-regions of the scanned volume (multiple isoplanatic patches) (Lindsey and Smith 2013).

8.3.2.3. *Descriptive methods trying to determine the medium geometry and estimate a sound speed map*

Instead of assuming that aberration is predominantly caused by a thin layer very near the transducer, it was proposed to describe aberration as being caused by a layer with a finite thickness in contact with the transducer (Smith et al. 1986; Lindsey and Smith 2014). The scanned volume is then described with two homogeneous layers with different sound speeds. The advantage compared to the near-field phase screen model is that refraction through the aberrating layer is taken into account. In fact, this approach aimed to solve the problem of isoplanatic patch of near-field phase screen techniques (see section 8.3.2.2). However, these first attempts had limited success, likely because the thickness of the aberrating layer was assumed constant and its value is predetermined by the operator. The sound speed in the aberrating layer was also predetermined by the operator. In addition, the aberrating layer was considered parallel to the surface of the transducer and in contact with the transducer.

Recently, this approach was extended to an aberrating layer whose thickness was not assumed constant and parallel to the transducer. The near and far surfaces of the aberrating layer were searched during the image reconstruction. Each layer was assumed homogeneous, and the sound speed was estimated in each layer with a technique similar to the approach described in section 8.3.2.1. As a result, refraction is more accurately modeled. The approach was applied to intraosseous ultrasound imaging for imaging the central part of a long bone (Renaud et al. 2018) and transcranial ultrasound imaging through the temporal window (Mozaffarzadeh et al. 2022a, 2022b, 2022c). Figure 8.12 shows an example of in vivo images of the cortex of the central part of a human tibia.

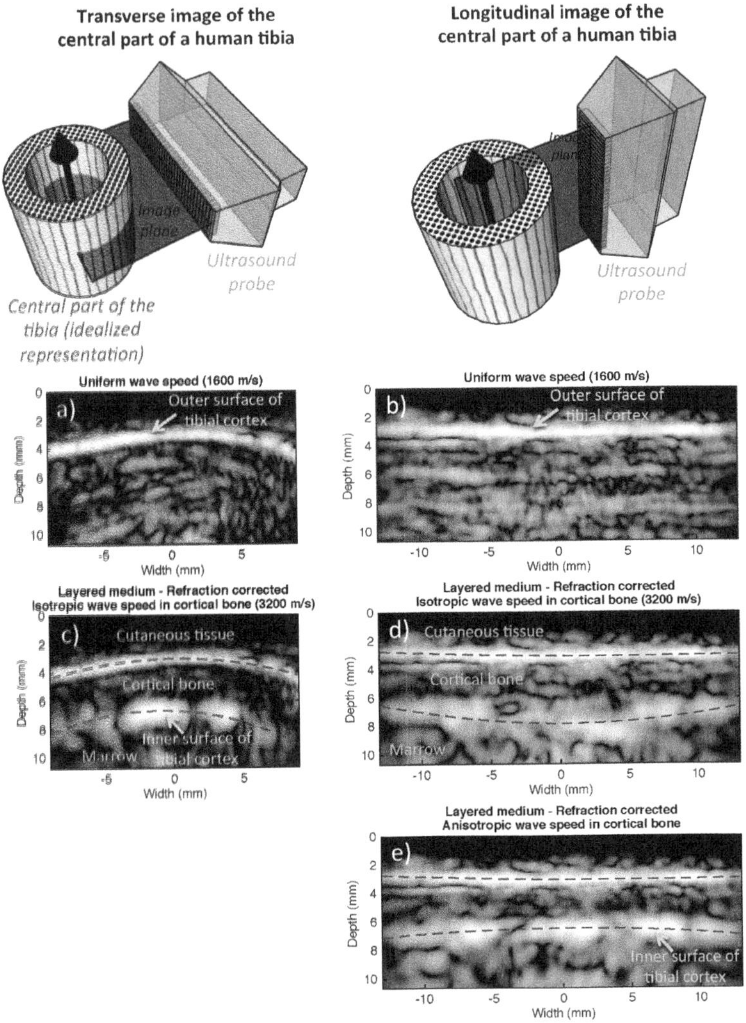

Figure 8.12. *In vivo images of the cortex of the central part of a human tibia obtained with synthetic aperture imaging. A phased array transducer with 96 elements was used, and the center frequency of the transmit short burst was 2.5 MHz. (a) and (b) Transverse and longitudinal images as obtained with traditional image reconstruction (uniform wave speed) are shown. (c) and (d) Transverse and longitudinal images obtained are shown when the medium is described with two layers (cutaneous tissue and cortical bone). The wave speed in cortical bone is isotropic. (e) The correction of wave speed anisotropy demonstrates improved image of the bone cortex. The displayed dynamic range is 40 dB*

Finally, a last family of techniques (Jaeger et al. 2015; Sanabria et al. 2018) attempts to recover a sound speed map of the scanned region similarly to ultrasound tomography (Wiskin et al. 2019), which required dedicated equipment capable of transmitting and receiving ultrasound waves all around the scanned object, but with single-sided pulse-echo ultrasound imaging.

8.3.3. *Correction of anisotropic elasticity in bone*

The anisotropic elasticity of cortical bone makes ultrasound image reconstruction more challenging in a region including the bone than in a region consisting only of heterogeneous soft tissues. The transmission of a plane wave, scattering by a small point target at 14 mm depth, and recording with a 2.5 MHz phased-array transducer, was simulated numerically with SimSonic software (Bossy et al. 2002). The wave speed anisotropy in cortical bone was modeled with the parameters used to plot Figure 8.7. Figure 8.13 compares the PSF in (a) an ideal uniform medium with a wave speed of 1.5 mm/µs, (b) cortical bone with wave speed anisotropy modeled during image reconstruction and (c) cortical bone with wave speed anisotropy ignored during image reconstruction. A significant degradation of the PSF occurs in cortical bone if wave speed anisotropy is ignored. Figure 8.14 similarly shows the degradation of the PSF in a region of soft tissue separated from the transducer by a layer of cortical bone (5 mm thick). The images in Figures 8.13(b) and 8.14(b) are reconstructed with the approach described in Renaud et al. (2018, 2020), which can take into account refraction and wave speed anisotropy in a layered medium.

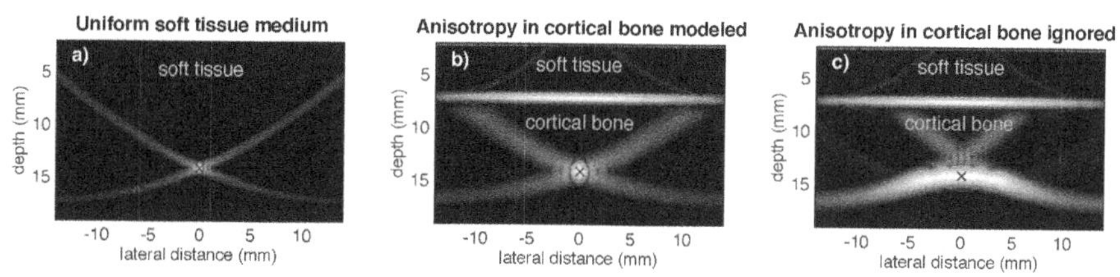

Figure 8.13. *Illustration of the importance of wave speed anisotropy in cortical bone with in silico data. PSF obtained from a point target at a 14-mm depth (shown by a red cross) in (a) a uniform medium with isotropic wave speed (1.5 mm/µs), (b) cortical bone with wave speed anisotropy modeled during image reconstruction (using the characteristics shown in Figure 8.7) and (c) cortical bone with wave speed anisotropy ignored during image reconstruction (an isotropic wave speed of 3 mm/µs is used). The displayed dynamic range is 60 dB*

With these idealized two-dimensional in silico datasets, ignoring wave speed anisotropy in cortical bone does not seem to degrade the image of the far surface of the cortical bone layer (see 10 mm depth in Figure 8.14(c)). However, Figure 8.12(e) shows that the correction of wave speed anisotropy significantly improves the detection of the inner surface of the tibial cortex with in vivo data. Equation [8.9] was used with $V_P^{axial} = 4$ mm/μs, $V_P^{radial} = 3.2$ mm/μs and $\xi = 1.6$.

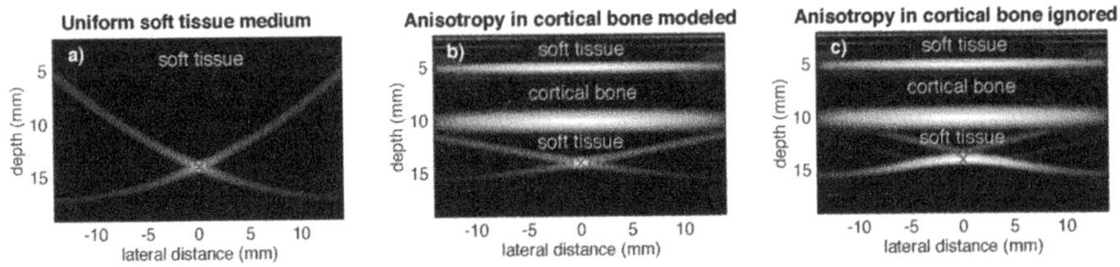

Figure 8.14. *Illustration with in silico data of the importance of wave speed anisotropy when imaging a layer of soft tissue separated from the transducer by a layer of cortical bone. The point spread function obtained from a point target at 14 mm depth (shown by a red cross) in (a) a uniform medium with isotropic wave speed (1.5 mm/μs), (b) soft tissue under a layer of cortical bone with wave speed anisotropy in the bone layer modeled during image reconstruction (using the characteristics shown in Figure 8.7) and (c) soft tissue under a layer of cortical bone with wave speed anisotropy in the bone layer ignored during image reconstruction (an isotropic wave speed of 3 mm/μs is used). The displayed dynamic range is 60 dB*

8.3.4. *Reduction of multiple scattering with tissue harmonic imaging*

Tissue harmonic imaging demonstrated improved image quality in transcranial ultrasound imaging (Puls et al. 2000) and ultrasound echocardiography (Spencer et al. 1998). In addition to improving the spatial lateral resolution in the ultrasound image and reducing clutter signal caused by the side lobes and grating lobes of the transmit beam, tissue harmonic imaging reduces clutter signal caused by reverberation occurring in heterogeneous tissue layers close to the transducer.

Tissue harmonic imaging relies on nonlinear ultrasound propagation. Nonlinear propagation distorts the waveform output by the transducer. This distortion progressively builds up as the wave propagates. If analyzed in the frequency domain, this progressive distortion corresponds to the generation of new frequency components that were absent in the waveform generated by the transducer. The largest new component is created at twice the ultrasound frequency generated by the transducer, which is often called the second harmonic component (sometimes also called first harmonic). For a transmit focused or unfocused beam, there exist two phases. During the first phase, between the transducer and a certain distance, the amplitude of the second harmonic component increases from zero to a maximum value. During the second phase, for larger distances, the amplitude of the second harmonic component decays progressively because the effect of attenuation overwhelms the effect of nonlinear propagation. In the first approximation, the amplitude of the second harmonic component is proportional to the squared amplitude at the transmit frequency. It is worth noting that linear backward propagation of echoes can be assumed because they have small amplitude. Therefore tissue harmonic imaging reduces reverberation clutter in transmit only (forward propagation), not during backward propagation of echoes.

Tissue harmonic imaging is now implemented in most clinical ultrasound scanners. The use of dedicated pulse sequences, like pulse inversion or amplitude modulation, enables the extraction of the second harmonic component.

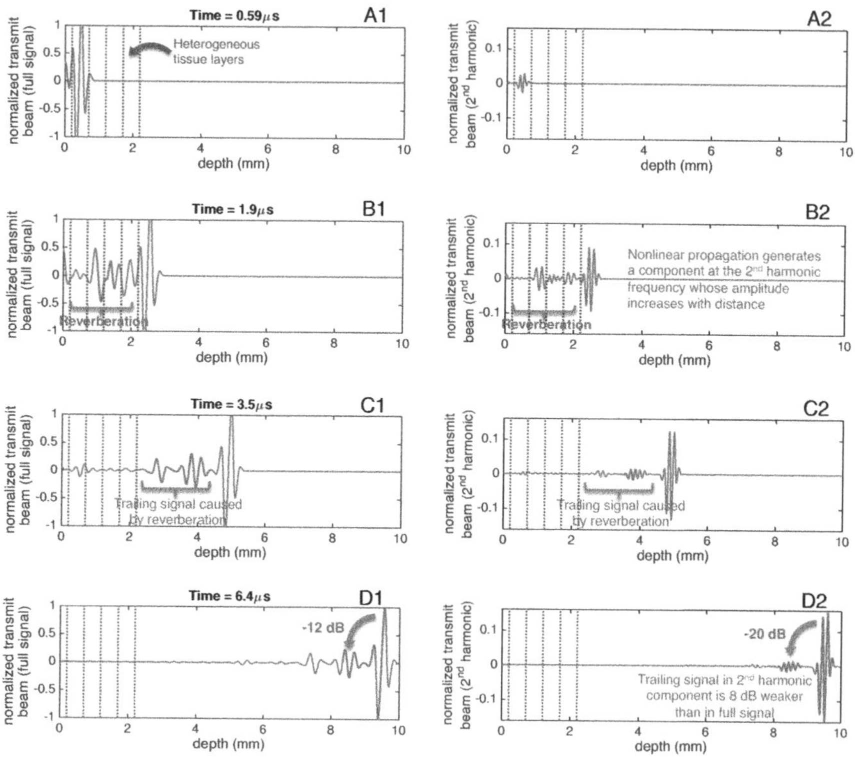

Figure 8.15. *Illustration of tissue harmonic imaging with a numerical simulation in a one-dimensional space. A 5-MHz short pulse is generated by a source located at depth = 0. Four heterogeneous layers are placed near the source. Panels (A1), (B1), (C1) and (D1) are snapshots at four different instants showing the full waveform. (A2), (B2), (C2) and (D2) are snapshots at the same four instants, showing the second harmonic component (10 MHz) extracted from the full waveform with pulse inversion*

Harmonic imaging can circumvent reverberation clutter as a mechanism for image degradation because of its low amplitude in the near field, where most of the reverberations occur. Trailing clutter can also potentially be reduced, given it is generated in the near field, because of its low amplitude, which makes it less prone to nonlinear distortion compared to the main pulse. Most of the energy in the pulse tail will remain in the fundamental frequency with propagation and will not appear in the harmonic image (Pinton et al. 2009b).

Figure 8.15 illustrates the reduction of near-field reverberation clutter achieved with tissue harmonic imaging. Using a numerical wave solver (k-wave (Treeby et al. 2012)), nonlinear propagation of a plane wave was computed through heterogeneous tissue layers located near the transducer. It can be seen that the relative magnitude of the trailing signal caused by reverberation in the second harmonic component is smaller than that in the full signal. As a result, reconstructing an ultrasound image with the second harmonic component produces an image with reduced reverberation clutter. The improvement is larger with transmit focused beams because the second harmonic component starts to build up at a distance deeper than the tissue layers (near the probe) that are responsible for reverberations (this distance is determined by the transmit focus depth and depth of field).

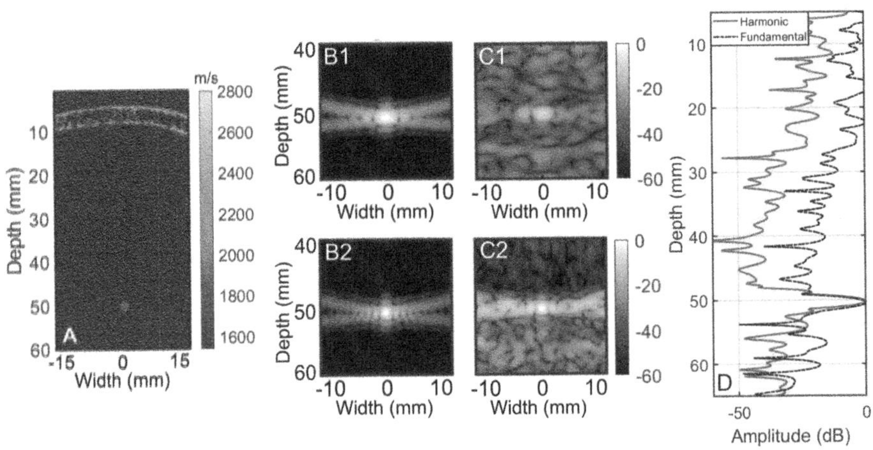

Figure 8.16. *Simulation derived B-mode images for a 1.25 MHz emission in a homogeneous medium (B1,B2) and transcranially (C1,C2) for the fundamental at 1.25 Hz (B1,C1) and the second harmonic frequency at 2.5 MHz (B2,C2). A two-cycle single-focus transmit focusing at 50 mm is used. (A) shows the sound speed map of the human skull slice used to generate images (C1) and (C2). Target size is exaggerated. In (D), the midline of (C1) and (C2) as a function of depth is plotted*

Figure 8.16 illustrates the improvement in the PSF/ambient clutter ratio in 2D in transcranial imaging. A 1.25 MHz single-focus transmit at 50 mm is used to generate images of a point target in a homogeneous medium (panels (B1) and (B2)) and transcranially (panels (C1) and (C2)) through the sound speed map shown in panel (A). In panel (D), the midline in images (C1) and (C2) as a function of depth illustrates how harmonic imaging decreases the relative amplitude of the ambient clutter around the target by about 20 dB in the transcranial image.

Instead of reducing the importance of multiple scattering during the acquisition as in tissue harmonic imaging, advanced signal post-processing was also proposed to remove multiple reflections from the recorded echo signals (Lambert et al. 2020).

8.4. Current limitations for correcting the sources of image degradation and future

8.4.1. *Need for matrix arrays and high computational power*

Most clinical transducers for 2D ultrasound imaging are still one-dimensional arrays, where the height of the elements (in the elevation dimension, i.e. the dimension normal to the image plane) is typically between 5 and 15 mm. These transducers are unable to correct for phase aberration in the elevation dimension because they do not spatially sample the recorded echo wavefronts in this dimension. Therefore, early work on aberration correction has advertised the need for two-dimensional arrays. Research has suggested that an elevation pitch that is at least 75%, but perhaps as fine as 25 to 30% of the aberration correlation length may be needed for effective aberration measurements and therefore the correction of phase aberration (Lacefield and Waag 2001). Two-dimensional arrays are becoming more and more available. An additional requirement for phase aberration correction is access to raw echo signals on each individual element of the array. This often represents a large amount of data, which needs to be processed with high-performance computers.

8.4.2. *Real-time versus offline aberration correction*

Until recently, real-time implementations of phase aberration correction on ultrasound scanners have achieved rather low imaging rates between 0.5 and 8.5 frames per second (Dahl et al. 2006), because phase aberration correction requires advanced strategies and signal processing. In 2022, GE Healthcare released a phase aberration correction, based on a near-field phase screen approach, operating in real time at $\sim$100 frames per second with a matrix array transducer (Masoy et al. 2022). When image degradation is strong, with two-dimensional arrays becoming more and more available, handheld 2D ultrasound imaging may shift towards 4D (3D+time) ultrasound imaging, with the transducer being held static in front of the region of interest with dedicated equipment. In these very challenging situations, the future ultrasound scanner may first acquire volumetric ultrasound data for a few seconds, likely including iterative strategies to characterize and mitigate the sources of image degradation during the acquisition, and reconstruct high-quality images in a second step, after post-processing of the acquired data.

8.4.3. *Blood flow quantification*

Ultrasound characterization of blood flow is commonly achieved by analyzing the non-stationary components of the ultrasound image, which correspond to moving red blood cells. Ultrasound contrast agents made of gas microbubbles are also used as a surrogate for the blood signal. Both red blood cells and microbubbles are much smaller than the ultrasound wavelength; therefore, they can be seen as point targets. Thus, the image of a single red blood cell or microbubble is a point spread function. Just like image quality, blood flow quantification is corrupted if the point spread function is degraded by aberration or multiple scattering. In particular, a degraded PSF results in degraded spatial specificity of the information on blood flow. Consequently, the correction of aberration and the reduction of multiple scattering are crucial because they improve both image quality and blood flow quantification.

8.5. References

Alexander, S.L., Rafaels, K., Gunnarsson, C.A., Weerasooriya, T. (2019). Structural analysis of the frontal and parietal bones of the human skull. *Journal of the Mechanical Behavior of Biomedical Materials*, 90, 689–701.

Ashman, R., Cowin, S., Van Buskirk, W., Rice, J. (1984). A continuous wave technique for the measurement of the elastic properties of cortical bone. *Journal of Biomechanics*, 17(5), 349–361.

Bernard, S., Schneider, J., Varga, P., Laugier, P., Raum, K., Grimal, Q. (2016). Elasticity–density and viscoelasticity–density relationships at the tibia mid-diaphysis assessed from resonant ultrasound spectroscopy measurements. *Biomechanics and Modeling in Mechanobiology*, 15(1), 97–109.

Bossy, E., Talmant, M., Laugier, P. (2002). Effect of bone cortical thickness on velocity measurements using ultrasonic axial transmission: A 2D simulation study. *The Journal of the Acoustical Society of America*, 112(1), 297–307.

Dahl, J.J., Mcaleavey, S.A., Pinton, G.F., Soo, M.S., Trahey, G.E. (2006). Adaptive imaging on a diagnostic ultrasound scanner at quasi real-time rates. *IEEE Transactions on Ultrasonics, Ferroelectrics, and Frequency Control*, 53(10), 1832–1843.

Demené, C., Robin, J., Dizeux, A., Heiles, B., Pernot, M., Tanter, M., Perren, F. (2021). Transcranial ultrafast ultrasound localization microscopy of brain vasculature in patients. *Nature Biomedical Engineering*, 5(3), 219–228.

Freiburger, P.D., Sullivan, D.C., LeBlanc, B.H., Smith, S.W., Trahey, G.E. (1992). Two dimensional ultrasonic beam distortion in the breast: In vivo measurements and effects. *Ultrasonic Imaging*, 14(4), 398–414.

Granke, M., Grimal, Q., Saied, A., Nauleau, P., Peyrin, F., Laugier, P. (2011). Change in porosity is the major determinant of the variation of cortical bone elasticity at the millimeter scale in aged women. *Bone*, 49(5), 1020–1026.

Gyöngy, M. and Kollár, S. (2015). Variation of ultrasound image lateral spectrum with assumed speed of sound and true scatterer density. *Ultrasonics*, 56, 370–380.

Hinkelman, L.M., Liu, D.-L., Metlay, L.A., Waag, R.C. (1994). Measurements of ultrasonic pulse arrival time and energy level variations produced by propagation through abdominal wall. *The Journal of the Acoustical Society of America*, 95(1), 530–541.

Hinkelman, L.M., Liu, D., Waag, R.C., Zhu, Q., Steinberg, B.D. (1995). Measurement and correction of ultrasonic pulse distortion produced by the human breast. *The Journal of the Acoustical Society of America*, 97(3), 1958–1969.

Hoskins, P.R., Martin, K., Thrush, A. (2019). *Diagnostic Ultrasound: Physics and Equipment*, 3rd edition. CRC Press, Boca Raton, FL.

Ivancevich, N.M., Pinton, G.F., Nicoletto, H.A., Bennett, E., Laskowitz, D.T., Smith, S.W. (2008). Real-time 3-D contrast-enhanced transcranial ultrasound and aberration correction. *Ultrasound in Medicine & Biology*, 34(9), 1387–1395.

Jaeger, M., Robinson, E., Akarcay, H.G., Frenz, M. (2015). Full correction for spatially distributed speed-of-sound in echo ultrasound based on measuring aberration delays via transmit beam steering. *Physics in Medicine & Biology*, 60(11), 4497–4515.

Lacefield, J. and Waag, R. (2001). Time-shift estimation and focusing through distributed aberration using multirow arrays. *IEEE Transactions on Ultrasonics, Ferroelectrics, and Frequency Control*, 48(6), 1606–1624.

Lagravere, M., Fang, Y., Carey, J., Toogood, R., Packota, G., Major, P. (2006). Density conversion factor determined using a cone-beam computed tomography unit NewTom QR-DVT 9000. *Dentomaxillofacial Radiology*, 35(6), 407–409.

Lambert, W., Cobus, L.A., Frappart, T., Fink, M., Aubry, A. (2020). Distortion matrix approach for ultrasound imaging of random scattering media. *Proceedings of the National Academy of Sciences*, 117(26), 14645–14656.

Lindsey, B.D. and Smith, S.W. (2013). Pitch-catch phase aberration correction of multiple isoplanatic patches for 3-D transcranial ultrasound imaging. *IEEE Transactions on Ultrasonics, Ferroelectrics, and Frequency Control*, 60(3), 463–480.

Lindsey, B.D. and Smith, S.W. (2014). Refraction correction in 3D transcranial ultrasound imaging. *Ultrasonic Imaging*, 36(1), 35–54.

Liu, D.-L. and Waag, R.C. (1994). Correction of ultrasonic wavefront distortion using backpropagation and a reference waveform method for time-shift compensation. *The Journal of the Acoustical Society of America*, 96(2), 649–660.

Liu, D.-L. and Waag, R.C. (1995). A comparison of ultrasonic wavefront distortion and compensation in one-dimensional and two-dimensional apertures. *IEEE Transactions on Ultrasonics, Ferroelectrics, and Frequency Control*, 42(4), 726–733.

Liu, D.-L., Sutcliffe, P., McDermott, B., Lazenby, J., von Behren, P., Kim, J. (2000). Adaptive ultrasonic imaging using SONOLINE Elegra/sup TM. *2000 IEEE Ultrasonics Symposium Proceedings*, 2, 1655–1658.

Mallart, R. and Fink, M. (1994). Adaptive focusing in scattering media through sound-speed inhomogeneities: The van Cittert Zernike approach and focusing criterion. *The Journal of the Acoustical Society of America*, 96(6), 3721–3732.

Marquet, F., Pernot, M., Aubry, J.-F., Montaldo, G., Marsac, L., Tanter, M., Fink, M. (2009). Non-invasive transcranial ultrasound therapy based on a 3D CT scan: Protocol validation and in vitro results. *Physics in Medicine and Biology*, 54(9), 2597–2613.

Marsac, L., Chauvet, D., Greca, R.L., Boch, A.-L., Chaumoitre, K., Tanter, M., Aubry, J.-F. (2017). Ex vivo optimisation of a heterogeneous speed of sound model of the human skull for non-invasive transcranial focused ultrasound at 1 MHz. *International Journal of Hyperthermia*, 33(6), 635–645.

Masoy, S.-E., Denarie, B., Sornes, A., Holte, E., Grenne, B., Espeland, T., Berg, E.A.R., Rindal, O.M.H., Rigby, W., Bjastad, T. (2022). Aberration correction in 2D echocardiography. Preprint, 1–10.

Montaldo, G., Tanter, M., Fink, M. (2011). Time reversal of speckle noise. *Physical Review Letters*, 106, 054301.

Mozaffarzadeh, M., Verschuur, E., Verweij, M.D., de Jong, N., Renaud, G. (2022a). Accelerated 2-D real-time refraction-corrected transcranial ultrasound imaging. *IEEE Transactions on Ultrasonics, Ferroelectrics, and Frequency Control*, 69(9), 2599–2610.

Mozaffarzadeh, M., Verschuur, E., Verweij, M.D., de Jong, N., Renaud, G. (2022b). Comparison of phase-screen and geometry-based phase aberration correction techniques for real-time transcranial ultrasound imaging. *Applied Sciences*, 12(19), 10183.

Mozaffarzadeh, M., Verschuur, E., Verweij, M.D., Daeichin, V., de Jong, N., Renaud, G. (2022c). Refraction-corrected transcranial ultrasound imaging through the human temporal window using a single probe. *IEEE Transactions on Ultrasonics, Ferroelectrics, and Frequency Control*, 69(4), 1191–1203.

Napolitano, D., Chou, C., McLaughlin, G., Ji, T., Mo, L., DeBusschere, D., Steins, R. (2006). Sound speed correction in ultrasound imaging. *Ultrasonics*, 44(Supplement), e43–e46.

Ng, G., Worrell, S., Freiburger, P., Trahey, G. (1994). A comparative evaluation of several algorithms for phase aberration correction. *IEEE Transactions on Ultrasonics, Ferroelectrics, and Frequency Control*, 41(5), 631–643.

Nock, L., Trahey, G.E., Smith, S.W. (1989). Phase aberration correction in medical ultrasound using speckle brightness as a quality factor. *The Journal of the Acoustical Society of America*, 85(5), 1819–1833.

O'Donnell, M. and Flax, S. (1988a). Phase-aberration correction using signals from point reflectors and diffuse scatterers: Measurements. *IEEE Transactions on Ultrasonics, Ferroelectrics, and Frequency Control*, 35(6), 768–774.

O'Donnell, M. and Flax, S. (1988b). Phase aberration measurements in medical ultrasound: Human studies. *Ultrasonic Imaging*, 10(1), 1–11.

Peterson, J. and Dechow, P.C. (2003). Material properties of the human cranial vault and zygoma. *The Anatomical Record Part A: Discoveries in Molecular, Cellular, and Evolutionary Biology*, 274A(1), 785–797.

Philips-Healthcare (2008). Results of a technically difficult patient study – Six sites in North America and Europe. White paper, 1–8.

Phillips, D., Smith, S., von Ramm, O., Thurstone, F. (1975a). A phase compensation technique for B-mode echoencephalography. In *Ultrasound in Medicine*, White, D.N. (ed.). Plenum Press, New York.

Phillips, D., Smith, S., von Ramm, O., Thurstone, F. (1975b). Sampled aperture techniques applied to B-mode echoencephalography. In *Acoustical Holography*, Booth, N. (ed.). Springer, Boston, MA.

Pinton, G.F., Dahl, J.J., Rosenzweig, S., Trahey, G.E. (2009a). A heterogeneous nonlinear attenuating full-wave model of ultrasound. *IEEE Transactions on Ultrasonics, Ferroelectrics, and Frequency Control*, 56(3), 474–488.

Pinton, G.F., Dahl, J.J., Trahey, G.E. (2009b). Clutter and sources of image degradation in fundamental and harmonic ultrasound imaging. *2009 IEEE International Ultrasonics Symposium*, 2300–2303.

Pinton, G.F., Trahey, G.E., Dahl, J.J. (2011). Sources of image degradation in fundamental and harmonic ultrasound imaging using nonlinear, full-wave simulations. *IEEE Transactions on Ultrasonics, Ferroelectrics, and Frequency Control*, 58(4), 754–765.

Puls, I., Berg, D., Mäurer, M., Schliesser, M., Hetzel, G., Becker, G. (2000). Transcranial sonography of the brain parenchyma: Comparison of B-mode imaging and tissue harmonic imaging. *Ultrasound in Medicine & Biology*, 26(2), 189–194.

Rachlin, D. (1990). Direct estimation of aberrating delays in pulse-echo imaging systems. *The Journal of the Acoustical Society of America*, 88(1), 191–198.

Renaud, G., Kruizinga, P., Cassereau, D., Laugier, P. (2018). In vivo ultrasound imaging of the bone cortex. *Physics in Medicine & Biology*, 63(12), 125010.

Renaud, G., Clouzet, P., Cassereau, D., Talmant, M. (2020). Measuring anisotropy of elastic wave velocity with ultrasound imaging and an autofocus method: Application to cortical bone. *Physics in Medicine & Biology*, 65(23), 235016.

Rigby, K., Chalek, C., Haider, B., Lewandowski, R., O'Donnell, M., Smith, L., Wildes, D. (2000). Improved in vivo abdominal image quality using real-time estimation and correction of wavefront arrival time errors. *IEEE Ultrasonics Symposium Proceedings*, 2, 1645–1653.

Salles, S., Shepherd, J., Vos, H.J., Renaud, G. (2021). Revealing intraosseous blood flow in the human tibia with ultrasound. *JBMR Plus*, e10543.

Sanabria, S.J., Ozkan, E., Rominger, M., Goksel, O. (2018). Spatial domain reconstruction for imaging speed-of-sound with pulse-echo ultrasound: Simulation and in vivo study. *Physics in Medicine & Biology*, 63(21), 215015.

Shung, K. (2015). *Diagnostic Ultrasound: Imaging and Blood Flow Measurements*, 2nd edition. CRC Press/Taylor & Francis Group, Boca Raton, FL.

Smith, S., Trahey, G., Von Ramm, O. (1986). Phased array ultrasound imaging through planar tissue layers. *Ultrasound in Medicine & Biology*, 12(3), 229–243.

Soulioti, D.E., Espíndola, D., Dayton, P.A., Pinton, G.F. (2020). Super-resolution imaging through the human skull. *IEEE Transactions on Ultrasonics, Ferroelectrics, and Frequency Control*, 67(1), 25–36.

Spencer, K., Bednarz, J., Rafter, P., Korcarz, C., Lang, R. (1998). Use of harmonic imaging without echocardiographic contrast to improve two-dimensional image quality. *The American Journal of Cardiology*, 82(6), 794–799.

Sumino, Y. and Waag, R.C. (1991). Measurements of ultrasonic pulse arrival time differences produced by abdominal wall specimens. *The Journal of the Acoustical Society of America*, 90(6), 2924–2930.

Szabo, T. (2013). *Diagnostic Ultrasound Imaging: Inside Out*, 2nd edition. Academic Press, Amsterdam.

Tanter, M., Thomas, J.-L., Fink, M. (1998). Focusing and steering through absorbing and aberrating layers: Application to ultrasonic propagation through the skull. *The Journal of the Acoustical Society of America*, 103(5), 2403–2410.

Thomsen, L. (1986). Weak elastic anisotropy. *Geophysics*, 51(10), 1954–1966.

Trahey, G., Zhao, D., Miglin, J., Smith, S. (1990). Experimental results with a real-time adaptive ultrasonic imaging system for viewing through distorting media. *IEEE Transactions on Ultrasonics, Ferroelectrics, and Frequency Control*, 37(5), 418–427.

Trahey, G., Freiburger, P., Nock, L., Sullivan, D. (1991). In vivo measurements of ultrasonic beam distortion in the breast. *Ultrasonic Imaging*, 13(1), 71–90.

Treeby, B.E., Varslot, T., Zhang, E., Laufer, J., Beard, P. (2011). Automatic sound speed selection in photoacoustic image reconstruction using an autofocus approach. *Journal of Biomedical Optics*, 16(9), 090501.

Treeby, B.E., Jaros, J., Rendell, A.P., Cox, B.T. (2012). Modeling nonlinear ultrasound propagation in heterogeneous media with power law absorption using a k-space pseudospectral method. *Journal of the Acoustical Society of America*, 131(6), 4324–4336.

Vignon, F., Aubry, J.F., Tanter, M., Margoum, A., Fink, M. (2006). Adaptive focusing for transcranial ultrasound imaging using dual arrays. *The Journal of the Acoustical Society of America*, 120(5), 2737–2745.

Vignon, F., Shi, W., Burcher, M., Powers, J. (2008). Determination of temporal bone isoplanatic patch sizes for transcranial phase aberration correction. *2008 IEEE Ultrasonics Symposium*, 1286–1289.

Wiskin, J., Malik, B., Natesan, R., Lenox, M. (2019). Quantitative assessment of breast density using transmission ultrasound tomography. *Medical Physics*, 46(6), 2610–2620.

Yoon, H.S. and Lawrence Katz, J. (1976). Ultrasonic wave propagation in human cortical bone II. Measurements of elastic properties and microhardness. *Journal of Biomechanics*, 9(7), 459–464.

9

Tomography and Spectroscopy: Photoacoustics

Théotim LUCAS[1,2] and Jérôme GATEAU[1]

[1] *CNRS, INSERM, Laboratoire d'Imagerie Biomédicale (LIB), Sorbonne Université, Paris, France*

[2] *CNRS, Laboratoire Matière et Systèmes Complexes (MSC), Université Paris Cité, France*

9.1. Combining ultrasound with optical waves

This chapter presents a biomedical hybrid imaging method, called photoacoustic imaging (PAI) or optoacoustic imaging, that uniquely combines ultrasound and optical waves. These two kinds of waves are very different by nature. Optical waves are transverse electromagnetic waves with a wavelength on the order of 400 nm–1,000 nm in the visible and near-infrared (NIR) range used in biomedical optics. They interact with molecules and can bring molecular compounds to higher energy levels upon absorption. This energy can then be dispersed by non-radiative relaxation (heat of the solvent) or radiative relaxation (fluorescence, for example). Optical waves can transport energy to a depth of up to a few centimeters in biological tissue, but they experience strong multiple scattering as soon as they penetrate to depths of 0.1 mm to 1 mm in most biological tissues. On the other hand, ultrasound waves used in medical ultrasonography are longitudinal acoustic waves with a wavelength on the order of 100 µm–1,000 µm in the MHz range. They

For a color version of all the figures in this chapter, see www.iste.co.uk/bridal/innovative.zip.

Innovative Ultrasound Imaging Techniques,
coordinated by S. Lori BRIDAL.

interact with a tissue's mechanical microstructure and propagate with only a weak level of scattering to depths of several centimeters. The multi-wave imaging strategy of PAI combines these two kinds of waves to provide a unique image that aims to provide a more interesting contrast and resolution than that offered by either ultrasound or optical imaging alone. In PAI, the optical wave provides the contrast and the ultrasound wave provides the spatial resolution. In this first section, we compare the properties of biological tissues for these two kinds of waves in terms of wave propagation and interactions, and then we introduce the different possible interactions between optical and ultrasound waves.

9.1.1. *Optical properties of biological tissue*

During its propagation inside biological tissue, light interacts with tissue structures through two main mechanisms: scattering and absorption (Jacques 2013). Scattering results from interactions with cellular structures that can deviate the photons (particles that correspond to optical waves) from their straight trajectory without loss of energy. The accumulation of multiple scattering events results in a gradual randomization of the propagation direction. The scattering strength is expressed with the so-called reduced scattering coefficient μ_s', which incorporates the scattering coefficient and the anisotropy and enables modeling of the diffusion of photons as a random walk of step size of $1/\mu_s'$. In biological tissues, $\mu_s' = 10–50\ cm^{-1}$. The propagation direction becomes randomized compared to the direction of the incident beam over a distance on the order of $1/\mu s' \sim 1$ mm for optical waves in the visible to near-infrared (NIR) range (Ntziachristos 2010). As a result, the optical path cannot be known and the achievable spatial resolution of optical imaging strongly degrades for depths above 1 mm. Absorption corresponds to a loss of energy of the optical beam through its transformation into the internal energy of the absorber. Absorption is quantified by the absorption coefficient μ_a, which is the sum of contributions from all absorbing chromophores within the tissue (Jacques 2013). In the visible and NIR range, the main endogenous absorbing chromophores are hemoglobin, water and melanin. At 806 nm, the contribution of blood to the tissue absorption is $\mu_a = 0.04\ cm^{-1}$ (Jacques 2013). Hemoglobin strongly limits the penetration depth of light for wavelengths below 600 nm and water limits penetration for wavelengths above 1,300 nm. Thereby, light has a maximum depth of penetration in tissue for the wavelength range between 630 nm and 1,300 nm, which is called the near-infrared window in biological tissue. In this window, optical energy can reach a centimeter of depth for incident light fluence on the skin within the limits imposed by the maximum permissible exposure safety limits.

Ultrasound waves also interact with biological tissues through scattering and absorption. However, in the MHz range used for medical ultrasound, the typical scattering and absorption distances are several orders of magnitude longer than for optical waves. The attenuation coefficient of ultrasound waves is approximately 0.7 dB/cm/MHz in soft tissue (O'Brien 2007). Thereby, at 5 MHz, the attenuation length (distance where the wave intensity has dropped to 1/e) is on the order of 2 cm for ultrasound waves compared to 1 mm for optical waves in the NIR. The weak scattering of acoustic waves in biological tissues enables the ultrasound path to be retraced to thus obtain a spatial resolution on the order of the ultrasound wavelength at centimetric depths.

9.1.2. *Interaction between optical and ultrasound waves*

Inside biological tissues, energy transfer between optical and ultrasound waves can occur through two main modes of interaction: acousto-optics and photoacoustics. In acousto-optics, the waves are generated externally. For example, an optical wave is generated with a laser and an ultrasonic wave is emitted using a transducer so that the generated beams overlap within the tissue. The acousto-optic interaction results in an ultrasonic modulation of the incident light, which effectively "tags" the photons interacting with the ultrasound wave in the tissue. By scanning the ultrasound beam from one position to another within the medium and then by assessing the absorption or scattering properties of the tissue from the tagged photons alone, optical properties of the medium can be mapped out (Gunther and Andersson-Engels 2017). Photoacoustics is a "light in and sound out" interaction. Optical energy is transiently deposited within tissue through optical absorption of the incident light, which leads to the generation of ultrasonic waves (see section 9.2.1). Ultrasound signals captured outside of the tissue enable image reconstruction of the optical absorption with an ultrasonic resolution. In the following sections, we focus on photoacoustics, which is currently the most investigated mode of interaction for biomedical imaging. More precisely, we focus on photoacoustic tomography, as opposed to photoacoustic microscopy. In the latter, the photoacoustic image is probed point-by-point by a focused illumination or detection at shallow depths (Jeon et al. 2019), whereas, in photoacoustic tomography, the image reconstruction is obtained by an acoustic inverse problem from the ultrasound signals recorded at several locations around the imaged object, and can reach ultrasonic resolution at depths of up to a few centimeters.

In addition to the development of photoacoustics to evaluate interactions inside tissue, work is advancing rapidly to develop better devices for the optical generation (Zhao et al. 2018) and detection (Wissmeyer et al. 2018) of ultrasonic waves. Compared to piezoelectric transducers such as those described in Chapter 2, such optical technology generally has a broader bandwidth and enables miniaturization of the detector as the optical beam that probes or emits the ultrasound can be focused down to a few hundred nanometers.

9.2. Generation and tomographic detection of ultrasound in photoacoustic imaging

9.2.1. *Optical generation of ultrasound waves in biological tissues*

Most photoacoustic imaging setups use a pulsed optical excitation with a pulse duration on the order of a few nanoseconds. This illumination regime ensures negligible heat leakage and stress leakage during the optical generation of ultrasound. These conditions, also known as heat and stress confinement, result in efficient conversion of absorbed optical energy into ultrasonic energy. In soft tissue, the generation of ultrasound waves comes from the following sequence: (1) light deposits heat up in the optical absorption zone, (2) the subsequent transient temperature change induces an initial pressure rise and (3) pressure waves propagate from the initial pressure distribution.

The initial pressure rise p_0 at a spatial position **r** can be written as:

$$p_0(\boldsymbol{r}) = \Gamma \cdot \mu_a(\boldsymbol{r}) \cdot \Phi(\boldsymbol{r}) \qquad [9.1]$$

where Γ is known as the Grüneisen coefficient, a dimensionless thermodynamic constant that describes the conversion efficiency of heat energy to pressure. The optical parameters are $\mu_a(\boldsymbol{r})$, the local absorption coefficient, and $\Phi(\boldsymbol{r})$, the local incident optical fluence expressed in units of energy per unit area.

In the case of a lossless and acoustically homogeneous infinite medium excited with a very short laser pulse (delta function heating pulse), the propagation of the pressure wave $p(\boldsymbol{r},t)$ obeys the photoacoustic wave equation (Wang 2017):

$$\frac{\partial^2 p(\boldsymbol{r},t)}{\partial t^2} - c_0^2 \, \Delta p(\boldsymbol{r},t) = p_0(\boldsymbol{r}) \frac{d\delta(t)}{dt} \qquad [9.2]$$

where c_0 denotes the constant sound speed value and $\delta(t)$ denotes the one-dimensional Dirac delta function corresponding to the optical heating pulse. Equation [9.2] is a classical wave equation with a source term. The spatial and temporal components of this source term (right-hand side of equation [9.2]) can be separated here. The temporal component $\frac{d\delta(t)}{dt}$ is linked to the heating pulse and the spatial component $p_0(\boldsymbol{r})$ to the spatial distribution of the optical absorption and light fluence (see equation [9.1]).

The ultrasonic pressure field observed at the position ***r'*** and at the time *t* (*t* > 0, where t = 0 is the time of light pulse emission) can then be written as:

$$p\,(\boldsymbol{r}',t) = \frac{1}{4\pi {c_0}^2}\int_V \quad d^3\boldsymbol{r}\; p_0(\boldsymbol{r})\frac{1}{|r-r\prime|}\frac{d}{dt}\delta\left(t-\frac{|r-r\prime|}{c_0}\right) \qquad [9.3]$$

where *V* is the volume comprising the pressure distribution p_0. Equation [9.3] describes the interference of spherical wavelets with a temporal shape equal to the time derivative of the heating pulse. It should be noted that this temporal shape is not only positive, but also has positive and negative parts such that destructive or constructive interference can occur. Since the speed of light in tissue is several orders of magnitude larger than the speed of sound, all the spherical acoustic wavelets are emitted essentially simultaneously on the time scale of interest for ultrasonic wave transmission. The ultrasound field that builds up as a result of the wavelet interferences has both a temporal frequency content and a spatial frequency content that strongly depend on the distribution of the optical absorption within the tissue. In the last part of this section, we illustrate the influence of the size and geometry of absorbing structures on the ultrasound field by considering two simple structures: a sphere and a rod that are homogeneously absorbing and uniformly illuminated.

For an absorbing sphere (ball, three-dimensional monopole) of diameter *D* centered at the origin of the spatial coordinate system, and which has acoustic properties that are identical to those of the surrounding medium, the PA pressure waveform can be derived analytically (Wang 2017):

$$p\,(\boldsymbol{r}',t) = \frac{D\cdot\Gamma\cdot\mu_a\cdot\Phi}{2\cdot r\prime}(1-\tau)\,\Theta_{0,2}(\tau) \qquad [9.4]$$

where τ is the retarded time expressed as:

$$\tau = \frac{2.c_0}{D}\left(t-\frac{|r\prime|-D/2}{c_0}\right) \qquad [9.5]$$

and $\Theta_{0,2}(\tau)$ is a boxcar function such that $\Theta_{0,2}(\tau) = 1$ if $\tau \in [0,2]$ and 0 otherwise.

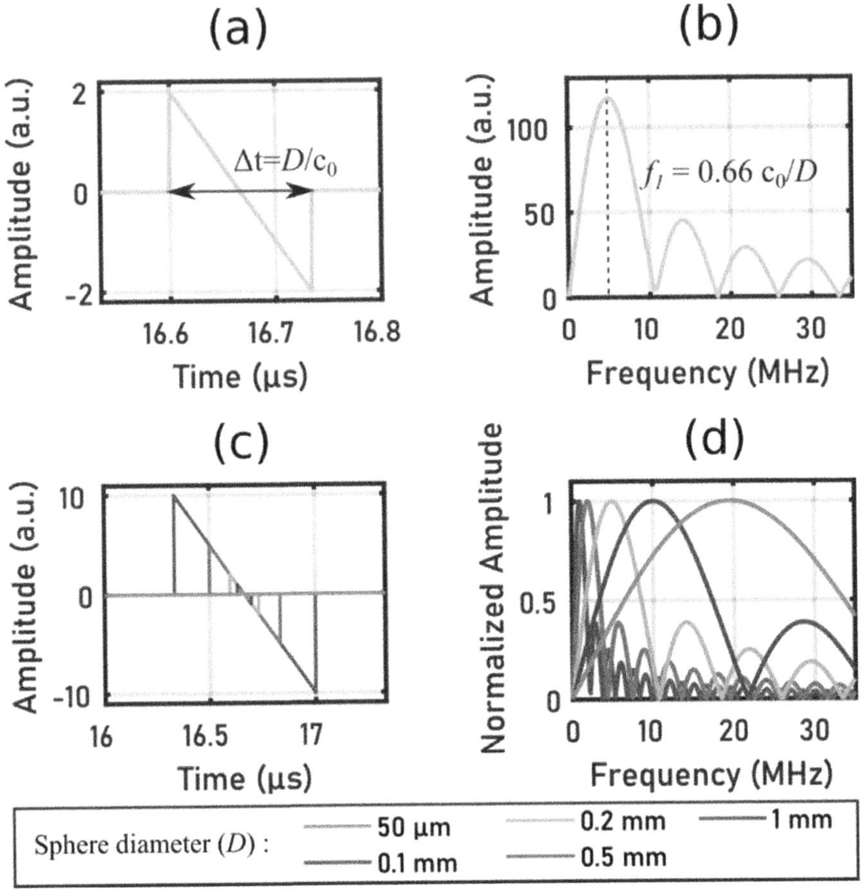

Figure 9.1. *Photoacoustic signals for spheres (balls) that are uniformly illuminated and homogeneously absorbing. The point detector is located at a distance of r = 25 mm from the center of the sphere, and the speed of sound is: c_0 = 1.5 mm.μs^{-1}. (a) Ultrasound signal in the time domain that has a typical N-shape, and (b) the magnitude of its spectrum for a sphere of diameter D = 0.2 mm. The first peak of the spectrum is located at $f^1 \approx$ 5 MHz. (c) Ultrasound signals for spheres composed of the same absorbing material, but with diameters ranging from 50 μm to 1 mm and (d) the corresponding spectra. For the sake of readability, the amplitude of each spectrum is normalized to the first peak. The influence of the sphere diameter on the spectrum is clearly visible*

The pressure waveform of equation [9.4] has a typical N-shape (see Figure 9.1(a)). Several properties of the ultrasound signal generated with the photoacoustic effect can be deduced from this analytical expression. First, the amplitude of the signal is directly proportional to the optical absorption coefficient and the incident light fluence, which are optical parameters. In addition, the signal is also proportional to the linear dimension of the object *D*, which implies that the size of an object will influence its detectability. For materials with identical optical properties (same μ_a), smaller objects require more sensitive detectors (see Figure 9.1(c)). Second, the emitted PA pressure signals are short, which implies that their spectrum is broadband. The frequency spectrum of the N-shape signal is illustrated in Figure 9.1(b) and shows a first peak at a frequency of $f_1 \sim 0.66\ c_0/D$ followed by harmonics of decaying amplitude. This peak falls in the typical frequency bandwidth of medical ultrasound [1 MHz–20 MHz] for spheres of diameter: [50 μm–1 mm] (see Figure 9.1(d)). As a result, if large objects are imaged with a high-frequency photoacoustic system (lower cutoff frequency $f_L > 3 \cdot f_1$, for example, $f_L > 1$ MHz for $D > 3$ mm), only the edges of the objects (corresponding to the high-frequency part of the signals) are well reconstructed on the PA image. Conversely, for small objects imaged with a low-frequency system (upper cutoff frequency $f_U < 2 \cdot f_1$, for example, $f_U < 10$ MHz for $D < 0.2$ mm), the reconstructed amplitude of p_0 may be underestimated. Since biological tissues comprise absorbing structures in a broad range of sizes, such as, for example, human blood vessels ranging from a diameter of 2 cm for the aorta to 8 μm for capillaries, the photoacoustic signal emitted by structures of very different sizes is expected to be broadband. The wide ultrasound bandwidth of the PA emissions and the dependence of the frequency content of the emitted field on the tissue composition and organization are two major differences between ultrasonography and photoacoustic imaging.

Spheres are isotropic objects; however, biological tissues contain many elongated, optically absorbing structures such as blood vessels. For an elongated object, the interference of the spherical wavelets, as described by equation [9.3], leads to directionality of the ultrasound emission. For optically absorbing rods shaped as finite-length cylinders with hemispherical ends, detected ultrasound signals due to the photoacoustic effect were estimated numerically for a set of point (isotropic) detectors arranged along a half-circle (see Figure 9.2(a)). Different aspect ratios for the rod were simulated to compare the angular dependence of the generated ultrasound waves, as illustrated in Figures 9.2(b) and (c). In particular, the peak-to-peak amplitude of each signal and the frequency f_1 of the first peak of the signal's spectrum are displayed as a function of the angular coordinate. As expected, the sphere (aspect ratio 1:1) displays an isotropic signal amplitude and an isotropic frequency peak position f_1. For an aspect ratio of 2:1, the generated ultrasound field becomes anisotropic with a maximum amplitude and maximum f_1 value in the direction $\theta = 90°$. The directivity, i.e. the concentration of the ultrasound emission in a single direction, increases with the anisotropy of the aspect ratio. The frequency f_1 decreases as θ deviates from 90°. The angular dependency of f_1 further shows that the geometry of the absorbing object influences the spectrum of the emitted ultrasound field. At $\theta = 0°$, f_1 is approximately inversely proportional to the length L.

IMPORTANT. –Ultrasound wave fields generated with short optical pulses have two very important properties. First, in terms of frequency bandwidth of the emitted ultrasound signals, they are broadband and their spectrum has a first and main peak with a peak frequency that is roughly inversely proportional to the linear dimension of the optically absorbing object. Second, the wave field has a directivity that results from the shape of the absorbing structure, and directivity increases as the aspect ratio is more highly anisotropic.

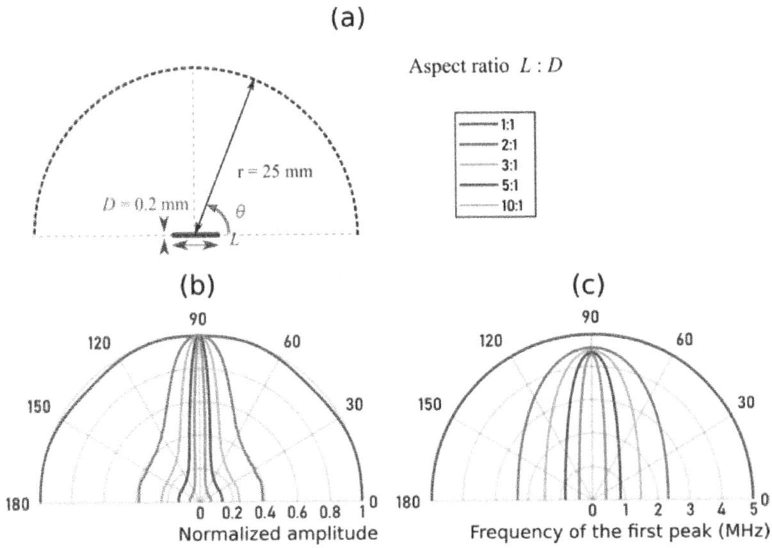

Figure 9.2. *Directivity of photoacoustic signals generated by finite-length cylinders. Ultrasound signals resulting from the photoacoustic effect were simulated for rods with hemispherical ends with aspect ratios from 1:1 to 10:1. (a) The detection geometry: point detectors are arranged along a half-circle centered on the position of a rod of length L and diameter D (aspect ratio L:D). (b) Polar plot of the peak-to-peak amplitude of the generated photoacoustic signals. (c) Polar plot of the frequency of the first peak in the spectrum of the signals*

9.2.2. *Tomographic ultrasound detection*

9.2.2.1. *Ideal detection configuration*

The acoustic inverse problem in photoacoustic imaging (PAI) consists of reconstructing an image of the initial pressure distribution p_0 from ultrasound signals created via the photoacoustic effect and recorded at several locations around the imaged object. This mode of imaging is called photoacoustic tomography (PAT). The acoustic inverse problem in PAT can benefit from the ensemble of information conveyed by the ultrasonic pressure field $p(\boldsymbol{r},t)$. To achieve this, the individual properties of the ultrasound detectors should be chosen with respect to the expected imaged object, in particular their frequency bandwidth and detection directivity should be well adapted to be sensitive to the structures of interest. Additionally, the spatial distribution of the detectors should be tailored to the directivity of the generated ultrasound field.

From the simulations presented in section 9.2.1 for the characteristics of the photoacoustic signals from spheres and rods, two rules of thumb can be inferred for the optimal PAI detection of optically absorbing objects:

– The frequency bandwidth of the detectors should be adapted to the expected size of the absorbers. For absorbers with a linear dimension D, the frequency $0.6 \cdot c_0/D$ should be in the ultrasound bandwidth of the detector. For the detection of small objects, this criterion calls for the detection of high frequencies. However, the acoustic attenuation is stronger for high frequencies than for low ones so that ultrasonic waves with ultrasound frequencies above 30 MHz originating from sources deeper than about 1 cm cannot be efficiently detected. Thus, the acoustic attenuation imposes a physical limit on the detection of the photoacoustic signal from small objects at frequencies above 10 MHz. Imaging large objects requires the detection of low frequencies. The expected spatial resolution of the image is linked to the upper cutoff frequency of the bandwidth. Therefore, for detectors with a small fractional bandwidth, a compromise may have to be found between the sensitivity to large objects and the spatial resolution of the sharp edges. For example, a 1 cm diameter sphere would require a −6 dB lower cutoff frequency below 100 kHz, while the resolution of its edges with a 100 μm resolution would impose an upper cutoff frequency around 8 MHz. This corresponds to a fractional bandwidth of 200%, which is not feasible, in general, for piezoelectric ultrasound detectors.

– Because of the directivity of the generated waves, a condition for “good visibility” of an absorbing object in PAT is that, for each of the object’s interfaces, at least one detector probes the object along the direction perpendicular to this interface (Wang 2017). If this rule is not satisfied for one interface, this interface will appear blurred, and if the rule is not satisfied for any of the interfaces, then the object will not be detected. Additionally, the ultrasound detectors have their own directivities that should be considered to efficiently cover the desired detection directions.

According to these two rules, an ideal tomographic ultrasound detection system would be comprised of detectors with an ultrawide bandwidth and a high sensitivity, especially to high frequencies, and the detectors would be distributed all over a closed surface (sphere, infinite cylinder or infinite plane) surrounding the imaged object and with a spatial sampling adapted to the highest recorded ultrasound frequency. However, practical limitations and realistic detector geometries cannot fulfill all of these criteria. This results in a so-called limited view artifact in the image, which mainly blurs some interfaces and renders some objects invisible.

9.2.2.2. *Practical implementations of PA scanners*

To build a system that is able to image a large variety of absorber orientations, it is necessary to enclose the imaged object as completely as possible with a surface filled with detectors. In fact, many parts of the human body are too large to be efficiency surrounded by ultrasound detectors, and even if some zones, like fingers or breasts, can be encircled, the number of available detectors and acquisition channels used in PA scanners is usually too low to ensure a satisfying spatial sampling. Determining the adequate spatial sampling is not trivial because of its dependence on both the aperture and the frequency bandwidth of the detectors. However, the order of magnitude required for adequate sampling can be determined using the Nyquist sampling theorem. If the detectors can be considered as point-like (small compared to the smallest recorded acoustic wavelength, Λ), then they would be ideally spaced if they are separated by a distance of $\Lambda/2$. For a half-sphere of radius $r = 25$ mm and detectors with a −6 dB upper cutoff frequency of 5 MHz (resulting in $\Lambda = 0.3$ mm), the number of detectors should then be around 4×10^4. By comparison, current detection systems typically have between 128 and 1,024 channels. For finite-size detectors, in the case of planar detection geometry, it has been shown that the sampling should be several times smaller than the detector length (Cox et al. 2007). Spatial under-sampling often results in streak artifacts in the image, and this artifact is common in PAI. A common strategy to increase the number of detection positions is to scan one or several detectors over the detection surface using a mechanical displacement of the detectors. To record the same ultrasound field for all the scanned detector positions, the optical excitation must be repeated for each scanned position and the imaged object must be stable over time, both in terms of its spatial position, and in terms of its optical and acoustic properties.

Among the various approaches used by PAI systems, we have chosen to present two different strategies that ensure an efficient coverage of absorber orientations and have promising clinical applications: (1) the use of a hemispherical or planar detection geometry for 3D PAI and (2) handheld 2D PAI that ensures flexible orientation of the detector array by the medical practitioner with real-time feedback.

For the first strategy, dedicated ultrasound detection systems have been developed for PAT with hemispherical or planar geometries. Within this category, hemispherical arrays have the largest angular aperture, especially if the imaged region is placed inside the hemisphere (see Figures 9.3(a) and (b)). These arrays were developed primarily for imaging the vasculature of breast tissue using the optical absorption of hemoglobin to detect breast cancer (see Figure 9.3(c)) (Manohar and Dantuma 2019), and were also recently used to image the function response of the human brain (Na et al. 2021). Typical configurations have a radius on the order of 10 cm and consist of ultrasound detectors arranged on a hemispherical shell covering at least a 90° arc. The array is scanned by rotation around the main axis to ensure an adequate spatial sampling. These arrays operate at frequencies below 6 MHz and have a resolution on the order of 0.3 mm and an imaging depth of 2–4 cm below the skin on each side. The planar detection geometry also has promising clinical applications. In a typical implementation of this geometry, a small or a spherically focused detector is raster-scanned across a detection plane, as shown in Figures 9.3(d) and (e). This imaging configuration is particularly adapted for superficial and high-frequency imaging. It has clinical applications in dermatology (Hindelang et al. 2019) and vascular imaging (Huynh et al. 2020) at imaging depths up to about 1 cm. Two dedicated detection systems based on different detector technologies have been extensively studied for the planar detection geometry. First, a 2D ultrasound detector based on an optical Fabry–Pérot cavity and interrogated by a raster-scanned laser beam has been developed by Zhang et al. (2008). The small size of the interrogating laser beam ensures a low directivity of the ultrasound sensor and thereby a wide angular aperture. Consequently, a 100 μm resolution could be achieved at depths up to 10 mm (see Figure 9.3(f)). Another implementation is based on the use of a spherically focused piezoelectric detector with the reception of signals from both inside and outside the focal zone. Raster scanning a spherically focused transducer is common in photoacoustic imaging, but this approach has been revitalized by the development (Omar et al. 2014) and commercialization (iThera Medical GmbH) of a high-frequency scanner based on this strategy. The scanner provides a maximum penetration depth of 5 mm coupled with a resolution on the order of 20 μm and is particularly adapted to imaging of skin pathologies (see Figure 9.3(g)). While for the first strategy with a dedicated detection geometry, the position and orientation of the scanned detectors are pre-defined and predominantly independent of the imaged object, the second strategy relies on real-time imaging and the ability of the medical practitioner to angle a detector array to visualize the structures of interest. This strategy requires a handheld imaging device containing both the illumination and the detection systems (Schellenberg and Hunt 2018). This approach is similar to 2D ultrasonography. However, for PAI, the practitioner must compensate for the directivity of the ultrasound emission by positioning the detectors perpendicular to the interface of the object of interest. In practice, many

PAI handheld systems use conventional ultrasound linear arrays on which a laser illumination system is attached (see Figures 9.3(h) and (i)), and combine 2D PAI and ultrasonography for dual-mode imaging (see Figure 9.3(j)) (Kuniyil Ajith Singh et al. 2016). Clinical applications of handheld PAI are focused on the evaluation of vascular disease and intraoperative imaging such as the guidance of metal needles for biopsies or injections.

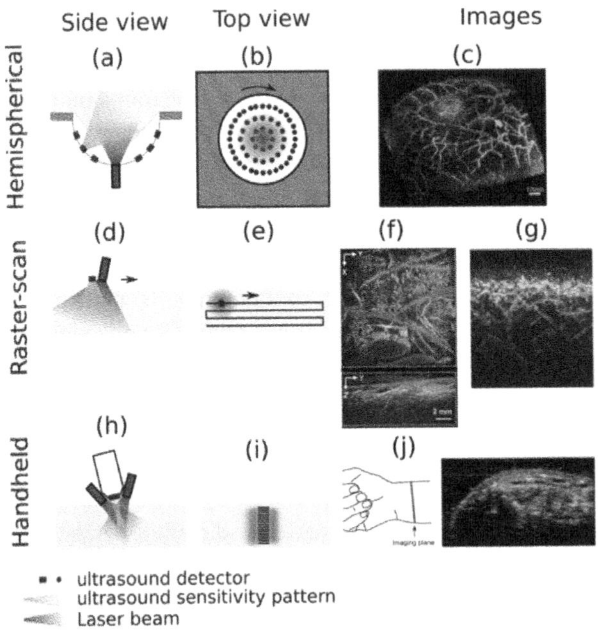

Figure 9.3. *Schematic drawings of PAI scanners and images illustrating their performance. (a–c) Hemispherical array for breast imaging, the array is rotated around its axis. (c) Maximum intensity projection (MIP) image of the vasculature of a healthy breast with a color map coding for depth information (reproduced from Toi et al. (2017)). The largest depth from the skin (orange arrow) is 24 mm. (d–g) Planar geometry with a raster-scanned ultrasound detector. The illumination is presented as mobile, but may be broader and fixed. (f) MIP images of the vasculature of a human placenta (reproduced from Maneas et al. (2020)). The color map code for depth information with a maximum depth of 7 mm. (g) MIP image of the skin microvasculature of the arm of a healthy volunteer (reproduced from Berezhnoi et al. (2018)). The maximum imaging depth is 1 mm. 40–120 MHz frequency components are depicted in green and 10–40 MHz frequency components are depicted in red. (h–j) Handheld configuration based on a linear ultrasound array with the illumination mounted on the side. (j) Overlaid photoacoustic (red color scale) and ultrasound (gray color scale) images of a wrist of a human volunteer (reproduced from Xia et al. (2018)). The imaging depth is 2 cm*

Once the detector configuration has been defined, it is necessary to ensure that the detectors have a high sensitivity over a wide spectral bandwidth. Different ultrasound detection technologies are being investigated to provide sensitive detection of photoacoustic signals: conventional piezoelectric transducers, micromachined transducers (e.g. Capacitive Micromachined Ultrasonic Transducer, CMUT) and optical ultrasound detectors (Manwar et al. 2020). Compared to conventional piezoelectric transducers, micromachined transducers have a wider bandwidth and a higher sensitivity, while optical ultrasound detectors have a higher sensitivity and a strong capability for miniaturization. While promising, these technologies are still emerging and, most commonly, conventional piezoelectric transducers are used in PAI. Dedicated piezoelectric transducer arrays have been designed, for example, in hemispherical or arc arrays. Transducer arrays designed for ultrasonography have also advantageously been adapted for PAI, especially linear arrays. In the following paragraphs, we focus on PAI systems using linear ultrasound arrays and present strategies that have been developed to mitigate the limitations of these detector arrays (Wang et al. 2020): limited angular aperture and limited bandwidth.

Linear transducer arrays comprise between 128 and 256 transducers distributed along a line. Cylindrical focus in the elevation direction provides a cross-sectional imaging plane (see Figure 9.4(a)). The weak elevation focusing results in a small angular aperture and a strongly limited view. As discussed above, a handheld approach can be applied, but it is strongly operator dependent. We developed a rotate-translate scanning scheme that systematically scans the transducer array around the object, to probe the ultrasound field from different orientations (Gateau et al. 2013a, 2015). In this approach, a larger-elevation aperture is synthesized from all the scanned orientations and 3D images are reconstructed with an enhanced view and a gain in resolution of at least a factor 3 as compared to a simple translational scan of the array (see Figure 9.4(b)). This approach was first developed in a configuration where the imaged object was surrounded by tomographic positions, but this configuration limited the object size to approximately twice the focal distance of the array (Gateau et al. 2013a). A second configuration with a planar detection geometry enabled single-side access (Gateau et al. 2015) (see Figure 9.4(b)). Recently, the rotate-translate scan has been applied using a linear array in pulse-echo ultrasound imaging mode and we demonstrated high-contrast and -resolution 3D ultrasonography (Lucas et al. 2021). This result opens the door to 3D dual PA and US high-quality imaging with conventional linear piezoelectric transducer arrays. Linear transducer arrays are commercially available for a broad range of center frequencies, in particular high frequency (>10 MHz). Their fractional bandwidth is on the order of 60–80%. We showed that imaging the same object with two different arrays with overlapping frequency bandwidth (center frequency of 6 MHz and 24 MHz, respectively) and combining the images results in an enhanced view of multiple vessel sizes (see Figure 9.4(f–h)).

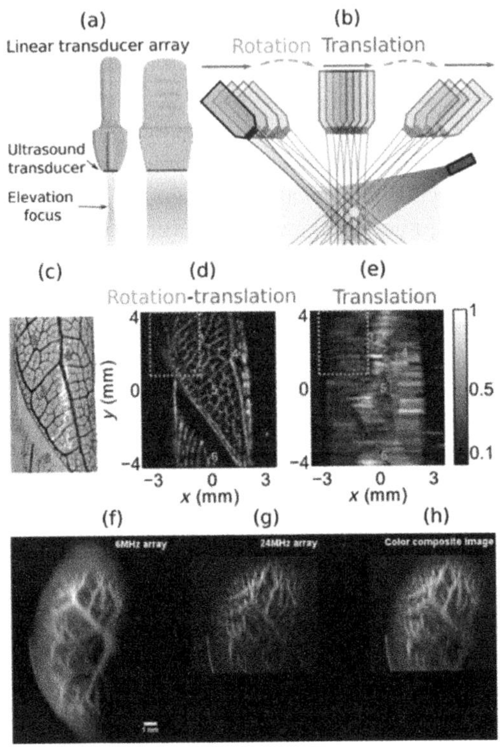

Figure 9.4. *Methods to improve the performance of linear ultrasound array in PAI. (a) Schematic drawing of a linear transducer: (left) side view of the focal zone, (right) front view of the imaging plane. (b) Schematic drawing of the rotate-translate scan with a single-side access. The array is rotated around the line of elements and the elevation focal zone is translated across the imaged region. Ultrasound signals from an isotropic object (yellow disk) are captured by one position for each of the scanned orientations. A larger-elevation angular aperture is synthesized. Ultrasound signals from a directional object would be captured on several positions with the same orientation but different translation positions. (c–e) Illustrations of the improvement of the resolution in the translation direction (x-axis) (reproduced with permission from Gateau et al. (2015) © SPIE). (c) Picture of a black stained tree leaf. (d) MIP image corresponding to a rotate-translate scan. (e) MIP image corresponding to a translation scan. (f–h) Illustration of the combination of images acquired with arrays that have different frequency bands. MIP images showing the vasculature of a mouse kidney ex vivo (adapted with permission from Gateau et al. (2013b) © The Optical Society). (f) MIP image acquired with a 6 MHz center frequency linear array, showing the large vessels and the absorption of the renal cortex. (g) MIP image acquired with a 24 MHz center frequency linear array enhancing the large vessels. (h) Combination of the two MIP images in red (f) and gray (g) color scales, respectively*

9.2.3. *Photoacoustic image reconstruction*

Once the ultrasound signals are recorded for multiple tomographic positions, the next step is the reconstruction of the photoacoustic image. As PAI has an optical absorption contrast, PA images would ideally map the optical absorption distribution $\mu_a(\boldsymbol{r})$ at a given optical wavelength. However, from equation [9.1], the reconstruction of $\mu_a(\boldsymbol{r})$ implies the quantitative determination of both the initial pressure distribution $p_0(\boldsymbol{r})$ and the light fluence distribution $\Phi(\boldsymbol{r})$. The evaluation of $\Phi(\boldsymbol{r})$ requires finding the solution to an optical inverse problem and, therefore, modeling the optical scattering and cumulative optical absorption during light propagation. Quantitative PAI faces multiple challenges (Cox et al. 2009), and we will focus here on the acoustic inverse problem: estimating the initial acoustic pressure distribution $p_0(\boldsymbol{r})$.

Theoretically, the initial pressure distribution $p_0(\boldsymbol{r})$ can be retrieved inside a closed surface S densely sampled by point-like detectors with an infinite bandwidth located at positions $\boldsymbol{r}_s$, using the analytical formula (Burgholzer et al. 2007):

$$p_0(\boldsymbol{r}) = -\frac{1}{2\pi}\int_S t\,\frac{\partial p(\boldsymbol{r}_s,t)}{\partial t}\Big|_{c_0 t=|\boldsymbol{r}_s-\boldsymbol{r}|}\,d\Omega_r(\boldsymbol{r}_s) \qquad [9.6]$$

where $d\Omega_r(\boldsymbol{r}_s)$ denotes the solid angle element corresponding to the detector surface element dS when viewed from $\boldsymbol{r}$ (see Figure 9.5(a)). This formula is valid in the far field of the detector, i.e. if the distance from the image to the detector is much larger than the recorded acoustic wavelengths. Otherwise, another term is added (Xu and Wang 2005). This analytical solution to the acoustic inverse problem is called the back-projection process, because it is based on the projection of the pre-processed acoustic signals onto 3D space in a way that is consistent with the time-of-flight principle. Let us examine equation [9.6] for the case of an absorbing sphere of diameter D centered on $\boldsymbol{r}_0$ and a spherical detection surface. For a spherical detection surface with a uniform distribution of detectors, $d\Omega_r(\boldsymbol{r}_s)$ can be considered constant. Given the N-shape of the photoacoustic signal (equation [9.4]), the term $-\frac{\partial p(\boldsymbol{r}_s,t)}{\partial t}$ is approximately a boxcar function of width D/c_0 centered on $t=\frac{|\boldsymbol{r}_s-\boldsymbol{r}_0|}{c_0}$ and the term t would compensate for the radial attenuation of the wave. The integral on the detection surface projects the signals on arcs of diameter $|\boldsymbol{r}_s-\boldsymbol{r}_0|$ and ensures a coherent summation inside a ball of diameter D centered on $\boldsymbol{r}_0$ to build up the image (see Figure 9.5(b)).

In practice, the theoretical conditions necessary to apply equation [9.6] are not met, as already mentioned in section 9.2.2.1. The high-pass filtering induced by the limited bandwidth of the detector can play a role similar to that of the time derivation, but other pre-processing may be required for noise removal. A very basic implementation of the back-projection process is often used: the delay and sum algorithm. This algorithm is similar to the beamforming process applied in reception for plane-wave ultrasound imaging. In brief, the pre-processed signal at each time instant t is projected in 3D space onto a sphere centered on the detector with a radius of $c_0 \bullet t$ (see Figure 9.5(b)). The signals from all detectors are added coherently and an envelope detection can be applied to obtain a non-negative image. This basic approach quantifies the location and size of simple photoacoustic sources, but cannot accurately quantify the amplitude of p_0.

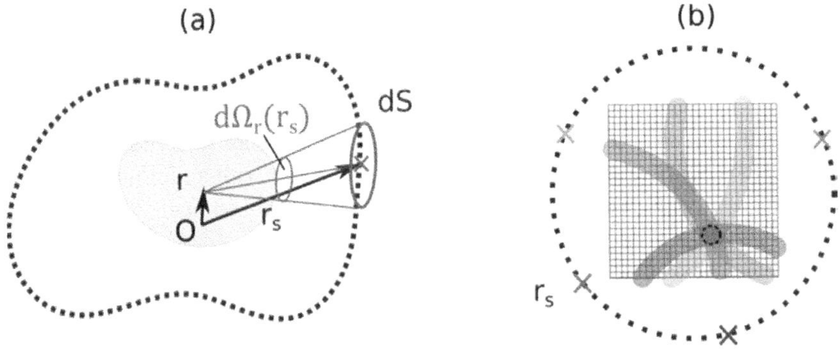

__Figure 9.5.__ Schematic drawings presenting the back-projection process. (a) Illustration of the infinitesimal solid solid-angle element $d\Omega_r(\boldsymbol{r}_s)$ in equation [9.6]. dS is the infinitesimal surface element of the detection surface. (b) Projection of the pre-processed signals onto the image grid for an absorbing sphere and four detector positions. The signals add at the location of the source to build up the image

More advanced acoustic inversion algorithms have been developed based on the inversion of a forward model (Rosenthal et al. 2013; Poudel et al. 2019). These algorithms are based on a discrete representation of the forward acoustic problem:

$$\boldsymbol{P} = \boldsymbol{M} \cdot \boldsymbol{P}_0 \qquad [9.7]$$

where $\boldsymbol{P}$ is a vector representing the acoustic signals measured at a set of positions and time instants, $\boldsymbol{P}_0$ is the vector representing the values of p_0 on the image grid and $\boldsymbol{M}$ is the model matrix. The image is obtained by inversion of equation [9.7]. The main advantage of this model-based approach is the ability to include any linear effect in the imaging system in $\boldsymbol{M}$. In particular, the spatial impulse response of the finite size detectors and a heterogeneity of the speed of sound can be included. Moreover, in many cases, the inversion problem is either ill-conditioned or ill-posed as, for example, in a limited view configuration where the detection geometry does not cover the full solid angle. The model-based approach enables the application of additional constraints on the solution to mitigate the effects of data incompleteness and measurement noise. However, model-based approaches are computationally demanding, which limits their use, in particular, for large image grids and large numbers of detector positions. Acceleration with parallel computing technologies such as graphical processing units (GPUs) has recently been proposed and may increase their use.

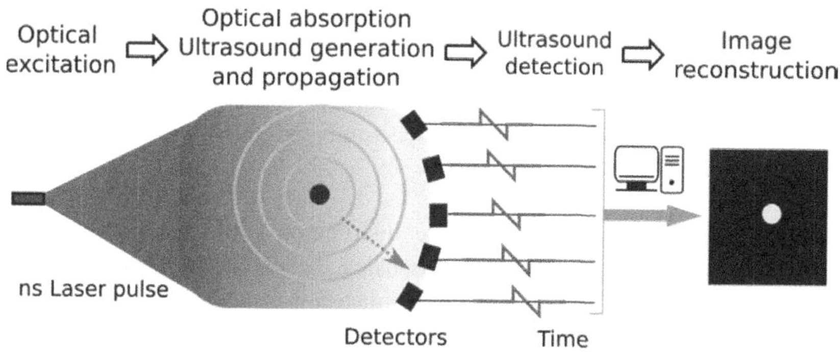

Figure 9.6. *Schematic drawing summarizing the different steps of photoacoustic imaging from the optical excitation to the image reconstruction*

9.3. Multispectral photoacoustic imaging

Section 9.2 mostly focused on the ultrasonic aspects of PAI. The steps to acquire and reconstruct an image with pixel values proportional to the optical absorption distribution $\mu_a(\boldsymbol{r}, \lambda)$ at the wavelength λ of the laser pulse were described (see Figure 9.6). However, several absorbing compounds could induce optical absorption at one wavelength. Successfully recording PA images of the same region at multiple and different wavelengths λ_i to add a spectral dimension to the images and to separate absorbers based on their respective spectra is referred to as multispectral PAI and will be developed in this section.

9.3.1. *Separation of optical absorbers with different absorption spectra*

According to the Beer–Lambert law, the absorption coefficient $\mu_a(\lambda)$ at the optical wavelength λ of a mix can be written as a weighted sum over its N absorbing compounds:

$$\mu_a(\lambda) = \sum_{i=1}^{N} c_i \cdot \varepsilon_i(\lambda) \qquad [9.8]$$

where c_i denotes the molar concentration of the compound i and $\varepsilon_i(\lambda)$ is its molar absorption coefficient (usually expressed in $mol.L^{-1}.cm^{-1}$) at the optical wavelength λ. If a compound can be isolated, its molar absorption coefficient can be measured over a range of optical wavelengths with optical spectroscopy. With the measured or tabulated molar absorption spectra $\varepsilon_i(\lambda)$, the respective concentrations c_i of all the compounds in a mix can be obtained from the measured absorption spectrum $\mu_a(\lambda)$ of the mix using a so-called unmixing method. The unmixing method quantifies the relative amount of each spectrum $\varepsilon_i(\lambda)$ in $\mu_a(\lambda)$ by solving an inverse problem. The accuracy of the unmixing method depends on the type of unmixing algorithm, but the accuracy usually decreases with an increasing number of expected compounds and the similarity of their spectra, and accuracy increases with the increasing number of optical wavelengths in the spectrum and the contrast-to-noise ratio (Tzoumas et al. 2013).

In PAI, the initial acoustic pressure distribution $p_0(\boldsymbol{r})$ can be sequentially measured at different optical wavelengths using a tunable laser or several lasers firing successively. Thereby, the spectral dimension can be added to the spatial dimensions to obtain maps of $p_0(\boldsymbol{r}, \lambda)$. Then, equation [9.1] can be modified:

$$p_0(\boldsymbol{r},\lambda) = \Gamma \cdot \Phi(\boldsymbol{r},\lambda) \cdot \sum_{i=1}^{N} c_i(\boldsymbol{r}) \cdot \varepsilon_i(\lambda) \qquad [9.9]$$

where Γ is the Grüneisen coefficient and $\Phi(\boldsymbol{r},\lambda)$ is the local optical fluence at the position $\boldsymbol{r}$ and the wavelength λ. The excitation wavelengths are usually chosen in the near-infrared range between 650 and 950 nm to allow centimetric penetration into biological tissues. However, as the absorption and scattering properties of tissue may vary with λ and the propagation path of the incident light, the optical fluence $\Phi(\boldsymbol{r},\lambda)$ is not uniform spatially and spectrally. The unmixing problem for equation [9.9] is therefore more complex than for equation [9.8] and requires nonlinear inversion strategies (Tzoumas and Ntziachristos 2017). Indeed, accurate quantification of the abundance of different compounds with PAI requires a simultaneous solution of an optical inverse problem and an unmixing problem. Because of this complexity, many studies use the approximation that the optical fluence is uniform in space and independent of the excitation wavelengths. With this simplification, straightforward linear spectral unmixing can be performed as for equation [9.8].

Multispectral PAI usually consists of two steps. First, the sequential acquisition and reconstruction of PA images is performed for the same area at n_λ different optical wavelengths to obtain $p_0(\boldsymbol{r}, \lambda)$, as explained in section 9.2 (see Figure 9.7, left). Then, an unmixing algorithm is applied on a pixel by pixel basis to convert the n_λ images to pixel values that are proportional to the optical absorption in N images, each of which displays pixel values that are proportional to the abundance of one type of absorbing compound (see Figure 9.7, right). The method yields images with a molecular contrast. The most common application of multispectral PAI is to separate oxygenated hemoglobin (HbO_2) from deoxygenated hemoglobin (Hb) to quantify the oxygen saturation of tissues or vessels at a sub-millimeter resolution.

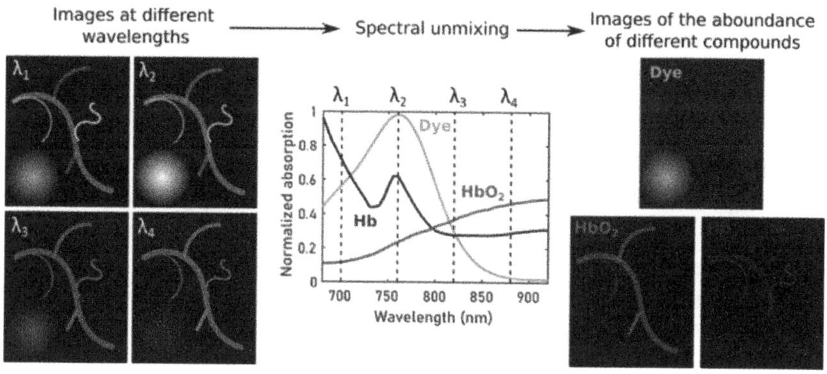

Figure 9.7. *Multispectral photoacoustic imaging. Images successively acquired at multiple optical wavelengths are combined with spectral unmixing algorithms to identify specific sources of contrast. This example shows the separation of oxyhemoglobin (HbO_2), deoxyhemoglobin (Hb) and an organic dye*

9.3.2. *Endogenous and exogenous absorbers*

Optical absorbers imaged with PAI can be divided into two groups: endogenous absorbers, which are naturally present in biological tissues, and exogenous absorbers, which are external contrast agents.

9.3.2.1. *PAI of endogenous absorbers and related clinical applications*

Endogenous absorbers are widely used in PAI because they can be imaged without any injection, which facilitates the clinical translation of the method. Moreover, the information provided by endogenous absorbers is already rich because it is both structural (architecture of blood vessels, for example) and functional (blood oxygenation, for example). The most common endogenous absorbers in the near-infrared range are hemoglobin, melanin, lipids and collagen. In the following paragraphs of this section, we detail the PAI of these four types of endogenous absorbers and give examples of clinical applications. For a review classified not by absorber types but by clinical application, the reader may refer to the review by Attia et al. (2019).

Hemoglobin, responsible for oxygen transport in red blood cells, is one of the most frequently called upon endogenous absorbers in PAI (Li et al. 2018). Indeed, blood oxygenation is a metabolic marker and tissue oxygenation is modified in many pathologies such as cancer. Changes in oxygenation can provide a relevant biomarker for the detection or therapy of cancer. Currently, one of the most advanced applications of PAI concerns the detection of breast cancer (Manohar and Dantuma 2019), since one of the characteristics of this cancer is the oxygenation and hemodynamic architecture of the tumor compared to the surrounding tissues. Treatment can also modify the oxygenation in peritumoral blood vessels in breast cancer (Toi et al. 2017). Muscular oxygenation may also be modified in degenerative or inflammatory muscle diseases and can be reproductively measured with multispectral PAI (Wagner et al. 2021). Blood oxygenation is usually quantified with the oxygen saturation, notated SO_2 and defined as the fraction of oxygen-saturated hemoglobin relative to total hemoglobin. SO_2 maps can be obtained from the unmixed multispectral PA images, by computing on a pixel by pixel basis the following ratio:

$$SO_2(\boldsymbol{r}) = \frac{c_{HbO_2}(r)}{c_{HbO_2}(r)+c_{Hb}(r)} \qquad [9.10]$$

where c_{HbO2} and c_{Hb} denote the estimated concentration of oxyhemoglobin and deoxyhemoglobin, respectively. The spectra of hemoglobin are illustrated in Figure 9.7.

Melanin is a pigment naturally present in the epidermis, the hair and the eyes. It plays an important role in the protection against the sun's radiation. Melanin absorbs over the entire near-infrared range with an absorption coefficient slowly decaying with the increasing wavelength. Because of its strong absorption, melanin can be easily detected with PAI. As for pathologies, melanin is produced by melanoma and metastatic melanoma cells, for example. Therefore, the main clinical application of the detection of melanin is the imaging of pigmented skin lesions and in particular, skin cancers (Li et al. 2021). One important parameter that PAI can reveal is the depth of the lesion.

Among endogenous absorbers with a lower absorption coefficient, lipids and collagen are of particular interest for clinical applications of PAI. The optical absorption of lipids becomes significant above 1,100 nm. The detection and characterization of lipids is of clinical interest for arterial tissue imaging and in particular lipid-rich atherosclerosis plaque imaged from the lumen (Jansen et al. 2014). The plaque composition could be revealed by multispectral PAI. Collagen is the main structural protein in the extracellular matrix found in connective tissues. Collagen mostly absorbs above 900 nm. Collagen is also present in atherosclerosis plaques and different types of collagen can be separated by multispectral PAI between 680 nm and 900 nm (Sethuraman et al. 2008). Collagen is also abundant in muscle tissue and its detection and quantification with multispectral PAI in the NIR range 680 nm–1,100 nm was found to be an imaging biomarker for Duchenne muscular dystrophy (Regensburger et al. 2019).

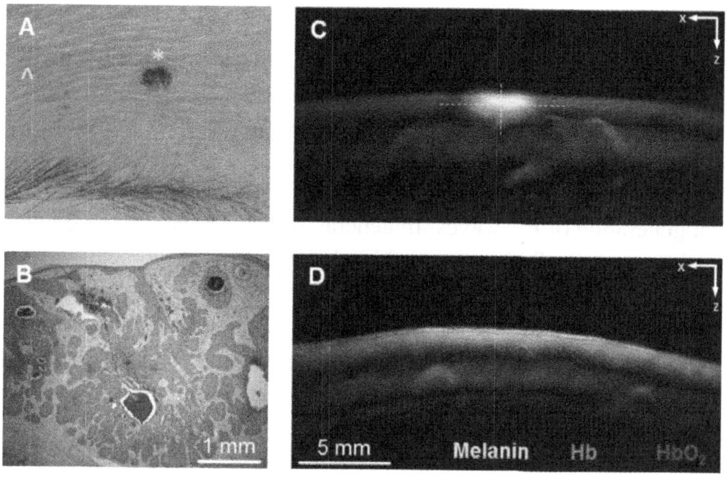

Figure 9.8. *Multispectral photoacoustic images of skin cancer (basal cell carcinoma), showing the spatial distribution of three different endogenous absorbers: melanin, oxy-hemoglobin (HbO_2) and deoxyhemoglobin (Hb). (A) Picture of the lesion. (B) Histological image. (C) Multispectral PAI image of the lesion. (D) Multispectral PAI image of normal skin. The color scales of (C) and (D) do not match. Reproduced from Attia et al. (2017)*

9.3.2.2. *Exogenous absorbers in PAI*

Exogenous absorbers are used as external contrast agents to obtain information that is not provided by the endogenous absorbers. Such absorbers can be made to bind or accumulate (e.g. via lymphatic pumping) to specifically reveal biomolecules of interest or physiological compartments (e.g. lymphatic vessels) that are not detectable based on their endogenous absorption signature. These agents are chosen according to their optical absorption characteristics to display a strong molar absorptivity $\varepsilon_i(\lambda)$ and a spectral signature different from the endogenous absorbers. An absorption peak in the NIR window [650 nm–950 nm] is, for example, a welcome feature for exogenous absorbers. In addition to the absorption spectrum, it is necessary to consider several characteristics such as the biocompatibility, the temporal and chemical stability and the photostability, i.e. the resistance of the material to intense light illumination.

The large variety of exogenous absorbers can be divided into two main categories: small-molecule dyes and nanoparticles. In each category, we focus on a main class of absorber: organic dyes and plasmonic nanoparticles, respectively. Several excellent comprehensive reviews have been published recently that provide a broader view of PA contrast agents (Weber et al. 2016; Fu et al. 2018; Wu et al. 2021).

Organic dyes are molecular absorbers. Their optical properties depend on their chemical structures, and dyes used in PAI are usually selected or modified to have an absorption peak in the NIR. Molecular absorption of light results from the transition between electronic energy levels in the molecule and a subsequent non-radiative energy transfer to the solvent that produces thermal heating and the subsequent generation of PA waves. In general, organic dyes have several properties that offer advantages for PAI: very good biodegradability, biocompatiblity and small size (~0.5 nm) allowing effective tissue penetration for labeling extravascular targets. However, organic dyes can have a short circulation time in the body and may undergo processes that alter their optical absorption or modify their absorption spectrum, for example, due to interactions with other (bio)molecules or aggregation and photodegradation. An undesired modification of the optical properties during the imaging process will bias multispectral unmixing and quantification. Interactions with other molecules or aggregation of dyes may modify the energy levels and the optical properties compared to isolated molecules. Photodegradation is the permanent alteration of absorption properties after an exposure to intense light that causes a photochemical destruction. Organic dyes may be encapsulated in nanoparticles such as liposomes to improve their solubility in water and prolong their circulation duration. A few examples of organic dyes authorized for clinical application are given below and in Laramie et al. (2018). However, the development of other organic dyes is a highly active field and multiple dyes are currently being tested preclinically.

Several blue dyes with absorbances below 720 nm are commonly used in clinical practice, such as methylene blue. They are often used as a biological stain because they are visible to the naked eye. For PAI, they are at the limit of detectability for many PAI scanners because their absorbance is in the lower part of the NIR wavelength range. Regardless of this limitation, methylene blue has been shown to be of interest for the PAI detection of sentinel lymph nodes in oncology, for example (Garcia-Uribe et al. 2015). Indocyanine Green (ICG) is a cyanine dye that has been FDA approved for human use since 1959. ICG has a peak absorption around 800 nm and is a fluorescent dye with a low quantum yield, which favors the conversion of optical energy into heat and in turn the creation of PA signal. ICG is a non-specific dye that can be used to enhance the signal of blood vessels or lymphatic vessels, and can also extravasate and accumulate in tumorous tissue (Okumura et al. 2018). However, the shape of the absorption spectrum of ICG strongly depends on the chemical environment and the concentration, which may bias the unmixing process of multispectral PAI.

A second major family of exogenous absorbers consists of plasmonic nanoparticles. They are composed of noble metals (most commonly silver or gold). Their optical absorption properties come from the surface plasmon resonance (SPR) phenomenon. A surface plasmon is a collective oscillation of electrons, occurring at the surface of the nanoparticle when exposed to light. At the plasmonic resonance frequency, the SPR results in an enhanced absorption and the conversion of light energy into heat that is transferred to the solvent or surrounding medium. This SPR frequency depends on the characteristics of the nanoparticle, such as its size, the material it is composed of and the surrounding dielectric medium. Plasmonic coupling of several nanoparticles can shift the SPR frequency. For example, an aggregation of single gold nanospheres that individually absorb at 520 nm may present a peak absorption shifted to the NIR. Gold nanorods and gold nanoshells (dielectric core, often silica, and nanometer-thick metallic shell) have an SPR in the NIR, and can be coated with polyethylene glycol (PEG) for biocompatibility. The NIR SPR wavelength of gold nanorods is influenced by their size and aspect ratio. With a width of 40 nm and a length of 120 nm, the SPR peak is around 790 nm (Knights et al. 2019). Gold nanorods can be conjugated to biomolecules as antibodies; however, they are unstable when illuminated with high-intensity laser pulses (Manohar et al. 2011). Nanoshells have been proven to be optically robust. They have been applied to increase the contrast of blood vessels in the rat brain (Wang et al. 2004). Both nanorods and nanoshells tend to passively accumulate in tumorous tissue via the enhanced permeability and retention (EPR) effect. The EPR effect has been imaged in cancer animal models. Furthermore, these particles can be used to induce hyperthermia of the tissue using photothermal therapy: illumination with a continuous laser to induce a local temperature rise sufficient to exert a therapeutic effect. However, PAI with gold nanoparticles is currently limited to preclinical studies because their injection in humans is not authorized. The regulation issue strongly limits the emergence of contrast-enhanced clinical PAI.

9.3.2.3. *Characterization of exogenous absorbers in PAI*

PA contrast agents are usually characterized with a spectrophotometer that measures μ_a by computing the ratio between the incident and transmitted light energy for a continuous illumination regime. However, this assessment of the absorption spectrum may differ from the spectrum measured in PAI due to light scattering by the solution (Pelivanov et al. 2018), or the fact that a pulsed illumination regime is used in PAI, rather than a continuous one (Fuenzalida Werner et al. 2020). Moreover, equation [9.1] assumes full conversion of the absorbed energy into heat, while other phenomena such as fluorescence can provide competitive de-excitement pathways, in particular for organic dyes. Consequently, it is strongly preferable to characterize PA contrast agents directly with a photoacoustic system.

In the case of a scattering contrast agent (e.g. plasmonic nanoparticles) measured with a spectrophotometer operating in transmission, the part of the incident light that is not transmitted to the sensor is either absorbed by the sample or scattered away from the initial propagation path. The measured spectrum is a mix of the absorption and scattering spectra and is called the extinction spectrum. The extinction spectrum only corresponds to the absorption spectrum for non-scattering solutions. To directly measure the photoacoustic properties of agents, we have developed a calibrated photoacoustic spectrometer based on a photoacoustic imaging system. The samples are injected in small tubes. The calibration is performed with a reference solution of copper sulfate that enables the determination of the conversion factor between p_0 in the PAI images and the spectroscopic units of μ_a (Lucas et al. 2022).

9.4. Conclusion and perspectives

This chapter introduced photoacoustic imaging, a multi-wave imaging modality combining optical excitation and ultrasound detection to reveal an optical absorption contrast at centimetric depths in biological tissue with sub-millimetric ultrasonic resolution. In the first part, we compared the propagation properties of optical and ultrasound waves in biological tissues and explained how the interaction between the two kinds of waves can be exploited for hybrid imaging. Then, we focused on photoacoustic imaging. In the second part of the chapter, we explained, from an ultrasound perspective, the different phases of the photoacoustic imaging process: the optical generation of ultrasound, tomographic ultrasound detection and image reconstruction. Several implementations of PA scanners were presented. Finally, in the third part, we explained other important aspects of the PAI process: the importance of the optical wavelength and the absorption spectra of different optical absorbers. We explained how multispectral imaging can be used to separate different kinds of absorbers and the aim to be able to quantify the abundance of different types of absorbers with multispectral PAI. Finally, we reviewed intrinsic absorbers in tissues and corresponding promising applications for PAI, as well as some contrast agents.

Compared to ultrasound imaging, photoacoustic imaging is still emerging and only a few scanners are currently available commercially for clinical trials. However, we can expect that, because of its ability to offer a unique molecular contrast and functional contrasts such as blood oxygenation, PAI will take its place in the conventional radiological armamentarium. Clinical trials are currently being conducted to evaluate several pathologies and demonstrate the relevance of PAI. PAI brings a new contrast, as well as new technical challenges for ultrasonic detection including, among others, a need for enhanced sensitivity and different arrangements of detectors. The simultaneous registration of the two complementary modalities (PAI and ultrasound imaging) can give access to new physiological and functional information. Due to the light attenuation in tissue, the penetration depth of PAI is usually lower than for ultrasound imaging, especially for ultrasound frequencies of a few MHz. This property limits the applications to superficial targets and may require minimally invasive procedures to obtain internal illumination and thereby increase the optical energy at depth (Zhao et al. 2019). The approval of contrast agents is another important challenge ahead. Currently, only a few dyes have been formally approved for clinical use with PAI. In the meantime, the research domain is very active, from hardware development to preclinical studies that will provide new knowledge in biology and on the capabilities of this modality.

9.5. References

Attia, A.B.E., Chuah, S.Y., Razansky, D., Ho, C.J.H., Malempati, P., Dinish, U.S., Bi, R., Fu, C.Y., Ford, S.J., Lee, J.S.S. et al. (2017). Noninvasive real-time characterization of non-melanoma skin cancers with handheld optoacoustic probes. *Photoacoustics*, 7, 20–26. doi: 10.1016/j.pacs.2017.05.003.

Attia, A.B.E., Balasundaram, G., Moothanchery, M., Dinish, U.S., Bi, R., Ntziachristos, V., Olivo, M. (2019). A review of clinical photoacoustic imaging: Current and future trends. *Photoacoustics*, 16(July), 100144. doi: 10.1016/j.pacs.2019.100144.

Berezhnoi, A., Schwarz, M., Buehler, A., Ovsepian, S.V., Aguirre, J., Ntziachristos, V. (2018). Assessing hyperthermia-induced vasodilation in human skin in vivo using optoacoustic mesoscopy. *Journal of Biophotonics*, 11(11), 1–8. doi: 10.1002/jbio.201700359.

Burgholzer, P., Matt, G.J., Haltmeier, M., Paltauf, G. (2007). Exact and approximative imaging methods for photoacoustic tomography using an arbitrary detection surface. *Physical Review E – Statistical, Nonlinear, and Soft Matter Physics*, 75(4). doi: 10.1103/PhysRevE.75.046706.

Cox, B.T., Arridge, S.R., Beard, P.C. (2007). Photoacoustic tomography with a limited-aperture planar sensor and a reverberant cavity. *Inverse Problems*, 23(6), S95–S112. doi: 10.1088/0266-5611/23/6/S08.

Cox, B.T., Laufer, J.G., Beard, P.C. (2009). The challenges for quantitative photoacoustic imaging. *Photons Plus Ultrasound: Imaging and Sensing*, 7177, 717713. doi: 10.1117/12.806788.

Fu, Q., Zhu, R., Song, J., Yang, H., Chen, X. (2018). Photoacoustic imaging: Contrast agents and their biomedical applications. *Advanced Materials*, 1805875. doi: 10.1002/adma.201805875.

Fuenzalida Werner, J.P., Huang, Y., Mishra, K., Janowski, R., Vetschera, P., Heichler, C., Chmyrov, A., Neufert, C., Niessing, D., Ntziachristos, V. et al. (2020). Challenging a preconception: Optoacoustic spectrum differs from the optical absorption spectrum of proteins and dyes for molecular imaging. *Analytical Chemistry*, 92(15), 10717–10724. doi: 10.1021/acs.analchem.0c01902.

Garcia-Uribe, A., Erpelding, T.N., Krumholz, A., Ke, H., Maslov, K., Appleton, C., Margenthaler, J.A., Wang, L.V. (2015). Dual-modality photoacoustic and ultrasound imaging system for noninvasive sentinel lymph node detection in patients with breast cancer. *Scientific Reports*, 5(1), 15748. doi: 10.1038/srep15748.

Gateau, J., Caballero, M.A.A., Dima, A., Ntziachristos, V. (2013a). Three-dimensional optoacoustic tomography using a conventional ultrasound linear detector array: Whole-body tomographic system for small animals. *Medical Physics*, 40(1), 013302. doi: 10.1118/1.4770292.

Gateau, J., Chekkoury, A., Ntziachristos, V. (2013b). Ultra-wideband three-dimensional optoacoustic tomography. *Optics Letters*, 38(22), 4671–4674. doi: 10.1364/OL.38.004671.

Gateau, J., Gesnik, M., Chassot, J.-M.J.-M., Bossy, E. (2015). Single-side access, isotropic resolution, and multispectral three-dimensional photoacoustic imaging with rotate-translate scanning of ultrasonic detector array. *Journal of Biomedical Optics*, 20(5), 056004. doi: 10.1117/1.JBO.20.5.056004.

Gunther, J. and Andersson-Engels, S. (2017). Review of current methods of acousto-optical tomography for biomedical applications. *Frontiers of Optoelectronics*, 10(3), 211–238. doi: 10.1007/s12200-017-0718-4.

Hindelang, B., Aguirre, J., Schwarz, M., Berezhnoi, A., Eyerich, K., Ntziachristos, V., Biedermann, T., Darsow, U. (2019). Non-invasive imaging in dermatology and the unique potential of raster-scan optoacoustic mesoscopy. *Journal of the European Academy of Dermatology and Venereology*, 33(6), 1051–1061. doi: 10.1111/jdv.15342.

Huynh, N.T., Francies, O., Soteriou, K., Allen, T.J., Pham, K., Noimark, S., Bodian, S., Desjardins, A., Zhu, J., Abeyakoon, O. et al. (2020). High resolution 3D photoacoustic scanner for clinical vascular imaging applications (Conference Presentation). *Photons Plus Ultrasound: Imaging and Sensing*, 11240. doi: 10.1117/12.2549559.

Jacques, S.L. (2013). Optical properties of biological tissues: A review. *Physics in Medicine and Biology*, 58(11). doi: 10.1088/0031-9155/58/11/R37.

Jansen, K., Wu, M., van der Steen, A.F.W., van Soest, G. (2014). Photoacoustic imaging of human coronary atherosclerosis in two spectral bands. *Photoacoustics*, 2(1), 12–20. doi: 10.1016/j.pacs.2013.11.003.

Jeon, S., Kim, J., Lee, D., Baik, J.W., Kim, C. (2019). Review on practical photoacoustic microscopy. *Photoacoustics*, 15(February), 100141. doi: 10.1016/j.pacs.2019.100141.

Knights, O.B., Ye, S., Ingram, N., Freear, S., McLaughlan, J.R. (2019). Optimising gold nanorods for photoacoustic imaging in vitro. *Nanoscale Advances*, 1(4), 1472–1481. doi: 10.1039/C8NA00389K.

Kuniyil Ajith Singh, M., Steenbergen, W., Manohar, S. (2016). Handheld probe-based dual mode ultrasound/photoacoustics for biomedical imaging. In *Frontiers in Biophotonics for Translational Medicine: In the Celebration of Year of Light (2015)*, Olivo, M. and Dinish, U.S. (eds). Springer, Singapore. doi: 10.1007/978-981-287-627-0_7.

Laramie, M., Smith, M., Marmarchi, F., McNally, L., Henary, M. (2018). Small molecule optoacoustic contrast agents: An unexplored avenue for enhancing in vivo imaging. *Molecules*, 23(11), 2766. doi: 10.3390/molecules23112766.

Li, M., Tang, Y., Yao, J. (2018). Photoacoustic tomography of blood oxygenation: A mini review. *Photoacoustics*, 10, 65–73. doi: 10.1016/j.pacs.2018.05.001.

Li, D., Humayun, L., Vienneau, E., Vu, T., Yao, J. (2021). Seeing through the skin: Photoacoustic tomography of skin vasculature and beyond. *JID Innovations*, 1(3), 100039. doi: 10.1016/j.xjidi.2021.100039.

Lucas, T., Quidu, I., Bridal, S.L., Gateau, J. (2021). High-contrast and -resolution 3-D ultrasonography with a clinical linear transducer array scanned in a rotate-translate geometry. *Applied Sciences*, 11(2), 493. doi: 10.3390/app11020493.

Lucas, T., Sarkar, M., Atlas, Y., Linger, C., Renault, G., Gazeau, F., Gateau, J. (2022). Calibrated photoacoustic spectrometer based on a conventional imaging system for in vitro characterization of contrast agents. *Sensors*, 22(17), 6543. https://doi.org/10.3390/s22176543.

Maneas, E., Aughwane, R., Huynh, N., Xia, W., Ansari, R., Kuniyil Ajith Singh, M., Hutchinson, J.C., Sebire, N.J., Arthurs, O.J., Deprest, J. et al. (2020). Photoacoustic imaging of the human placental vasculature. *Journal of Biophotonics*, 13(4), 1–10. doi: 10.1002/jbio.201900167.

Manohar, S. and Dantuma, M. (2019). Current and future trends in photoacoustic breast imaging. *Photoacoustics*, 16(February), 100134. doi: 10.1016/j.pacs.2019.04.004.

Manohar, S., Ungureanu, C., Van Leeuwen, T.G. (2011). Gold nanorods as molecular contrast agents in photoacoustic imaging: The promises and the caveats. *Contrast Media & Molecular Imaging*, 6(5), 389–400. doi: 10.1002/cmmi.454.

Manwar, R., Kratkiewicz, K., Avanaki, K. (2020). Overview of ultrasound detection technologies for photoacoustic imaging. *Micromachines*, 11(7), 1–24. doi: 10.3390/mi11070692.

Na, S., Russin, J.J., Lin, L., Yuan, X., Hu, P., Jann, K.B., Yan, L., Maslov, K., Shi, J., Wang, D.J. (2021). Massively parallel functional photoacoustic computed tomography of the human brain. *Nature Biomedical Engineering*. doi: 10.1038/s41551-021-00735-8.

Ntziachristos, V. (2010). Going deeper than microscopy: The optical imaging frontier in biology. *Nature Methods*, 7(8), 603–614. doi: 10.1038/nmeth.1483.

O'Brien, W.D. (2007). Ultrasound-biophysics mechanisms. *Progress in Biophysics and Molecular Biology*, 93(1–3), 212–255. doi: 10.1016/j.pbiomolbio.2006.07.010.

Okumura, K., Yoshida, K., Yoshioka, K., Aki, S., Yoneda, N., Inoue, D., Kitao, A., Ogi, T., Kozaka, K., Minami, T. et al. (2018). Photoacoustic imaging of tumour vascular permeability with indocyanine green in a mouse model. *European Radiology Experimental*, 2(1), 5. doi: 10.1186/s41747-018-0036-7.

Omar, M., Soliman, D., Gateau, J., Ntziachristos, V. (2014). Ultrawideband reflection-mode optoacoustic mesoscopy. *Optics Letters*, 39(13), 3911–3914. doi: 10.1364/OL.39.003911.

Pelivanov, I., Petrova, E., Yoon, S.J., Qian, Z., Guye, K., O'Donnell, M. (2018). Molecular fingerprinting of nanoparticles in complex media with non-contact photoacoustics: Beyond the light scattering limit. *Scientific Reports*, 8(1), 1–13. doi: 10.1038/s41598-018-32580-2.

Poudel, J., Lou, Y., Anastasio, M.A. (2019). A survey of computational frameworks for solving the acoustic inverse problem in three-dimensional photoacoustic computed tomography. *Physics in Medicine & Biology*, 64(14), 14TR01. doi: 10.1088/1361-6560/ab2017.

Regensburger, A.P., Fonteyne, L.M., Jüngert, J., Wagner, A.L., Gerhalter, T., Nagel, A.M., Heiss, R., Flenkenthaler, F., Qurashi, M., Neurath, M.F. et al. (2019). Detection of collagens by multispectral optoacoustic tomography as an imaging biomarker for Duchenne muscular dystrophy. *Nature Medicine*, 25(12), 1905–1915. doi: 10.1038/s41591-019-0669-y.

Rosenthal, A., Ntziachristos, V., Razansky, D. (2013). Acoustic inversion in optoacoustic tomography: A review. *Current Medical Imaging Reviews*, 9(4), 318.

Schellenberg, M.W. and Hunt, H.K. (2018). Hand-held optoacoustic imaging: A review. *Photoacoustics*, 11(July), 14–27. doi: 10.1016/j.pacs.2018.07.001.

Sethuraman, S., Amirian, J.H., Litovsky, S.H., Smalling, R.W., Emelianov, S.Y. (2008). Spectroscopic intravascular photoacoustic imaging to differentiate atherosclerotic plaques. *Optics Express*, 16(5), 3362. doi: 10.1364/OE.16.003362.

Toi, M., Asao, Y., Matsumoto, Y., Sekiguchi, H., Yoshikawa, A., Takada, M., Kataoka, M., Endo, T., Kawaguchi-Sakita, N., Kawashima, M. et al. (2017). Visualization of tumor-related blood vessels in human breast by photoacoustic imaging system with a hemispherical detector array. *Scientific Reports*, 7(December 2016), 1–11. doi: 10.1038/srep41970.

Tzoumas, S. and Ntziachristos, V. (2017). Spectral unmixing techniques for optoacoustic imaging of tissue pathophysiology. *Philosophical Transactions of the Royal Society A: Mathematical, Physical and Engineering Sciences*, 375(2107), 20170262. doi: 10.1098/rsta.2017.0262.

Tzoumas, S., Deliolanis, N., Morscher, S., Ntziachristos, V. (2014). Unmixing molecular agents from absorbing tissue in multispectral optoacoustic tomography. *IEEE Trans. Med. Imaging*, 33, 48–60. doi:10.1109/TMI.2013.2279994.

Wagner, A.L., Danko, V., Federle, A., Klett, D., Simon, D., Heiss, R., Jüngert, J., Uder, M., Schett, G., Neurath, M.F. et al. (2021). Precision of handheld multispectral optoacoustic tomography for muscle imaging. *Photoacoustics*, 21, 100220. doi: 10.1016/j.pacs.2020.100220.

Wang, L.V. (ed.) (2017). *Photoacoustic Imaging and Spectroscopy*. CRC Press, Boca Raton, FL. doi: 10.1201/9781420059922.

Wang, Y., Xie, X., Wang, X., Ku, G., Gill, K.L., O'Neal, D.P., Stoica, G., Wang, L.V. (2004). Photoacoustic tomography of a nanoshell contrast agent in the in vivo rat brain. *Nano Letters*, 4(9), 1689–1692. doi: 10.1021/nl049126a.

Wang, Y., Zhan, Y., Tiao, M., Xia, J. (2020). Review of methods to improve the performance of linear array-based photoacoustic tomography. *Journal of Innovative Optical Health Sciences*, 13(2), 1–12. doi: 10.1142/S1793545820300037.

Weber, J., Beard, P.C., Bohndiek, S.E. (2016). Contrast agents for molecular photoacoustic imaging. *Nature Methods*, 13(8), 639–650. doi: 10.1038/nmeth.3929.

Wissmeyer, G., Pleitez, M.A., Rosenthal, A., Ntziachristos, V. (2018). Looking at sound: Optoacoustics with all-optical ultrasound detection. *Light: Science and Applications*, 7(1). doi: 10.1038/s41377-018-0036-7.

Wu, Y., Zeng, F., Zhao, Y., Wu, S. (2021). Emerging contrast agents for multispectral optoacoustic imaging and their biomedical applications. *Chemical Society Reviews*, 50(14), 7924–7940. doi: 10.1039/D1CS00358E.

Xia, W., Singh, M.K.A., Maneas, E., Sato, N., Shigeta, Y., Agano, T., Ourselin, S., West, S.J., Desjardins, A.E. (2018). Handheld real-time LED-based photoacoustic and ultrasound imaging system for accurate visualization of clinical metal needles and superficial vasculature to guide minimally invasive procedures. *Sensors (Basel, Switzerland)*, 18(5). doi: 10.3390/s18051394.

Xu, M. and Wang, L.V (2005). Universal back-projection algorithm for photoacoustic computed tomography. *Physical Review E*, 71(1), 16706. doi: 10.1103/PhysRevE.71.016706.

Zhang, E., Laufer, J., Beard, P. (2008). Backward-mode multiwavelength photoacoustic scanner using a planar Fabry-Perot polymer film ultrasound sensor for high-resolution three-dimensional imaging of biological tissues. *Applied Optics*, 47(4), 561. doi: 10.1364/AO.47.000561.

Zhao, T., Su, L., Xia, W. (2018). Optical ultrasound generation and detection for intravascular imaging: A review. *Journal of Healthcare Engineering*, 2018(April). doi: 10.1155/2018/3182483.

Zhao, T., Desjardins, A.E., Ourselin, S., Vercauteren, T., Xia, W. (2019). Minimally invasive photoacoustic imaging: Current status and future perspectives. *Photoacoustics*, 16(September), 100146. doi: 10.1016/j.pacs.2019.100146.

Glossary

A-mode: a single scan line describing the relative amplitudes of the echoes returned to the ultrasonic probe along a specific line of sight.

Aberration: a defect in the ultrasound image that is caused by an inaccurate description of ultrasound propagation.

Aberrator: any sub-region in the scanned region of interest that causes an aberration.

Acoustic coupling: see impedance matching (acoustical).

Acoustic impedance: see impedance; characteristic acoustic impedance and impedance; specific acoustic impedance.

Acoustic radiation force: a unidirectional force that can be applied to absorbing and reflecting targets that results from the transfer of momentum from the acoustic wave to the target. It can be used to create a displacement in a medium.

Acoustic window: a location on the body where the transducer can be placed to make a scan through an unobstructed pathway for sound propagation.

Acousto-optics: mode of interaction for which both optical and acoustic waves are generated externally and the ultrasonic wave modulates the incident light to "tag" photons.

Amplitude aberration: a departure of the performance of the ultrasound imaging system caused by an altered amplitude of recorded ultrasound wavelets.

Angular frequency: an angular displacement per unit time in units of radians per second.

Anisotropic properties: the characteristic of a material that depends on the direction.

Aperture: the number of adjacent array elements that are used to electrically focus or steer the acoustic beam.

ARFI (acoustic radiation force impulses): mimics the palpation by a physician using acoustic radiation force to directly measure the elastic modulus in a medium based on the relation between the applied force and the observed deformation, which is known as the spring ratio.

Artifacts: see section 7.3.3.

Attenuation: the attenuation describes what fraction of the signal is lost as a function of the propagation distance through a medium. In biological media, higher ultrasonic frequencies are more strongly attenuated than lower ones. Attenuation limits the depth than can be imaged.

Attenuation heterogeneity: see section 8.2.6.

AUC: area under the indicator dilution curve, which can be related to blood flow and contrast dose after the bolus injection of an ultrasound contrast agent.

Axial resolution: spatial resolution along the propagation direction.

B-flow imaging: tracks flow of red blood cell scatterers by extracting acoustic speckle scattered by the blood with high-frame-rate imaging.

B-mode image or brightness-mode image: echo amplitudes are presented on a log-compressed scale in an image with lateral and depth axes.

Back-projection process: in photoacoustic tomography, analytical solution to the acoustic inverse problem based on the projection of the pre-processed acoustic signals onto 3D space in a way that is consistent with the time-of-flight principle.

Backing layer: material adhered to the rear side of each PZT element to absorb waves propagating within the transducer housing and to dampen the resonance.

Backscatter cross-section: the part of the power scattered by an object that is within a limited solid angle oriented back toward the transmitting transducer expressed relative to the incident intensity.

Bandwidth: range of significant frequency response of a probe or of transmit or receive circuits.

Beam steering: orientation of the direction of an ultrasonic beam by applying transmit delays along the individual elements of a transducer array.

Beer–Lambert law: principle that the optical absorption coefficient at a specific optical wavelength from a mixture can be written as a weighted sum of that for its N absorbing compounds.

Buckling behavior: effect arising at high pressures for lipid-coated micro bubbles as the surface of the bubble shrinks such that lipids can no longer remain distributed across the reduced, available surface area.

Bulk piezoelectric transducers: transducers produced by mechanically dicing and stacking different material layers.

Cadence contrast pulse sequencing: contrast-agent specific imaging sequence exploiting the nonlinear behavior of the microbubbles through a sequence of phase- and amplitude-modulated ultrasonic pulses.

Cardiac cycle: a series of contractions and relaxations during the course of one complete sequence of filling and ejection from the cardiac chambers occurring over a single heartbeat.

Casorati matrix: see section 7.2.2.

Cavitation: formation of pockets of gas in a medium due to a strong change in pressure. This mechanical bio effect is evaluated based on the mechanical index. The term cavitation is also used to describe the oscillation and violent collapse of gas bubbles (ultrasound contrast agents) subjected to ultrasound.

Clutter: diffuse signals due to reverberations in heterogeneous tissue layers or multiple diffuse scattering or echoes from side lobes, which can interfere with visualization and analysis of signals returned from structures of interest, for example.

Color flow imaging: flow mapping modality based on evaluating pulsed Doppler signals in range gates that are swept across the imaged region.

Compound imaging, compounding: superposition of raw imaged data acquired from slightly different points of view. It improves image quality.

Compressibility: property of a medium describing the relationship between the change in pressure and the change in the medium's density.

Compression: application of force along an axis leading to local particle displacement such that particles are closer than at equilibrium and the local pressure is increased.

Compression zones: regions of a medium where the molecules are closer together than at equilibrium due to the passage of a longitudinal acoustic wave. This leads to higher local density and pressure.

Compressional wave speed: speed of the "curl free" wave, meaning that no rotation occurs during propagation; that it only results in local volumic changes. Around 1,500 m/s in soft biological tissue.

Continuous-wave Doppler: measures blood flow using the classical Doppler effect, which refers to a shift in the acoustic frequency perceived by a target due to the motion of either the source or the target (or both). CW Doppler ultrasound can examine time-varying, pulsatile flow dynamics inside the vasculature.

Contrast resolution: ability to discriminate a structure presenting a different average intensity than the background.

Contrast-to-noise ratio, CNR: local intensity variation divided by the standard deviation of the averaged background intensity.

Crossed electrode arrays: 2D arrays that behave as two overlapped, orthogonal 1D arrays.

Damping (acoustic or mechanical): reduction of wave or oscillation amplitude. Can be achieved with material that absorbs or dissipates vibrations, for example.

Delay and sum algorithm: preprocessed signal at each time instant is projected in 3D space at a distance from the detector equal to the speed of sound times the time of flight. Signals from all detectors are added coherently.

Density, ρ: mass per unit volume.

Diffraction: waves from a finite source interfere with each other constructively and destructively as a function of the field position.

Direct piezoelectric effect: squeezing a piezoelectric material creates a minute displacement of electrical charges within it. This results in the creation of an electric potential across opposite faces of the material.

Dispersion of shear waves: differences in the propagation speed of shear waves as function of frequency.

Diverging waves: a defocused wave originating from a virtual point-source.

Doppler aliasing: fast blood flow is incorrectly rendered as slow flow moving in the reversed direction when the slow-time sampling frequency determined by the pulse repetition frequency undersamples the pulsed Doppler signal.

Doppler echocardiography: evaluation of blood flow in the heart that can reveal abnormal blood flow patterns or valve function.

Doppler effect: discovered by Christian Doppler in 1842, this effect refers to a relative-motion-induced change in the perceived wave frequency.

Doppler mode: ultrasound imaging mode that tracks the movement of red blood cells.

Doppler power: qualitative representation of the total power of Doppler signals returned from moving structures in a region.

Doppler resolution: the frequency bin size that determines the uncertainty range in the pulsed Doppler frequency spectrum and thus determines the minimum detectable flow velocity.

Doppler shift: the total extent of frequency change resulting from the two Doppler events in the typical CW Doppler ultrasound measurement scenario.

Dynamic contrast-enhanced ultrasound: dynamic ultrasound scan capturing the time-evolution of the ultrasound-contrast-agent concentration.

Dynamic range: see section 8.2.4.

Echo ranging: mapping of echoes using depths estimated based on the average speed of sound propagation in the medium and the lapse of time between signal emission and echo reception.

Echo time delay, Δt_echo: the lapse of time between the emission of the ultrasound pulse and echo reception. See equation [1.1].

Elastography: a field of medical imaging calling upon a variety of different techniques to map out the elastic properties of biological tissues and organs.

Electrical impedance: a measure of the opposition that a transducer presents to the flow of electric current when a voltage is applied across its electrodes. It describes the electro-mechanical energy conversion capacity of a transducer in conjunction with the imaging system's electronic circuits.

Electro-acoustic conversion: application of the direct and indirect (or inverse) piezoelectric effects to generate and receive ultrasonic signals.

Electro-acoustic response: transducer characteristic that quantifies its capability to generate an acoustic pressure in response to an electrical excitation and vice versa.

Elevation direction: see sections 1.5.7 and 2.1.1.2.

Endogenous absorbers (optical): intrinsic optical absorbers that are naturally present in biological tissue.

Enhancement (due to attenuation heterogeneity): see section 8.2.6.

Equivalent circuit model: an arrangement of R, L, C components in a circuit to simulate the properties of an oscillating system such as an ultrasonic transducer.

Erlang model: the model describing the dilution of contrast agent as the transport through a series of *n* compartments.

Exogenous absorbers (optical): optical absorbers that must be introduced into the body; photo acoustic contrast agents.

Extinction spectrum: the spectrum describing losses due both to the absorption and scattering in a medium.

Fast time: timescale of the signal acquired as echoes return to the ultrasonic probe along a specific line of sight.

Flow vector estimation: any of several flow vector estimation approaches that provide information on both flow speed and the flow direction to better describe complex flow.

Fourier ring correlation method: see section 7.3.2.

Frame rate: number of images recorded per unit time, typically the number of frames per second.

Frequency (or linear frequency): number of oscillatory cycles per second measured in hertz, Hz. Within the MHz range for medical ultrasonic imaging.

Graphical processing units (GPUs): see sections 1.5.4 and 2.3.1.2.

Grating lobes: sound energy that is not aligned along the primary beam path. Grating lobes are strong when element spacing is too large.

Grüneisen coefficient: a dimensionless thermodynamic constant that describes the conversion efficiency of heat energy to pressure.

Harmonics: frequency content arising from nonlinear behavior such as nonlinear micro bubble oscillation or nonlinear wave propagation.

High-frame-rate ultrasound imaging, HFR (also called ultrafast ultrasound imaging): techniques based on the transmission of unfocused or multi-line transmission beams with advanced beam forming strategies to provide frame rates (1,000s of frames per second) much higher than possible with conventional, focused ultrasound imaging.

Hooke's law: the principle stating that stress is proportional to strain through a constant called the elastic modulus.

Image contrast: refers to differences in the image brightness perceived between one region and another.

Impedance; characteristic acoustic impedance, Z: the property of a medium defined by the material's density multiplied by the speed of sound in the material. It is expressed in units of Rayl.

Impedance; specific acoustic impedance, z: the complex ratio of the acoustic pressure and acoustic particle velocity. For a plane wave propagating in an infinite medium, the specific acoustic impedance is numerically and dimensionally equivalent to the characteristic acoustic impedance.

Impedance matching (acoustical): selection of properties at an interface to optimize the transfer from one medium to another. Matching layers of materials are used to optimize transmission of the ultrasonic pulse at the interface between the transducer material and the body. Ultrasonic gel is placed on the body to ensure that no air impedes transmission from the probe to the body.

Impedance matching (electrical): electrical impedance is matched to adapt the properties of the imaging system's electronic circuits to the transducer's electrical impedance for optimization of its electro-mechanical energy conversion capacity.

Intracardiac echocardiography (ICE): cardiac imaging performed using an ultrasound transducer at the tip of a catheter, which is inserted through a vein and advanced towards the heart.

Intravascular ultrasound: imaging of the vessel walls from within the vessels using a transducer at the tip of a catheter, which is inserted through a vein and advanced to the site to image.

Inverse (or indirect) piezoelectric effect: applying an electric field across the opposite faces of a piezoelectric material results in a global deformation of the material's thickness.

Isoimpedance medium: medium where aberration is present, but multiple scattering is absent.

Isovelocity medium: medium where multiple scattering is present, but sound speed inhomogeneity is artificially absent.

Kerf: distance along the azimuth of a transducer array that separates adjacent array elements.

Lamé coefficient: the natural elastic moduli, 5 and μ, applied in wave physics that describe the two different elastic waves that travel in any solid: the compressional wave and the shear wave.

Lateral resolution: spatial resolution in the direction perpendicular to the beam axis and along the lateral axis of the transducer array.

M-mode: side-by-side display of consecutive scan lines along a single line of sight. Each scan line is at the same position but acquired at times separated by the pulse repetition interval.

Matching layer: layers of material with carefully selected thickness and acoustic impedance values that are placed on the face of the transducer to optimize transmission of ultrasound from the PZT elements into biological tissues.

Matrix array: see sections 1.2.2, 5.3.2 and 8.4.1.

Maximum intensity projection: representation obtained by retaining the maximum intensity value for each pixel over time.

Mechanical index (MI): imaging safety limit to determine the peak negative pressure ensuring that no significant cavitation is created during ultrasonic imaging.

Micromachined transducers: transducers produced using fabrication techniques used to make semiconductors. Different approaches (CMUT, PMUT) have been developed.

Molecular imaging: for ultrasound imaging, molecular imaging requires the injection of a functionalized contrast agent with specific affinity to a biological marker expressed in the body.

MTT: mean transit time of contrast micro bubbles estimated based on analysis of the time–intensity curve.

Multi-wave imaging: imaging modality that makes use of different types of wave physics. Photoacoustic imaging and Shear Wave Elastography are examples of multi-wave imaging.

Multiple scattering (reverberation): echoes arising from multiply scattered waves that can occur, for example, when the propagation medium consists of multiple layers of different types of tissues with large impedance mismatches. It produces clutter in the ultrasound image.

Nanoparticles: submicron-sized particles, usually on the order of a few hundreds of nanometers in diameter for nanoparticles developed for use with ultrasound or photoacoustic imaging.

Near-infrared window: optical wavelength range between 630 and 1300 nm for which light has a maximum depth of penetration in biological tissue.

Optical absorption: loss of energy of the optical beam through transformation into internal energy of the absorber.

Optical absorption coefficient: see section 9.3.1.

Optoacoustic imaging: same as photoacoustic imaging.

Passive elastography: imaging and characterization of elasticity based on shear waves generated by innate, natural vibrations within the body.

Period of oscillation, τ: time necessary for a complete oscillatory vibration. It is the inverse of the frequency of vibration.

Phase aberration: wave front delay or distortion due to propagation through layered media with variable thickness and different speed of sound.

Photoacoustic imaging: optical energy is transiently deposited in tissue. Optical absorption of the incident light leads to the generation of ultrasonic waves.

Piezoelectric plate: the piezoelectric material that is connected to electrodes and dimensioned according to the application.

Pitch: the distance along the azimuth between the center of adjacent transducer array elements.

Point-spread function: spatial impulse response of the imaging system.

Poisson's ratio: the second normalized coefficient that is associated with the Young's modulus to describe the elasticity of a cylinder. It assesses the component of the cylinder's elastic properties related to the lateral strain that characterizes the change of the cylinder's cross-sectional diameter. Soft biological tissues are nearly incompressible so the Poisson's ratio is very close to 0.5.

Pressure (acoustic): refers to localized change in pressure due to the interaction of a medium with an acoustic wave. It is expressed relative to the equilibrium pressure in units of Pascal (Pa) so that it is positive in zones that are compressed by the sound wave and negative in zones that are rarefied by the sound wave.

Pulse duration: the time between the beginning and the end of the ultrasound pulse.

Pulse repetition interval: separation in time between the emissions of consecutive pulses. The pulse repetition interval must at least provide the time necessary for propagation of the pulse from the transducer to the deepest region of the explored region and the return of echoes from this region to the transducer.

Pulsed-wave Doppler: a multi-pulse echo-sensing mechanism in which blood flow velocities are estimated from time of flight changes between consecutive pulse echoes. Pulsed Doppler ultrasound does not make use of the classical Doppler effect.

Rarefaction zones: regions of a medium where the molecules are farther apart than at equilibrium due to the passage of a longitudinal acoustic wave. This leads to lower local density and pressure.

Rayleigh–Plesset equation: see section 6.2.

Real time (noun), real-time (adjective): in actual time; refers to the immediate updating of data and images acquired with many ultrasonic techniques.

Receive beam former: field programmable gate arrays (FPGAs) that adjust the receive delays relative to the time-range equation to focus echoes returned from each point in the imaged plane. A Delay-and-Sum (DAS) algorithm is applied to RF channels to produce an echo scan line.

Refraction: change in propagation direction for an ultrasonic wave at an interface between two media with different acoustic impedance when the beam is not perfectly perpendicular to the interface.

Resolution-to-acquisition time trade-off: see section 7.3.3.

Resonance frequency: value of the frequency at which resonance occurs.

Resonant frequency: a specific frequency providing optimized reverberation.

Scan conversion: projection of received scan lines onto a rectangular grid for image display.

Scattering, scattering structures: structures on the order of or smaller than the wavelength of the interrogating ultrasound that have a different acoustic impedance from the surrounding medium. Incident ultrasonic intensity is redirected or scattered along many directions.

Scattering cross-section: parameter describing how much power is redirected or scattered in all directions by an object relative to the incident intensity.

Shadowing (due to attenuation heterogeneity): see section 8.2.6.

Shear elastic modulus: the Lamé coefficient μ extracted from the shear wave speed, which, within the ultrasonic frequency range, is the tissue elasticity that would be felt through physical palpation of a tissue. It is one-third of the value of the Young's modulus for the same isotropic solid.

Shear wave elastography (SWE): ultrasound is focused on multiple points at successively deeper regions to generate (through acoustic radiation force) a shear wave front as a Mach cone. To accomplish this, the ultrasonic focal spot must be displaced at a faster rate than the shear wave propagation velocity in the medium. The shear wave front is detected with an ultrafast ultrasound imaging system so that the measurement is based on the characterization of the propagation of the transient shear wave front and not on the local displacement induced by the shearing radiation force impulses.

Shear wave speed: speed of the "divergent free" wave which characterizes any shape changes other than volumic changes. The shear wave speed is in the range of 1–20 m/s.

Signal linearization: the process applied to image-based video intensity to reverse transformations applied to the raw RF signals before image display.

Signal-to-noise ratio: describes the amplitude of the useful signal relative to the background noise.

Singular value decomposition (SVD): see section 7.2.2.

Slow time: a sampled time axis formed by extracting each echo's desired fast-time point of interest and remapping them such that adjacent sampled time points differ in absolute time by one pulse repetition period.

Sparse arrays: 2D phased arrays with a reduced number of small transducer elements distributed across a large area.

Spatial pulse length: number of cycles in the pulse times the wavelength.

Spatial resolution: minimum separation between two different objects that allows them to be discriminated from each other.

Speckle-tracking echocardiography (STE): quantifies regional motion or deformation of the heart using speckle tracking.

Spectrogram (Doppler): a frequency–time plot that shows the measured Doppler shifts along the vertical axis and time along the horizontal axis.

Speed of sound propagation in a medium, c: the speed at which individual waves travel through a medium. The average value can be expressed in m/s. It is related to the density and compressibility of the medium (see section 1.3.3).

Structure insonification microscopy: super-resolution technique based on shaping the emission patterns so that the frequency content is shifted in the Fourier space and higher-frequency components will get through the diffraction window.

Super-resolution imaging: an imaging method that surpasses the classical diffraction limit in resolving power, generally, for distinguishing individual objects

Thermal index (TI): imaging safety limit to determine the peak power output level ensuring that no significant heating is created during ultrasonic imaging.

Thickness-mode resonance frequency: central frequency of the electro-acoustic response of a piezoelectric plate determined by its thickness and the way it is mechanically and acoustically coupled to the surrounding media. A piezoelectric plate will resonate along the orientation of its thickness when the round-trip time of vibration is equal to the speed of sound in the material times the period required for one cycle of vibration.

Time–intensity curves: data acquired after the injection of an ultrasound contrast agent that describes the acoustic intensity as a function of time. Information related to blood flow can be estimated from these curves based on indicator dilution theory.

Time gain compensation: increased gain applied more strongly for signals returning from deeper zones that have suffered greater attenuation. It provides a more uniform brightness over the full imaged depth.

Time resolution: related to the signal acquisition or imaged frame rate; this parameter determines that capacity to evaluate dynamic phenomena.

Tissue Doppler imaging: movement-based signal analysis to follow myocardial wall motion during the cardiac cycle.

Tissue harmonic imaging: relies on the detection of new frequency components generated by the distortion of the transmitted wave fore by nonlinear ultrasound propagation.

Tomography: image reconstruction obtained by an acoustic inverse problem from the ultrasound signals recorded at several locations around the imaged object.

Transducer array: a geometrical arrangement of individual transducer elements that are independently connected to the imaging system; allows electronic control of transmission and reception of acoustic beams for focusing or steering.

Transesophageal echocardiography (TEE): cardiac imaging performed using a small probe mounted on a catheter introduced through the esophagus.

Transmit beam former: usually uses Field Programmable Gate Arrays (FPGAs) that apply delays to transmitted signals to control focusing.

Transthoracic echocardiography (TTE): ultrasonic imaging through the thoracic wall to provide real-time ultrasonic images of the beating heart.

Ultrasonic probe: the device used to transmit and receive ultrasound including the physical housing, acoustic matching and backing layers, PZT elements and electrical connections.

Ultrasonic speckle: the grainy pattern of ultrasound images due to the constructive and destructive interference patterns produced by random variations in the arrangement of scattering structures within biological tissue that are much smaller than the acoustic wavelength.

Ultrasonic transducer: a device that converts electrical energy into acoustic energy and vice versa using the electro-acoustic conversion that operates at acoustic frequencies above the audible range.

Ultrasound contrast agents: solutions of gas-filled micro bubbles encapsulated in a biocompatible shell with a diameter distribution from 1 to 10 μm. Once injected intravascularly, their strong and nonlinear acoustic response makes them excellent tracers for blood flow.

Ultrasound localization microscopy: super-resolution technique based on the isolation and localization of individual punctual sources with a precision better than the diffraction limit.

Unmixing method: see section 9.3.1.

Wavelength: the wavelength of an acoustic wave is the distance between positions where the particle displacement is at the same point in the cyclic motion (distance between the two closest points along the propagation direction where the phase and amplitude of the particle motion is matched).

Young's modulus: the quantity describing the elasticity measured along a cylinder of a homogeneous, isotropic material when uniaxial loading is applied.

List of Authors

Enrico BONI
Department of Information Engineering
University of Florence
Italy

S. Lori BRIDAL
CNRS
INSERM
Laboratoire d'Imagerie Biomédicale (LIB)
Sorbonne Université
Paris
France

Stefan CATHELINE
Laboratory of Therapeutic Applications of Ultrasound (LabTAU)
INSERM
University of Lyon
France

Peiran CHEN
Eindhoven University of Technology
The Netherlands

Olivier COUTURE
CNRS
INSERM
Laboratoire d'Imagerie Biomédicale (LIB)
Sorbonne Université
Paris
France

Jan D'HOOGE
Katholieke Universiteit Leuven
Belgium

Ahmed EL KAFFAS
Stanford Medicine
California
USA

Jérôme GATEAU
CNRS
INSERM
Laboratoire d'Imagerie Biomédicale (LIB)
Sorbonne Université
Paris
France

Bruno GIAMMARINARO
Laboratory of Therapeutic Applications of Ultrasound (LabTAU)
INSERM
University of Lyon
France

Vincent HINGOT
CNRS
INSERM
Laboratoire d'Imagerie Biomédicale (LIB)
Sorbonne Université
and
ResolveStroke SAS
Paris
France

Théotim LUCAS
CNRS
INSERM
Laboratoire d'Imagerie Biomédicale (LIB)
Sorbonne Université
and
CNRS
Laboratoire Matière et Systèmes Complexes (MSC)
Université Paris Cité
France

Andrej LYSHCHIK
Thomas Jefferson University Hospital
Philadelphia
USA

Massimo MISCHI
Eindhoven University of Technology
The Netherlands

Sjoerd NOOIJENS
Katholieke Universiteit Leuven
Belgium

Marta ORLOWSKA
Katholieke Universiteit Leuven
Belgium

Konstantina PAPANGELOPOULOU
Katholieke Universiteit Leuven
Belgium

Gianmarco PINTON
Joint Department of Biomedical Engineering
University of North Carolina at Chapel Hill and North Carolina State University
USA

Alessandro RAMALLI
Department of Information Engineering
University of Florence
Italy

Guillaume RENAUD
Department of Imaging Physics
Delft University of Technology
The Netherlands

Alessandro Stuart SAVOIA
Department of Industrial, Electronic and Mechanical Engineering
Roma Tre University
Rome
Italy

Danai E. SOULIOTI
Joint Department of Biomedical Engineering
University of North Carolina at Chapel Hill and North Carolina State University
USA

Piero TORTOLI
Department of Information Engineering
University of Florence
Italy

Simona TURCO
Eindhoven University of Technology
The Netherlands

Alfred C.H. YU
Schlegel-UW Research
Institute for Aging
University of Waterloo
Ontario
Canada

Index

E, F

G, H

I, K

U, W

Printed and bound by CPI Group (UK) Ltd, Croydon, CR0 4YY

13/09/2026

14961069-0006